Andrology: Male Reproductive Health

Andrology: Male Reproductive Health

Editor: Lucy Mitchel

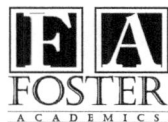

FA
FOSTER
ACADEMICS

www.fosteracademics.com

www.fosteracademics.com

FA FOSTER ACADEMICS

Cataloging-in-Publication Data

Andrology : male reproductive health / edited by Lucy Mitchel.
  p. cm.
Includes bibliographical references and index.
ISBN 978-1-63242-961-2
1. Andrology. 2. Generative organs, Male. 3. Male reproductive health.
4. Human reproduction--Endocrine aspects. 5. Men--Physiology. I. Mitchel, Lucy.
RC875 .A53 2020

612.6--dc23

Foster Academics,
118-35 Queens Blvd., Suite 400,
Forest Hills, NY 11375, USA

ISBN 978-1-63242-961-2 (Hardback)

Contents

Permissions

List of Contributors

Index

Preface

Over the recent decade, advancements and applications have progressed exponentially. This has led to the increased interest in this field and projects are being conducted to enhance knowledge. The main objective of this book is to present some of the critical challenges and provide insights into possible solutions. This book will answer the varied questions that arise in the field and also provide an increased scope for furthering studies.

Sexual health and function are important for a healthy life. The male reproductive system is responsible for the production, maintenance and transportation of sperms and semen, the discharge of sperm during sex, and for the production and secretion of male sex hormones. Male reproductive health depends on male hormones. The primary hormones involved are testosterone, follicle-stimulating hormone and luteinizing hormone. Testosterone is important for the development of male characteristics, such as muscle mass and strength, facial hair growth, sex drive, fat distribution, bone mass, etc. Follicle-stimulating hormone is involved in spermatogenesis, while luteinizing hormone stimulates testosterone production. The field of andrology deals with the anomalies and disorders of the male genitalia, and encompasses the diagnosis and treatment of these conditions. The objective of this book is to give a general view of the different areas of clinical andrology. It aims to shed light on some of the unexplored aspects of male reproductive health and the recent researches in this domain. The extensive content of this book provides the readers with a thorough understanding of the subject.

I hope that this book, with its visionary approach, will be a valuable addition and will promote interest among readers. Each of the authors has provided their extraordinary competence in their specific fields by providing different perspectives as they come from diverse nations and regions. I thank them for their contributions.

Editor

Oncologic outcomes in men with metastasis to the prostatic anterior fat pad lymph nodes

Young Suk Kwon[1†], Yun-Sok Ha[1,2†], Parth K. Modi[1], Amirali Salmasi[1], Jaspreet S. Parihar[1], Neal Patel[1], Izak Faiena[1], Michael May[3], David I. Lee[4], Elton Llukani[4], Tuliao Patrick[5], Koon Ho Rha[5], Thomas Ahlering[6], Douglas Skarecky[6], Hanjong Ahn[7], Seung-Kwon Choi[7], Sejun Park[8], Seong Soo Jeon[9], Yen-Chuan Ou[10], Daniel Eun[11], Varsha Manucha[12], David Albala[13], Ketan Badani[14], Bertram Yuh[15], Nora Ruel[15], Tae-Hwan Kim[2], Tae Gyun Kwon[2], Daniel Marchalik[16], Jonathan Hwang[16], Wun-Jae Kim[17] and Isaac Yi Kim[1*]

Abstract

Background: The presence of lymph nodes (LN) within the prostatic anterior fat pad (PAFP) has been reported in several recent reports. These PAFP LNs rarely harbor metastatic disease, and the characteristics of patients with PAFP LN metastasis are not well-described in the literature. Our previous study suggested that metastatic disease to the PAFP LN was associated with less severe oncologic outcomes than those that involve the pelvic lymph node (PLN). Therefore, the objective of this study is to assess the oncologic outcome of prostate cancer (PCa) patients with PAFP LN metastasis in a larger patient population.

Methods: Data were analyzed on 8800 patients from eleven international centers in three countries. Eighty-eight patients were found to have metastatic disease to the PAFP LNs (PAFP+) and 206 men had isolated metastasis to the pelvic LNs (PLN+). Clinicopathologic features were compared using ANOVA and Chi square tests. The Kaplan-Meier method was used to calculate the time to biochemical recurrence (BCR).

Results: Of the eighty-eight patients with PAFP LN metastasis, sixty-three (71.6 %) were up-staged based on the pathologic analysis of PAFP and eight (9.1 %) had a low-risk disease. Patients with LNs present in the PAFP had a higher incidence of biopsy Gleason score (GS) 8–10, pathologic N1 disease, and positive surgical margin in prostatectomy specimens than those with no LNs detected in the PAFP. Men who were PAFP+ with or without PLN involvement had more aggressive pathologic features than those with PLN disease only. However, there was no significant difference in BCR-free survival regardless of adjuvant therapy. In 300 patients who underwent PAFP LN mapping, 65 LNs were detected. It was also found that 44 out of 65 (67.7 %) nodes were located in the middle portion of the PAFP.

Conclusions: There was no significant difference in the rate of BCR between the PAFP LN+ and PLN+ groups. The PAFP likely represents a landing zone that is different from the PLNs for PCa metastasis. Therefore, the removal and pathologic analysis of PAFP should be adopted as a standard procedure in all patients undergoing radical prostatectomy.

Keywords: Lymph node metastases, Prostate anterior fat pad, Prostate cancer

* Correspondence: kimiy@cinj.rutgers.edu
†Equal contributors
[1]Section of Urologic Oncology, Rutgers Cancer Institute of New Jersey and Rutgers Robert Wood Johnson Medical School, The State University of New Jersey, 195 Little Albany Street, New Brunswick, NJ, USA
Full list of author information is available at the end of the article

Background

In men undergoing radical prostatectomy (RP), pelvic lymph node dissection (PLND) is the most accurate and reliable staging procedure for detecting lymph node (LN) metastasis in prostate cancer (PCa) [1–4]. Aside from providing clinicians with the most accurate LN staging, the therapeutic role of PLND in PCa has emerged as some have suggested that RP and removal of involved regional LNs has survival benefit [5–7]. Currently, an extended template for PLND has been accepted by many surgeons as the standard due to higher LN yield, increased removal of positive nodes, and fewer missed positive nodes [8, 9]. Nevertheless, the optimal extent of PLND that balances potential morbidity with therapeutic benefit remains controversial.

During RP, Ahlering et al. have proposed that the prostatic anterior fat pad (PAFP) should be dissected to aid in the identification of the puboprostatic ligaments and the anterior surface of the dorsal vein complex [10]. In addition, the potential oncologic rationale for the PAFP removal has been suggested initially by Kothari et al. in 2001 [11]. Since then, several groups have reported the presence of LNs in the PAFP and incidence of PAFP LN metastasis occurring in the range of 5.5 % to 17.0 % and 1.2 % to 2.5 %, respectively [12–16].

Most recently, we have reported the largest series on the pathologic analysis of LNs and LN metastasis in the PAFP after reviewing 4,261 patients from 8 institutions [17]. In this study, PAFP LNs were found in 11.9 % and 0.94 % harbored metastatic disease. More importantly, our initial study suggested that metastatic disease to the PAFP LN was associated with more favorable oncologic outcome than those that involve the PLNs. To further define the oncologic implications of PAFP LN metastasis, we have expanded the scope of the study to 8800 men from 11 international institutions.

Methods

Ethics statement

This study was approved by the institutional review board of all 13 participating institutions (see Additional file 1). Furthermore, the principles of the Helisinki Declaration were followed. Each board exempted informed consent because this was a retrospective study.

Study population

Prospectively maintained database approved by the institutional review board (IRB) at each institution was analyzed. Written informed consent was obtained from all study subjects during the study period between January of 2006 and February of 2014. In this study, only men who underwent PAFP excision and pathologic analysis during open retropubic radical prostatectomy (RRP)

or robot-assisted radical prostatectomy (RARP) were included. All patients routinely undergo PAFP excision and pathologic analysis from the thirteen participating institutions. Initially, the outcomes of 9510 PCa patients were reviewed [RARP, $N = 8747$ and RRP, $N = 763$]. Of these, 8800 PCa patients from eleven institutions with complete data were selected for analysis.

The participating thirteen institutions are as follows: Rutgers Cancer Institute of New Jersey (New Brunswick, NJ, USA), University of Pennsylvania (Philadelphia, PA, USA), Yonsei University (Seoul, Korea), University of California Irvine (Orange, CA, USA), Asan Medical Center (Seoul, Korea), Samsung Medical Center (Seoul, Korea), Taichung Veterans General Hospital (Taichung, Taiwan), Temple University (Philadelphia, PA, USA), Associated Medical Professionals (Syracuse, NY, USA), Icahn school of Medicine at Mount Sinai Hospital (New York, NY, USA), City of Hope National Medical Center (Duarte, CA, USA), Kyungpook National University Medical Center (Daegu, Korea), and Georgetown University (Washington, D.C., USA).

PAFP removal and pathologic evaluation

PAFP removal and pathological analysis were performed as described previously [17].

Statistical analysis

For comparison of variables, a student t test or analysis of variance (ANOVA) test and Pearson χ^2 test were used for analysis of each set of continuous and categorical data. Biochemical recurrence (BCR) was defined as 2 consecutive PSA increases with the last PSA 0.2 ng/ml or greater. Multivariate Cox regression analyses were performed to identify factors predictive of BCR. The time to BCR was used as the end point for the Kaplan-Meier model. The log-rank test was used for comparison with $p \leq 0.05$ considered statistically significant. All statistical analyses were performed using the SPSS v.18.0 (IBM Corp., Armonk, NY).

Results

From the eleven international institutions, 8800 patients underwent pathologic analysis of the PAFP (data not shown; see Additional file 2) because the number of patients with LNs present in the PAFP was not available due to an institutional procedure on not reporting negative LNs at two sites. Metastatic disease in the PAFP was detected in eighty-eight patients out of 8800 (0.93 %). The overall incidence of LNs present in the PAFP was 10.3 % (909/8800).

2835 out of 5260 (53.9 %) patients with available data on pelvic LNs underwent pelvic LN dissection, with varying institutional range from 23.2 % to 100.0 %. For these patients, the mean (median) number of dissected total pelvic LN was 6.1 (7) with values in the range of 1–45. Of the ones who underwent pelvic LN dissection, 4.4 % of patients had metastasis to pelvic LN.

Pre- and post-operative patient characteristics of 8800 men with known LN status in the PAFP is known are summarized in Table 1 with a median follow-up of 18.0 months (range 3.0-84.0 months). In this cohort, 7891 patients were found to have no LNs in the PAFP. Preoperatively, biopsy Gleason score (GS) was the only variable significantly different between the two groups. Specifically, patients with LNs present in the PAFP had more frequent biopsy GS of 8–10 than those with LNs absent in the PAFP. Regarding pathologic characteristics of the RP specimens, statistically significant differences were found for pathologic LN (N) stage ($P = 0.001$) and surgical margin status ($P < 0.001$).

Table 2 lists the clinicopathologic results of the patients with metastatic disease to the LNs stratified by

Table 1 Pre- and post-operative characteristics of patients with absence or presence of lymph nodes in PAFP

	LN absent in PAFP (N = 7891)	LN present in PAFP (N = 909)	P-value
Age, years: mean (SD)	62.7 (7.5)	62.9 (7.7)	0.413
BMI, kg/m^2 :mean (SD)	27.9 (3.7)	27.9 (4.2)	0.814
PSA, ng/ml: mean (SD)	8.84 (12.32)	10.00 (24.62)	0.107
Categorical PSA, ng/ml: %			0.814
0-3.9	20.0	22.0	
4-9.9	58.3	56.2	
10-20	15.1	14.0	
>20	6.7	7.8	
Biopsy GS: %			<0.001
6-7	82.8	78.3	
8-10	17.2	21.7	
Pathologic GS: %			0.307
6-7	83.8	82.1	
8-10	16.7	17.9	
Pathologic T stage: %			0.659
T2≥	67.5	66.8	
T3≤	32.5	33.2	
Pathologic N stage: %			0.001
N0/Nx	96.0	93.5	
N1	4.0	6.5	
Margin status: %			<0.001
Negative	82.3	78.1	
Positive	17.7	21.9	

PAFP, Prostate anterior fat pad; LN, Lymph node; BMI, Body mass index; PSA, Prostate-specific antigen; GS, Gleason score

Table 2 Differences in clinicopathologic results among the 3 groups stratified by the location of positive lymph nodes.

	Group 1, N = 206	Group 2, N = 63	Group 3, N = 25	P-value
Age, years: mean (SD)	63.3 (6.9)	63.3 (7.4)	64.4 (8.1)	0.744
PSA, ng/ml: mean (SD)	21.6 (36.0)	26.9 (85.5)	37.3 (66.5)	0.336
BCR-free survival, months: mean (range)	19.2 (0.7-77.7)	21.6 (1.0-76.3)	19.6 (2.6-60.0)	0.163
BCR: N (%)				0.073
No	145 (70.4)	35 (55.6)	15 (60.0)	
Yes	61 (29.6)	28 (44.4)	10 (40.0)	
D'Amico risk: N (%)				0.009
Low risk	29 (14.1)	7 (11.1)	1 (4.0)	
Intermediate risk	65 (31.6)	17 (27.0)	1 (4.0)	
High risk	112 (54.4)	39 (61.9)	23 (92.0)	
Biopsy GS: N (%)				<0.001
6-7	116 (56.5)	25 (41.0)	5 (20.0)	
8-10	89 (43.4)	36 (59.0)	20 (80.0)	
Pathologic GS: N (%)				0.021
6-7	113 (54.9)	29 (46.0)	8 (32.0)	
8-10	93 (45.1)	34 (54.0)	17 (68.0)	
Pathologic T stage: N (%)				0.005
T2	81 (39.3)	18 (28.6)	3 (12.0)	
T3a	48 (23.3)	22 (34.9)	6 (24.0)	
T3b	59 (28.6)	19 (30.2)	10 (40.0)	
T4	18 (8.7)	4 (6.3)	6 (24.0)	
Margin status: N (%)				0.043
Negative	69 (33.5)	37 (58.7)	9 (36.0)	
Positive	137 (66.5)	26 (41.3)	16 (64.0)	
Adjuvant therapy: N (%)				0.012
No	165 (80.1)	42 (66.7)	16 (64.0)	
Yes	41 (19.9)	21 (33.3)	9 (36.0)	

Group 1, Pelvic LN metastasis only; Group 2, PAFP LN metastasis only; Group 3, Both pelvic LN & PAFP LN metastasis; PSA, Prostate-specific antigen; BCR, Biochemical recurrence; GS, Gleason score

location. Group 1 had isolated metastasis to the pelvic LNs (PLNs) (n = 206). Group 2 had metastatic disease limited to the PAFP LNs (n = 63). Group 3 involved disease both in the pelvic and PAFP LNs (n = 25). Among the eighty-eight patients with metastasis to the PAFP LNs, eight (9.1 %) had low-risk disease based on the D'Amico criteria and sixty-three (71.6 %, Group 2) were up-staged as a result of the PAFP pathologic analysis. Compared to men with pelvic LNs metastasis only (group 1), patients with metastatic disease to the PAFP LNs (Group 2 and 3) had more aggressive features in biopsy and pathologic GS as well as pathologic stage.

Adjuvant therapy, including androgen deprivation (ADT), radiation, and chemotherapy was performed more frequently in men with PAFP LN involvement. 63 out of 71 patients (88.7 %) who were given adjuvant therapy received ADT with or without radiation and chemotherapy. The remaining 8 patients (11.3 %) did not receive ADT and received radiation, chemotherapy, or both. The median BCR-free survival period for PLN+, PAFP+, and PAFP+/PLN+ were 19.2, 21.6, and 19.6 months, respectively. Currently, fifty patients with PAFP LN metastasis remain free of BCR.

In order to check whether PAFP LN+ was a surrogate for extracapsular extension (ECE+), survival analysis of those with simultaneous ECE+ and PAFP LN+ was compared with that of individuals with ECE- or PAFP LN-. Although the relative frequency of BCR seemed different, the Kaplan-Meier analysis revealed no differences between the two groups: 46.3 % of ECE+/PAFP LN+ group had BCR with the median BCR free survival time of 18.0 months. On the other hand, 30.0 % of ECE- or PAFP- group had BCR with the median BCR free survival time of 15.4 months (P = 0.287). To determine the anatomic location of the LNs with in PAFP, LN mapping was carried out at one institution as reported previously [17]. From the cohort of 300 men, the total number of LNs detected was 65 (Table 3). Of these, 44 (67.7 %) were located in the middle packet. The numbers of LNs found in the left and right segments were 11 (16.9 %) and 10 (15.4 %), respectively.

The Multivariate Cox regression model suggested that higher preoperative PSA was predictive of higher recurrence rates in all patients (HR 1.005; 95 % CI 1.000-1.009; P = 0.042) and in the subgroup of patients with adjuvant therapy (HR 1.009; 95 % CI 1.001-1.016; P = 0.019). In addition, PLN+, PAFP LN+, and PLN+/PAFP LN+ demonstrated comparable risks of developing BCR (Table 4).

Kaplan-Meier curves were used to assess BCR according to the location of the metastatic LNs (Fig. 1). No statistically significant difference was found in the BCR when all three groups were compared (Fig. 1a). When stratified by the administration of adjuvant therapy, again no difference was observed among the three groups (Fig. 1b and c).

Discussion

Our international study spanning multiple institutions has demonstrated that in 8800 patients who underwent

Table 3 Location of lymph nodes within the PAFP

Total # Patients	300
Number of Nodes Detected	657
Middle (# of Nodes)	44
Left (# of Nodes)	11
Right (# of Nodes)	10

Table 4 Multivariate Cox regression analyses to identify predictors of biochemical recurrence

Variables	HR	95 % CI		P-value
		Lower	Upper	
All patients				
Age	1.008	.979	1.038	.604
Preoperative PSA	1.005	1.000	1.009	.042
Post-operative GS (≤7 vs. ≥8)	1.264	.822	1.943	.286
Pathologic stage (T2 vs. T3)	.931	.584	1.484	.763
Margin status (Negative vs. Positive)	1.159	.745	1.803	.514
Pelvic and PAFP LN metastasis status				
Group 1	1	-	-	-
Group 2	1.335	.821	2.169	.244
Group 3	1.288	.639	2.594	.479
Patients without adjuvant therapy				
Age	1.020	.985	1.055	.265
Preoperative PSA	1.003	.996	1.009	.423
Post-operative GS (≤7 vs. ≥8)	1.094	.648	1.848	.737
Pathologic stage (T2 vs. T3)	1.024	.601	1.746	.930
Margin status (Negative vs. Positive)	1.094	.648	1.848	.555
Pelvic and PAFP LN metastasis status				
Group 1	1	-	-	-
Group 2	1.350	.754	2.418	.312
Group 3	1.064	.406	2.792	.899
Patients with adjuvant therapy				
Age	.994	.933	1.059	.842
Preoperative PSA	1.009	1.001	1.016	.019
Post-operative GS (≤7 vs. ≥8)	1.925	.774	4.788	.159
Pathologic stage (T2 vs. T3)	.727	.250	2.117	.559
Margin status (Negative vs. Positive)	1.316	.467	3.711	.604
Pelvic and PAFP LN metastasis status				
Group 1	1	-	-	-
Group 2	1.633	.600	4.446	.337
Group 3	2.592	.857	7.842	.092

HR, hazard ratio; CI, confidence interval; Group 1, Pelvic LN metastasis only; Group 2, PAFP LN metastasis only; Group 3, Both pelvic LN & PAFP LN metastasis

RP, the overall incidence of metastasis in the PAFP LNs was 0.93 %. Simultaneously, the rate of LNs detected within the PAFP was 10.3 %. LN mapping within the PAFP demonstrated that 67.7 % of the LNs were located in the middle packet. Of the 88 patients with PAFP LN metastasis, 63 were upstaged as a result of the PAFP pathologic evaluation.

When clinicopathologic features were analyzed between men with and without LN in the PAFP, patients with LNs in the PAFP more frequently had biopsy GS 8–10, N1 disease pathologically, and positive surgical

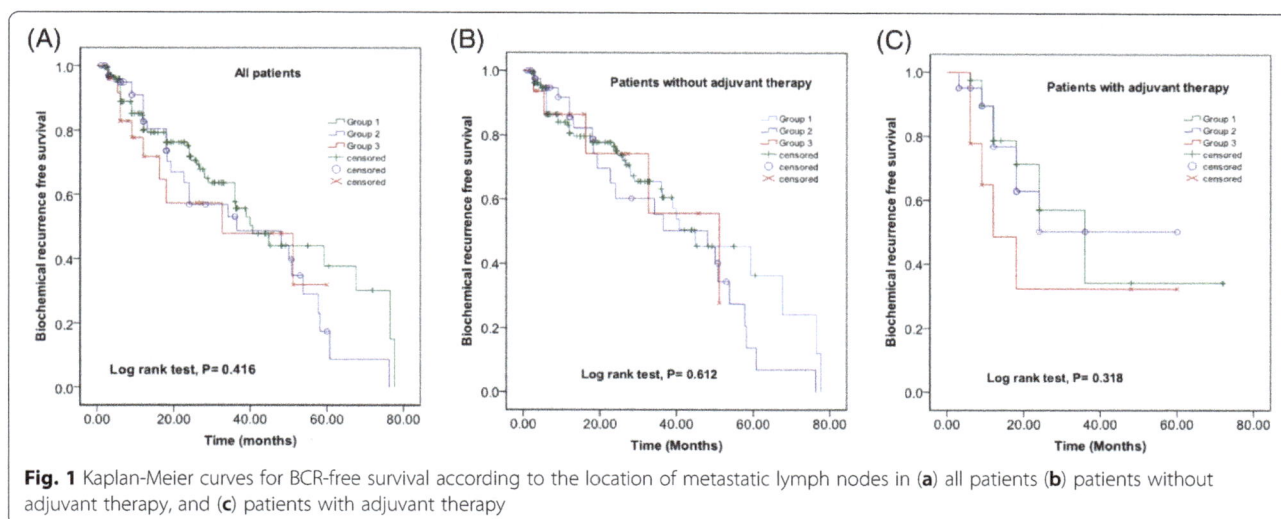

Fig. 1 Kaplan-Meier curves for BCR-free survival according to the location of metastatic lymph nodes in (**a**) all patients (**b**) patients without adjuvant therapy, and (**c**) patients with adjuvant therapy

margins. In comparison to the patients with isolated metastasis to the pelvic LNs, men with PAFP LNs metastasis had worse pathologic features. Yet, there was no significant difference in BCR free survival when the data were assessed based on the location of the metastasis (pelvic LN+, PAFP LN+, or pelvic LN+/PAFP LN+). Collectively, these observations suggest that the PAFP should be removed in all patients undergoing RP and that the oncologic implication of PAFP LN metastasis is equivalent to that of pelvic LN involvement in men with PCa.

Previously, our group reported on the detailed analysis of 40 patients with metastatic PCa to the PAFP LNs [17]. Because this original report was largely focused on the clinicopathologic features of men with PAFP LN metastasis, we designed the current study to assess the oncologic implications of PAFP LN involvement in men with PCa. To this end, we have increased the sample size to 9510 by increasing the number of participating institutions to thirteen. The study sites represent fourteen urologic surgeons from three different countries – USA, South Korea, and Taiwan.

A careful analysis of 8800 men after excluding patients with incomplete data revealed that men with LNs present in the PAFP were more likely to have aggressive disease as indicated by the higher frequency of biopsy GS 8–10 PCa, pathologic stage N1, and positive surgical margin. In a significantly smaller sample size of 356 men, Hansen et al. similarly reported that pathologic N1 disease was more frequently detected in patients who harbor LNs within the PAFP than those without LNs within the PAFP (21.1 % vs. 7 %, $P = 0.02$) [14]. In addition, it has been suggested that patients with LNs found in the PAFP were younger (60.5 vs. 65.0, $P = 0.002$) [13] while Jeong et al. noted that the mean preoperative PSA level was

significantly higher in patients with LNs present in the PAFP (7.70 vs. 6.01, $P = 0.039$) [15]. But in the present study, age and PSA did not show any differences between the two groups.

Clinically, the current study demonstrated that the outcome of men with metastatic PCa to the PAFP LNs is similar to that of patients with pelvic LN metastasis. To assess the oncologic significance of PAFP LN metastasis in men with PCa, we have compared the outcome based on the location of the positive LNs (pelvic LN only, PAFP LN only, and pelvic LN+/PAFP LN+) in both Cox regression model as well as Kaplan-Meier survival analysis. Pathologic analysis revealed that men with PAFP LN involvement, regardless of the pelvic LN status, had more aggressive features. Nevertheless, BCR free survival duration was not significantly different among the three groups. More importantly, this lack of difference in BCR free survival period was present regardless of adjuvant therapy ($P = 0.469$). Moreover, among 88 patients with PAFP LN+, there were 67 patients who had simultaneous ECE+ and PAFP LN+, illustrating a high level of correlation. The risk of BCR in the above group was highly elevated although no statistical difference was found when compared to those with ECE- or PAFP-: (31/67) 46.3 % vs. (68/227) 30.0 %, respectively ($P = 0.287$). Taken together, these findings suggest that PCa patients with metastasis to the PAFP LNs should be treated as those with pelvic LN metastasis.

Finally, results of the present study provide multiple reasons for the PAFP removal and pathologic analysis in all men undergoing RP. First, the PAFP LNs are likely an independent and separate anatomic landing zone for PCa metastasis. In our group's initial publication, we have reported that the LNs within the PAFP overwhelmingly mapped to the middle packet [17]. In this update, we have increased the sample size and carried out LN mapping in 300 patients. Again, a significant majority (67.7 %) of the LNs in PAFP were located in the middle packet. Accordingly, the detection of LNs within PAFP is not likely a result of an incomplete dissection of the obturator LNs. Second, the pathologic analysis of PAFP enhances the accuracy of staging. Of the 88 men with metastatic disease to the PAFP LNs, 63 were upstaged based on the PAFP LNs involvement. Third, there are no reliable preoperative parameters that predict the PAFP LN metastasis. Although no preoperative imaging is currently recommended for the detection of PAFP LN metastasis and for guidance in removing PAFP LN, the added surgical step in the absence of imaging modality will not likely compromise the quality of surgical outcomes. In our aforementioned initial multi-institution study that analyzed forty patients with PAFP LN disease, only three had a low-risk disease defined by the D'Amico criteria pre-operatively. Based on this observation, we suggested that the pathologic analysis of PAFP may not be necessary in men with low-risk PCa. However in the current study, 9.1 % had low-risk disease. Accordingly, all PAFP specimens should be analyzed pathologically. Fourth, there may be a therapeutic effect of PAFP removal. Of the 88 men with PAFP LN metastasis, fifty remain free of BCR. Taken together with the minimal surgical morbidity of PAFP dissection, we now contend that the removal and pathologic examination be a standard procedure in all patients undergoing RP.

Notwithstanding the strength of the largest sample size to date on this topic, our study is not without weaknesses. First, the number of men with PAFP LN metastasis was only 88. Given this small number of event, it is entirely possible that there is a unique oncologic implication of PAFP LN metastasis that requires a larger sample size to uncover. Indeed in this cohort, PAFP LN involvement, regardless of the pelvic LN status, had more aggressive pathologic features. Second, additional follow-up is necessary to evaluate cancer-specific and overall survival. Third, BCR comparisons among pelvic LN+, PAFP LN+, and PAFP LN+/Pelvic LN+ groups were likely confounded because a greater proportion of men with PAFP LN+ with and without pelvic LN+ (group 2 and 3) received adjuvant therapy than the men with pelvic LN+ only (group 1) (P = 0.012) (Table 2). Because adjuvant therapy may lower BCR, adjuvant therapy-adjusted BCR in group 2 and 3, may in fact, be higher. Hence, this finding may further support the substantial BCR risk associated with PAFP metastasis. We plan to continue increasing the overall sample size and track the patients with PAFP LN metastasis to determine the long-term oncologic outcome. In the meantime, the present study provides the relative confidence that PCa patients with PAFP LN metastasis should be treated as those with pelvic LN disease.

Conclusions

Metastasis to the PAFP LNs and pelvic LNs had equivalent duration of BCR free survival. Because the PAFP is likely an anatomically independent and separate landing zone of PCa metastasis, the PAFP should be removed and analyzed in all men undergoing RP.

Abbreviations

BCR: Biochemical recurrence; ECE: Extracapsular extension; GS: Gleason score; LN: Lymph node; PAFP: Prostatic anterior fat pad; PCa: Prostate cancer; PSA: Prostate-specific antigen; PAFP+: Metastasis to prostatic anterior fat pad lymph node; PNL+: Metastasis to pelvic lymph node; PLN: Pelvic lymph node; RARP: Robot-assisted radical prostatectomy; RRP: Retropubic radical prostatectomy.

Competing interests

None of the contributing authors have any conflicts of interest, including specific financial interests and relationships and affiliation relevant to the subject matter or materials discussed in the manuscript.

Authors' contributions

YSK and YSH reviewed the pertinent literature, analyzed the results, and drafted and edited the manuscript. IYK was responsible for the entire project. He designed the study concept, guided the study design, conducted data acquisition, and revised the manuscript critically for important intellectual content. PKM, AS, JSP, NP, IF, MM, DIL, EL, TP, KHR, TA, DS, HA, SKC, SP, SSJ, YCO, DE, VM, DA, KB, BY, NR, THK, TGK, DM, JH, and WJK collected data, analyzed data, and revised the manuscript. All authors read and approved the final manuscript.

Acknowledgements

This work was supported by a grant from the National Cancer Institute (P30CA072720), generous grants from the Tanzman Foundation, and a grant from the Korea Health Technology R&D Project through the Korea Health Industry Development Institute (KHIDI), funded by the Ministry of Health & Welfare, Republic of Korea (HI14C1642).

Author details

[1]Section of Urologic Oncology, Rutgers Cancer Institute of New Jersey and Rutgers Robert Wood Johnson Medical School, The State University of New Jersey, 195 Little Albany Street, New Brunswick, NJ, USA. [2]Department of Urology, School of Medicine, Kyungpook National University Medical Center, Daegu, Korea. [3]Department of Pathology, Robert Wood Johnson Medical School, New Brunswick, NJ, USA. [4]Division of Urology, University of Pennsylvania, Philadelphia, PA, USA. [5]Department of Urology, College of Medicine, Yonsei University, Seoul, Korea. [6]Department of Urology, UC Irvine School of Medicine, Orange, CA, USA. [7]Department of Urology, Asan Medical Center, University of Ulsan College of Medicine, Seoul, Korea. [8]Department of Urology, University of Ulsan College of Medicine, Ulsan University Hospital, Ulsan, Korea. [9]Department of Urology, Samsung Medical Center, Sungkyunkwan University School of Medicine, Seoul, Korea. [10]Prostate Disease Center, Taichung Veterans General Hospital, Taichung, Taiwan. [11]Department of Urology, Temple University School of Medicine, Philadelphia, PA, USA. [12]Department of Pathology, Temple University School of Medicine, Philadelphia, PA, USA. [13]Associated Medical Professionals, Syracuse, NY, USA. [14]Department of Urology, Icahn School of Medicine at Mount Sinai Hospital, New York, NY, USA. [15]Division of Urology and Urologic Oncology, City of Hope National Medical Center, Duarte, CA, USA. [16]Department of Urology, Georgetown University, Washington, DC, USA. [17]Department of Urology, Chungbuk National University College of Medicine, Cheongju, Korea.

References

1. Briganti A, Blute ML, Eastham JH, Graefen M, Heidenreich A, Karnes JR, et al. Pelvic lymph node dissection in prostate cancer. Eur Urol. 2009;55(6):1251–65.

2. Briganti A, Larcher A, Abdollah F, Capitanio U, Gallina A, Suardi N, et al. Updated nomogram predicting lymph node invasion in patients with prostate cancer undergoing extended pelvic lymph node dissection: the essential importance of percentage of positive cores. Eur Urol. 2012;61(3):480–7.

3. Briganti A, Abdollah F, Nini A, Suardi N, Gallina A, Capitanio U, et al. Performance characteristics of computed tomography in detecting lymph node metastases in contemporary patients with prostate cancer treated with extended pelvic lymph node dissection. Eur Urol. 2012;61(6):1132–8.

4. Joung JY, Cho I-C, Lee KH. Role of pelvic lymph node dissection in prostate cancer treatment. Korean J Urol. 2011;52(7):437–45.

5. Pound CR, Partin AW, Eisenberger MA, Chan DW, Pearson JD, Walsh PC. Natural history of progression after PSA elevation following radical prostatectomy. JAMA. 1999;281(17):1591–7.

6. Pagliarulo V, Hawes D, Brands FH, Groshen S, Cai J, Stein JP, et al. Detection of occult lymph node metastases in locally advanced node-negative prostate cancer. J Clin Oncol. 2006;24(18):2735–42.

7. Daneshmand S, Quek ML, Stein JP, Lieskovsky G, Cai J, Pinski J, et al. Prognosis of patients with lymph node positive prostate cancer following radical prostatectomy: long-term results. J Urol. 2004;172(6 Pt 1):2252–5.

8. Heidenreich A, Varga Z, Von Knobloch R. Extended pelvic lymphadenectomy in patients undergoing radical prostatectomy: high incidence of lymph node metastasis. J Urol. 2002;167(4):1681–6.

9. Bader P, Burkhard FC, Markwalder R, Studer UE. Disease progression and survival of patients with positive lymph nodes after radical prostatectomy. Is there a chance of cure? J Urol. 2003;169(3):849–54.

10. Ahlering TE, Eichel L, Edwards RA, Lee DI, Skarecky DW. Robotic radical prostatectomy: a technique to reduce pT2 positive margins. Urology. 2004;64(6):1224–8.

11. Kothari PS, Scardino PT, Ohori M, Kattan MW, Wheeler TM. Incidence, location, and significance of periprostatic and periseminal vesicle lymph nodes in prostate cancer. Am J Surg Pathol. 2001;25(11):1429–32.

12. Finley DS, Deane L, Rodriguez E, Vallone J, Deshmukh S, Skarecky D, et al. Anatomic excision of anterior prostatic fat at radical prostatectomy: implications for pathologic upstaging. Urology. 2007;70(5):1000–3.

13. Yuh B, Wu H, Ruel N, Wilson T. Analysis of regional lymph nodes in periprostatic fat following robot-assisted radical prostatectomy. BJU Int. 2012;109(4):603–7.

14. Hansen J, Budaus L, Spethmann J, Schlomm T, Salomon G, Rink M, et al. Assessment of rates of lymph nodes and lymph node metastases in periprostatic fat pads in a consecutive cohort treated with retropubic radical prostatectomy. Urology. 2012;80(4):877–82.

15. Jeong J, Choi EY, Kang DI, Ercolani M, Lee DH, Kim W-J, et al. Pathologic implications of prostatic anterior fat pad. Urol Oncol. 2013;31(1):63–7.

16. Aning JJ, Thurairaja R, Gillatt DA, Koupparis AJ, Rowe EW, Oxley J. Pathological analysis of lymph nodes in anterior prostatic fat excised at robot-assisted radical prostatectomy. J Clin Pathol. 2014;67(9):787–91.

17. Kim IY, Modi PK, Sadimin E, Ha Y-S, Kim JH, Skarecky D, et al. Detailed analysis of patients with metastasis to the prostatic anterior fat pad lymph nodes: a multi-institutional study. J Urol. 2013;190(2):527–34.

2

Clinical, molecular and cytogenetic analysis of 46, XX testicular disorder of sex development with *SRY*-positive

Qiu-Yue Wu[1], Na Li[1], Wei-Wei Li[1], Tian-Fu Li[1], Cui Zhang[1], Ying-Xia Cui[1], Xin-Yi Xia[1*] and Jin-Sheng Zhai[2*]

Abstract

Background: To review the possible mechanisms proposed to explain the etiology of 46, XX sex reversal by investigating the clinical characteristics and their relationships with chromosomal karyotype and the *SRY*(sex-determining region Y)gene.

Methods: Five untreated 46, XX patients with *SRY*-positive were referred for infertility. Clinical data were collected, and Karyotype analysis of G-banding in lymphocytes and Fluorescence in situ hybridization (FISH) were performed. Genomic DNA from peripheral blood of the patients using QIAamp DNA Blood Kits was extracted. The three discrete regions, AZFa, AZFb and AZFc, located on the long arm of the Y chromosome, were performed by multiplex PCRs(Polymerase Chain Reaction) amplification. The set of PCR primers for the diagnosis of microdeletion of the AZFa, AZFb and AZFc region included: sY84, sY86, sY127, sY134, sY254, sY255, SRY and ZFX/ZFY.

Results: Our five patients had a lower body height. Physical examination revealed that their testes were small in volume, soft in texture and normal penis. Semen analyses showed azoospermia. All patients had a higher follicle-stimulating hormone(FSH), Luteinizing Hormone(LH) level, lower free testosterone, testosterone level and normal Estradiol, Prolactin level. Karyotype analysis of all patients confirmed 46, XX karyotype, and FISH analysis showed that *SRY* gene were positive and translocated to Xp. Molecular analysis revealed that the *SRY* gene were present, and the AZFa, AZFb and AZFc region were absent.

Conclusions: This study adds cases on the five new 46, XX male individuals with *SRY*-positive and further verifies the view that the presence of *SRY* gene and the absence of major regions in Y chromosome should lead to the expectance of a completely masculinised phenotype, abnormal hormone levels and infertility.

Keywords: 46, XX testicular disorder of sex development (DSD), *SRY*-positive, Sexual hormone

Background

The 46, XX disorder of sex development (DSD) is a rare form of sex reversal in infertile men, that was first described by la Chapelle et al. in 1964 and occurred 1:20000 in newborn subjects [1]. By 1996, 150 patients with classical XX male syndrome had been reported, and more than 100 cases of this disorder have been discribed between 1996 and 2006 worldwide [2]. Clinical phenotypes about 46, XX DSD have been identified to three groups, including males with normal phenotype, males with genital ambiguities and males with true hermaphrodites [3]. Ovotesticular DSD, which is characterized by the presence of both testicular and ovarian tissue in the gonads of the same individual, and testicular DSD characterized by a full development of both gonads as testes without any evidence of ovarian tissue [4]. Approximately 80% of individuals with 46,XX testicular DSD present after puberty with normal pubic hair and normal penile size, but small testes, and sterility resulting from azoospermia [5].

The sex-determining region Y gene (*SRY*) locating in Y chromosome, plays a major role in encoding a testis determining factor (TDF) [6,7]. About 90% of these patients have Y chromosomal material including the *SRY* gene, that

* Correspondence: xinyixia78@gmail.com; Zhaijinshengnz@gmail.com
[1]Institute of Laboratory Medicine, Jinling Hospital, Nanjing University School of Medicine, 305 East Zhongshan Road, Nanjing 210002, PR China
[2]Department of Health Care, Jinling Hospital, Nanjing University School of Medicine, Nanjing 210002, PR, China

are usually translocated to the distal tip of the short arm of X chromosome or autosomal chromosomes. About 10% 46, XX males are negative for SRY gene, which could carry different degrees of masculinization [8,9].

There are several pathogenic mechanisms explaining 46, XX testicular DSD patients: 1. translocation of Y sequences, including the SRY gene, to an X chromosome or to an autosome; 2. a mutation in a gene in the testis-determining pathway triggering testis differentiation in SRY negative XX males; and 3. a hidden Y chromosome mosaicism limited to the gonad [10].

This study aimed to describing five 46, XX male DSD with SRY-positive, investigating the clinical characteristics and their relationships with chromosomal karyotype and the SRY gene.

Methods
Participant and Clinical data
We collected 5 untreated patients with SRY-positive 46, XX, that were referred for infertility. The physical examination included the measurement of height, potential gynecomastia and the inspection of external sex organs. Bilateral volume was calculated as the sum of the volume of both testes. According to guidelines of the World Health Organization, semen analysis was indicated to azoospermia after centrifugation of the ejaculate.

Serum levels of follicle-stimulating hormone (FSH), Luteinizing Hormone (LH), Estradiol, Prolactin, testosterone and free testosterone were assessed.

All procedures used in the study confirmed to the tenets of the Declaration of Helsinki. The Ethics Committee of Jinling Hospital approved the protocols used. All participants have known to participate in the study. Written informed consents were obtained from all participants.

Karyotype analysis of G-banding in lymphocytes and Fluorescence in situ hybridization (FISH)
Karyotypes were performed on peripheral blood lymphocytes in five patients respectively including 100 metaphase cells by conventional operating techniques. X chromosome, Y chromosome and SRY gene was located using FISH with probes of X chromosome centromere, Y chromosome centromere (CEP X with Spectrum Green, CEP Y with Spectrum Orange, Vysis, Downers Grove, IL; item no.32-111051) and SRY gene (SRY with Orange,Vysis, Downers Grove, IL; item no.30-190079).

Molecular analysis
Genomic DNA from peripheral blood of the patients using QIAamp DNA Blood Kits was extracted. The three discrete regions, AZFa, AZFb and AZFc, located on the long arm of the Y chromosome, were performed by multiplex PCRs(Polymerase Chain Reaction) amplification. The set of PCR primers for the diagnosis of

microdeletion of the AZFa, AZFb and AZFc region included: sY84, sY86, sY127, sY134, sY254, sY255, SRY and ZFX/ZFY.

Results
Our five patients had a lower body height. Physical examination revealed that their testes were small in volume, soft in texture and normal penis. No potential gynecomastia and congenital hypospadias were seen. And they all described that they had normal sexual function. Semen analyses showed azoospermia. Endocrinological data indicated that the patients had a higher FSH, LH level, lower free testosterone, testosterone level and normal Estradiol, Prolactin level. General characteristics and endocrine hormone levels are shown in Table 1.

Karyotype analysis of all patients confirmed 46, XX karyotype, and FISH analysis showed that SRY gene were positive and translocated to Xp (Figure 1). Molecular analysis revealed that the SRY gene was present, and the AZFa, AZFb and AZFc region were absent (Figure 2).

Discussion
46, XX male syndrome is a rare sex reversal syndrome characterized by a female karyotype in discordance with a male phenotype. 90% of 46, XX testicular DSD usually have a normal male phenotypic heterogeneity at birth and are diagnosed after puberty on genital ambiguities, or infertility [8]. Our research reported that five patients had a female karyotype but were phenotypically male (46, XX males). They had normal external genitalia and masculinization, but showed azoospermia. That might be that all males were SRY-positive, which translocated on the short arm of X chromosome, and absent of the spermatogenic factors encoding gene on Yq, such as AZFa, AZFb and AZFc region in Y chromosome.

SRY gene is located in the Y chromosome and encodes a high mobility group(HMG) domain, a conserved motif present in many DNA-binding proteins, which could regulate testicular differentiation [11,12]. SRY protein is expressed in the genital ridge before testis formation, and in the testis during the period of testicular formation early in fetal life, until the development of adult testis [13]. Molecular genetics analysis demonstrated that most 46, XX testicular DSD patients carry SRY gene which translocated to X chromosome [14-16]. There was a report that an SRY gene fragment translocated from Y chromosome to autosomal chromosome [17]. Some patients showed SRY negative, who always had external genital ambiguities and gynecomastia. Despite the fact that SRY gene is considered to be the main regulatory factor for testis determination, phenotypic variability showed in 46, XX sex reversed cases cannot be explained only by whether SRY gene is presented. And a number of other genes such as SOX9, DAX-1, WT1,

Table 1 General characteristics and endocrine hormone levels

Cases	Body height (cm)	Age at presentation, development of secondary sex (year)	Volume of teste (ml)	Stretched penile length (cm)	Testosterone (nmol/L)	Free testosterone (pmol/L)	FSH (IU/L)	LH (IU/L)	Estradiol (pmol/L)	Prolactin (mIU/L)
1	165	12	6	9	6.8	27.7	35.5	13.8	112	201
2	162	15	3	8	5.4	15.2	29.2	12.9	70	158
3	164	14	4	8.5	8.9	29.4	45.9	25.1	98	78
4	167	11	9	11	8.4	28.1	33.7	22.3	107	232
5	165	12	7	10	7.0	20.5	31.4	19.6	81	167
Normal ranges	≥169	12-14	12-20	8-18	9.4-37.0	30.9-147.6	1-7	2-10	0-250	0-400

WNT4, FGF9 and RSPO1 have been involved in the process of gonadal differentiation [8].

The phenotype of the XX male observed in *SRY* positive 46,XX individuals varies greatly, from normal internal and external male gonads to abnormal secondary sexual characteristics, small testes and hypospadias, to a true hermaphrodite. It has been suggested that the variation in phenotype is primarily dependent on two mechanisms: X chromosome inactivation(XCI) pattern and the amount of Y material including *SRY* gene that has been translocated to the X chromosome [18]. Reviewing the literature, 46,XX males with true hermaphrodites or gonadal ambiguity have a small portion of the Y chromosome material translocated to the X, presumably allowing for XCI spreading and inactivating the *SRY* gene [19]. A normal male phenotype is expected to result from a larger Yp *SRY* bearing fragment being translocated to the X chromosome, where the length of the Yp fragment may protect the *SRY* gene from silencing by the spread of XCI [19]. In our study, all five cases have

normal external genitalia and masculinization, which is expected that more Y chromosome material is present on the X, presumably protecting the *SRY* gene from the spread of inactivation. Because of the unavailable in specimens from the five cases to further study, we cannot do more molecular analysis to confirm the above point. Till now, both random and non-random XCI patterns have been reported in 46, XX males with a normal male phenotype [18,20]. It is indicated that the XCI pattern may be not associated with the XX male phenotype.

However, another mechaniam, known as the position effect, has been reported to explain the observed phenotypic differences. The phenotypic differences are dependent on the proximity of the breakpoint to the *SRY* gene as well as the presence or absence of cryptic rearrangements affecting the expression of the *SRY* gene [21]. The rearrangements, may result in transcriptional repression, probably by removing essential regulatory elements or alterations of local chromatin structure [22].

Additionally, phenotypic variability might be associated with variations in genetic polymorphisms and copy

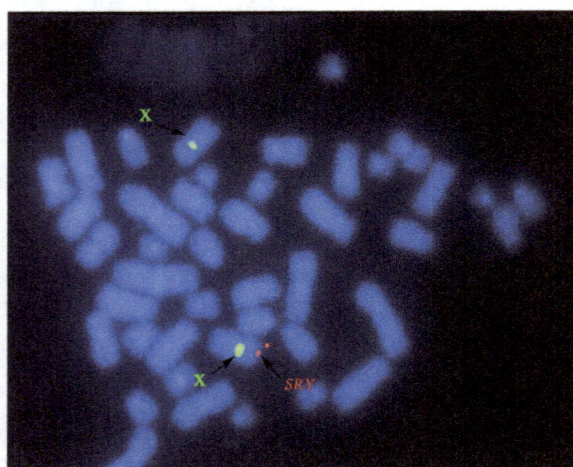

Figure 1 Fluorescent in situ hybridization (FISH) on metaphase chromosomes of second case with the LSI *SRY*(orange)/CEP X (green) probes. Metaphase spread showing a normal X chromosome (green signal for centromeric DXZ1 locus) and the *SRY* (orange) translocates to the distal end of short arm of chromosome X.

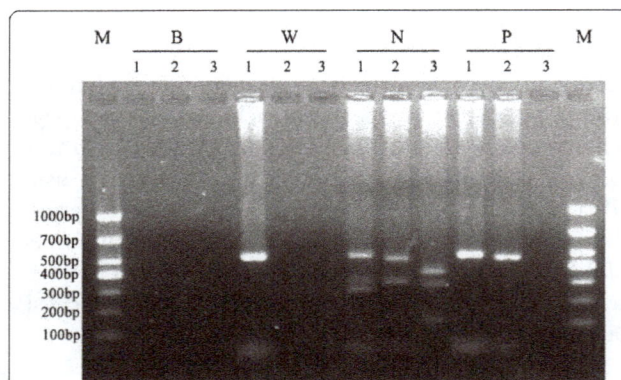

Figure 2 Result of multiplex polymerase chain reaction (PCR). Multiplex 1: ZFX/ZFY(690 bp), sY84 (320 bp), sY127 (274 bp); Multiplex 2: SRY (472 bp), sY86 (326 bp); Multiplex 3: sY254 (400 bp), sY134 (301 bp), sY255 (126 bp). M: DL1000 DNAMarker; W: a DNA sample from a woman as a negative control; N: a DNA sample fro-m a normal fertile man as a positive control; P: a DNA sample from the patient; B: a al-ank (water) control.

number variation of specific genes on the X chromosome, such as NROB1 and TAF7L [23,24].

Classical 46, XX male have normal testosterone level and free testosterone level during adolescence, but may decrease in adulthood, leading to hypergonadotropic hypogonadism [25]. Our cases had normal genitalia and were diagnosed for infertility after puberty. The level of testosterone and free testosterone is deficiency in five patients. In addition, high levels of FSH and LH are observed. This might explain that even though the 46, XX male have a normal external genitalia and masculinization, and they are lack of spermatogenesis.

The body heights of the patients we reported were all under 169 cm (the average height of Chinese male) and close to that of normal females. There are some phenotypic similarities between 46,XX men and those with Klinefelter syndrome, but 46,XX men tend to be shorter than men with KS [9]. Kirsch *et al.* indicated that the Y chromosome growth-control gene(*GCY*) which next to the centromere had a possible impact on growth [26]. And there were some papers indicating that *SHOX* gene (short stature homeobox) expression and *SHOX* enhancer regions played a role in the growth [27]. It has been suggested that specific growth genes in the Y chromosome cannot switched to the patients, which might make them to show a female stature. GH (growth hormone) therapy may have some statural effects in the SHOX haploinsufficiency and may be insufficient to prevent the development of skeletal lesions after puberty [28].

Conclusions

Our reports adds cases on the five new 46, XX male individuals with sex reversal and further verifies the view that the presence of *SRY* gene and the absence of major regions in Y chromosome should lead to the expectance of a completely masculinised phenotype, abnormal hormone levels and infertility.

Abbreviations
DSD: Disorder of sex development; *SRY*: Sex-determining region Y gene; TDF: testis determining factor; FISH: Fluorescence in situ hybridization; FSH: Follicle-stimulating hormone; LH: Luteinizing Hormone; PCR: Polymerase Chain Reaction; HMG: High mobility group; SOX9: SRY (sex determining region Y)-box 9 gene; *WT1*: Wilms tumor 1 gene, WNT4, wingless-type MMTV integration site family, member 4 gene; FGF9, fibroblast growth factor 9 gene; RSPO1: R-spondin 1 gene; GCY: Growth-control gene; SHOX: Short stature homeobox; GH: Growth hormone; XCI: X chromosome inactivation; KS: Klinefelter syndrome; NROB1(DAX-1): Nuclear receptor subfamily 0, group B, member 1 gene; TAF7L: TAF7-like RNA polymerase II gene.

Competing interests
The authors declare that they have no competing interests.

Authors' contributions
QW carried out the molecular genetic studies and drafted the manuscript. NL, WL, TL and CZ participated in the laboratory work. YC, JZ and XX conceived of the study, and participated in its design and coordination and helped to draft the manuscript. All authors read and approved the final manuscript.

Acknowledgements
This work was supported by the Natural Science Foundation of Jiangsu province (BK2011660), Key Foundation of Jiangsu Science and Technology Bureau (BM2013058) and the Natural Science Foundation of China (30901652). We thank all members of the family for their cooperation in the study.

References
1. Chapelle A, Hortling H, Niemi M, Wennström J: XX sex chromosomes in a human male. *Acta Medica Scandinavica* 1964, 175(Suppl 412):25–28.
2. Chiang HS, Wu YN, Wu CC, Hwang JL: Cytogenic and molecular analyses of 46, XX male syndrome with clinical comparison to other groups with testicular azoospermia of genetic origin. *J Formos Med Assoc* 2013, 112(2):72–78.
3. Lee GM, Ko JM, Shin CH, Yang SW: A Korean boy with 46,XX testicular disorder of sex development caused by SOX9 duplication. *Ann Pediatr Endocrinol Metab* 2014, 19(2):108–112.
4. Alves C, Braid Z, Coeli FB, Mello MP: 46, XX Male-Testicular Disorder of Sexual Differentiation (DSD): hormonal, molecular and cytogenetic studies. *Arq Bras Endocrinol Metabol* 2010, 54(8):685–689.
5. Vilain EJ: 46, XX testicular disorder of sex development. Washington University Press: Seattle (WA); 1993.
6. Anık A, Çatlı G, Abacı A, Böber E: 46, XX Male Disorder of Sexual Development: A Case Report. *J clin res pediatr endocrinol* 2013, 5(4):258–260.
7. Jain M, Chaudhary I, Halder A: The Sertoli Cell Only Syndrome and Glaucoma in a Sex–Determining Region Y (SRY) Positive XX Infertile Male. *J Clin Diagn Res* 2013, 7(7):1457–1459.
8. Ergun-Longmire B, Vinci G, Alonso L, Matthew S, Tansil S, Lin-Su K, McElreavey K, New MI: Clinical, hormonal and cytogenetic evaluation of 46, XX males and review of the literature. *J Clin Endocrinol Metab* 2005, 18(8):739–748.
9. Vorona E, Zitzmann M, Gromoll J, Schüring AN, Nieschlag E: Clinical, endocrinological, and epigenetic features of the 46, XX male syndrome, compared with 47, XXY Klinefelter patients. *Journal of Clinical Endocrinology & Metabolism* 2007, 92(9):3458–3465.
10. Zenteno-Ruiz JC, Kofman-Alfaro S, Méndez JP: 46, XX sex reversal. *Arch Med Res* 2001, 32(6):559–566.
11. Jiang T, Hou CC, She ZY, Yang WX: The SOX gene family: function and regulation in testis determination and male fertility maintenance. *Mol Biol Rep* 2013, 40(3):2187–2194.
12. Zhao L, Koopman P: SRY protein function in sex determination: thinking outside the box. *Chromosom Res* 2012, 20(1):153–162.
13. Sekido R: SRY: A transcriptional activator of mammalian testis determination. *Int J Biochem Cell Biol* 2010, 42(3):417–420.
14. Rizvi AA: 46, XX man with SRY gene translocation: cytogenetic characteristics, clinical features and management. *Am J Med Sci* 2008, 335(4):307–309.
15. Chernykh V, Kurilo L, Shilova N, Zolotukhina T, Ryzhkova O, Bliznetz E, Polyakov A: Hidden X chromosomal mosaicism in a 46, XX male. *Sex Dev* 2009, 3(4):183–187.
16. Beaulieu Bergeron M, Lemyre E, Lemieux N: Identification of new susceptibility regions for X; Y translocations in patients with testicular disorder of sex development. *Sex Dev* 2010, 5(1):1–6.
17. Dauwerse JG, Hansson KB, Brouwers AA, Peters DJ, Breuning MH: An XX male with the sex-determining region Y gene inserted in the long arm of chromosome 16. *Fertil Steril* 2006, 86(2):463. e461-463. e465.
18. Minor A, Mohammed F, Farouk A, Hatakeyama C, Johnson K, Chow V, Ma S: Genetic characterization of two 46, XX males without gonadal ambiguities. *J Assist Reprod Genet* 2008, 25(11–12):547–552.
19. Kusz K, Kotecki M, Wojda A, Szarras-Czapnik M, Latos-Bielenska A, Warenik-Szymankiewicz A, Ruszczynska-Wolska A, Jaruzelska J: Incomplete masculinisation of XX subjects carrying the SRY gene on an inactive X chromosome. *J Med Genet* 1999, 36(6):452–456.
20. Jakubowski L, Jeziorowska A, Constantinou M, Helszer Z, Baumstark A, Vogel W, Mikiewicz-Sygula D, Kaulzewski B: Xp; Yp translocation inherited from the father in anSRY, RBM, andTSPY positive true hermaphrodite with oligozoospermia. *J Med Genet* 2000, 37(10):E28.
21. Gunes S, Asci R, Okten G, Atac F, Onat OE, Ogur G, Aydin O, Ozcelik T, Bagci H: Two males with SRY-positive 46, XX testicular disorder of sex development. *Systems Bio Reprod Med* 2013, 59(1):42–47.

22. Sharp A, Kusz K, Jaruzelska J, Tapper W, Szarras-Czapnik M, Wolski J, Jacobs P: **Variability of sexual phenotype in 46, XX (SRY+) patients: the influence of spreading X inactivation versus position effects.** *J Med Genet* 2005, **42**(5):420–427.

23. White S, Ohnesorg T, Notini A, Roeszler K, Hewitt J, Daggag H, Smith C, Turbitt E, Gustin S, van den Bergen J, Miles D, Western P, Arboleda V, Schumacher V, Gordon L, Bell K, Bengtsson H, Speed T, Hutson J, Warne G, Harley V, Koopman P, Vilain E, Sinclair A: **Copy number variation in patients with disorders of sex development due to 46, XY gonadal dysgenesis.** *PLoS One* 2011, **6**(3):e17793.

24. Akinloye O, Gromoll J, Callies C, Nieschlag E, Simoni M: **Mutation analysis of the X-chromosome linked, testis-specific TAF7L gene in spermatogenic failure.** *Andrologia* 2007, **39**(5):190–195.

25. Velasco G, Savarese V, Sandorfi N, Jimenez SA, Jabbour S: **46, XX SRY-positive male syndrome presenting with primary hypogonadism in the setting of scleroderma.** *Endocr Pract* 2011, **17**(1):95–98.

26. Kirsch S, Weiss B, Schön K, Rappold GA: **The definition of the Y chromosome growth-control gene (GCY) critical region: relevance of terminal and interstitial deletions.** *Journal of pediatric endocrinology & metabolism: JPEM* 2002, **15**:1295–1300.

27. Chen J, Wildhardt G, Zhong Z, Röth R, Weiss B, Steinberger D, Decker J, Blum WF, Rappold G: **Enhancer deletions of the SHOX gene as a frequent cause of short stature: the essential role of a 250 kb downstream regulatory domain.** *J Med Genet* 2009, **46**(12):834–839.

28. Binder G: **Short stature due to SHOX deficiency: genotype, phenotype, and therapy.** *Horm Rese Paediatr* 2011, **75**(2):81–89.

3

The ProCaSP study: quality of life outcomes of prostate cancer patients after radiotherapy or radical prostatectomy in a cohort study

Nora Eisemann[1*], Sandra Nolte[2,3], Maike Schnoor[4], Alexander Katalinic[1,4], Volker Rohde[5,6] and Annika Waldmann[4]

Abstract

Background: This study describes and compares health-related quality of life (HRQOL) of prostate cancer patients who received either radical prostatectomy (nerve-sparing, nsRP, or non-nerve-sparing, nnsRP) or radiotherapy (external RT, brachytherapy, or both combined) for treatment of localised prostate cancer.

Methods: The prospective, multicenter cohort study included 529 patients. Questionnaires included the IIEF, QLQ-C30, and PORPUS-P. Data were collected before (baseline), three, six, twelve, and twenty-four months after treatment. Differences between groups' baseline characteristics were assessed; changes over time were analysed with generalised estimating equations (GEE). Missing values were treated with multiple imputation. Further, scores at baseline and end of follow-up were compared to German reference data.

Results: The typical time trend was a decrease of average HRQOL three months after treatment followed by (partial) recovery. RP patients experienced considerable impairment in sexual functioning. The covariate-adjusted GEE identified a significant - but not clinically relevant - treatment effect for diarrhoea (b = 7.0 for RT, p = 0.006) and PORPUS-P (b = 2.3 for nsRP, b = 2.2 for RT, p = 0.045) compared to the reference nnsRP. Most of the HRQOL scores were comparable to German norm values.

Conclusions: Findings from previous research were reproduced in a specific setting of a patient cohort in the German health care system. According to the principle of evidence-based medicine, this strengthens the messages regarding treatment in prostate cancer and its impacts on patients' health-related quality of life. After adjustment for baseline HRQOL and other covariates, RT patients reported increased symptoms of diarrhoea, and nnsRP patients decreased prostate-specific HRQOL. RP patients experienced considerable impairment in sexual functioning. These differences should be taken into account by physicians when choosing the best therapy for a patient.

Keywords: Prostatic neoplasms, Radiotherapy, Prostatectomy, Quality of life, Cohort study

Background

Prostate cancer has a very long period of latency of up to 15–20 years during which the disease is histologically present but has not yet become symptomatic. Autopsy studies have shown that a relevant proportion of men – depending on age and on ethnicity up to 83% (US whites, age group 71–80 years) – has an occult prostate cancer [1,2].

Despite the conflicting evidence of benefits and harms of PSA screening [3,4] and no coverage of costs by

statutory health insurance in Germany, testing on patient request is common practice (approx. 30% per year in men aged 45+) [5]. With the increasing use of PSA testing it can be assumed that nowadays a relevant proportion of former asymptomatic, occult cancer will be diagnosed. Today, prostate cancer is the most common malignancy in men in Germany with about 65,000 incident cases each year and a five-year prevalence of about 280,000 men [6].

As every screening test, including the PSA test, aims to detect occult cancers at an early stage, one can assume that a relevant proportion of screening detected prostate cancers would not have become symptomatic

* Correspondence: nora.eisemann@uksh.de
[1]Institute of Cancer Epidemiology, University of Luebeck, Ratzeburger Allee 160, 23562 Luebeck, Germany
Full list of author information is available at the end of the article

during life time and thus can be regarded as overdiagnosis. In these patients cancer treatment may have no benefit but may result in treatment associated morbidity [7]. As there is a moral imperative for treatment of cancer patients independent of tumour size, most young to middle-aged patients with non-metastatic prostate cancer receive some kind of invasive treatment. The main therapeutic strategies are radical prostatectomy (RP), external radiation, and interstitial brachytherapy. Each of above therapies can achieve a five-year cancer-specific survival of more than 90% [8]. Because of the favourable prognosis of early stage tumours and because of treatment morbidity, outcomes other than 'survival' are increasingly important [9].

As a result, many studies focus on middle-term or long-term health-related quality of life (HRQOL) outcomes. For example, non-nerve-sparing RP (nnsRP) has been shown to lead to a higher rate of incontinence and impotence. Nerve-sparing RP (nsRP) has been reported to have a positive impact on postoperative incontinence and impotence [10,11], and is preferred whenever possible. Examples of side effects of radiotherapy (RT) include irritable urinary and bowel problems, i.e. symptoms that can fundamentally compromise patients' overall well-being [12-14]. While it is desirable to detect early stages of prostate cancer and thus lower mortality rates of prostate cancer, these therapies can have substantial impact on the HRQOL of cancer patients.

In view of the high proportion of overdiagnosis in prostate cancer [15-17] and while there is 'no optimal way to treat localised prostate cancer' [18], the pros and cons of the available treatment options must be considered. The ProCaSP Study was an observational study aimed at comparing longitudinal HRQOL outcomes across a range of treatment groups for localised prostate cancer in real-world treatment situations. In detail, it was aimed at exploring inter-group differences between two prostatectomy and three radiotherapy groups: 1) nerve-sparing RP, 2) non-nerve-sparing RP, 3) brachytherapy (brachyRT), 4) external RT (externRT), and 5) combined external and brachytherapy (combRT). In addition, HRQOL of the cancer patients was compared to a reference population.

Methods
The ProCaSP Study
The Prostate Cancer, Sexuality, and Partnership (ProCaSP) Study was a German prospective multicenter study. ProCaSP was aimed at evaluating HRQOL outcomes of patients with localised prostate cancer treated with either radical prostatectomy or radiotherapy. Furthermore, the data included patients' perceptions on sexuality and partnership (data not reported) and their partners' HRQOL [19]. Inclusion criteria were stages

T1a to T3b according to the TNM-classification 5th edition [20], no transurethral prostate resection within the last six months, and prostate volume ≤50 ml. Exclusion criteria were positive skeletal scintigraphy, synchronic or metachronic secondary tumours, participation in another study, and insufficient capacity to contract. Patients were classified into different risk groups [21].

The choice of treatment was based on a shared decision between patient and urologist. The decision regarding nerve-sparing versus non-nerve-sparing procedure was made by the hospital surgeon during surgery.

Data collection
From 2002 to 2006, patients were recruited in ten German study locations. Follow-up was completed in 2008. Data were collected before (baseline), three, six, twelve, and twenty-four months after the start of treatment. Patients were asked to provide information on sociodemographic characteristics, treatment, sexual functioning, and HRQOL.

Cancer-specific HRQOL, prostate-specific HRQOL, and sexual functioning were measured by validated questionnaires (see below). Urinary functioning, which is of interest as it is often compromised after RT, was measured by the best available instrument in German language at that time, the Prostate Specific Module (PSM) [22]. However, in our study cohort the PSM was found to have insufficient psychometric properties for some of the PSM scales and the data was, therefore, not considered in this analysis.

European organisation of research and treatment in cancer quality of life questionnaire, core module (EORTC QLQ-C30)
The QLQ-C30 is a cancer-specific HRQOL measure. Version 3.0 comprises 30 items covering five functioning scales, three symptom scales, six symptom items, and two items on global HRQOL. Raw scores can be transformed to a range between 0 and 100, with higher functioning scores representing better functioning and higher scores for symptoms/problems representing worse conditions, respectively [23]. The minimal clinically important difference (MCID) was set at ten points [24].

Patient-oriented prostate utility scale (PORPUS)
The PORPUS questionnaire is a prostate-specific HRQOL instrument. The single HRQOL score, the PORPUS-P [25,26], ranges from 0 to 100, with higher values representing higher HRQOL. Differences of five points were interpreted as the MCID [25].

International index of erectile function (IIEF)

The IIEF-15 measures sexual functioning. The 15 items were summed up to a total score ranging between 5 and 75. Higher values correspond to higher functioning.

Ethics and consent

The study protocol was approved by the ethics committee of the Giessen University Hospital, Germany. All patients provided written informed consent.

Statistical analysis

Analyses were performed using R 3.0.2 [27]. First, patients' sociodemographic characteristics and their tumor-specific data were described with means (standard deviations), absolute and relative frequencies. Differences in patients' characteristics between the three main groups (nnsRP, nsRP, RT) were tested with Chi-square and F-tests, respectively. Statistical significance was defined as $p< =0.05$.

Second, time trends of mean HRQOL were presented graphically by main treatment groups (nnsRP, nsRP, RT) and by RT subgroups (brachyRT, externRT, and combRT). Although we did not consider sexual functioning as a main outcome, changes over time are shown to illustrate the different trends of the treatment group.

Third, the relationship between treatment (nnsRP, nsRP, RT) and HRQOL was analysed using generalised estimating equations (GEE) that account for the correlation between repeated HRQOL observations. The HRQOL observations of the follow-up period were modeled depending on respective treatment option, while adjusting for baseline characteristics (baseline HRQOL, age, having a partner (yes/no), highest education level (no graduation, 8–9 years ('Hauptschulabschluss'), 10–11 years ('Realschulabschluss'), >= 12 years high school ('(Fach-)Abitur'), working (yes/no), residence (rural/urban), tumour stage (T-category of the TNM-classification), pre-therapeutic Gleason score, pre-therapeutic PSA score, and sexual functioning at baseline (IIEF total scale)). Regression coefficients of treatment options with their confidence intervals and Wald tests for testing the effect of treatment option are reported. The analysis was repeated after splitting the RT group into the three subgroups brachyRT, externRT, and combRT.

Most HRQOL domains and some patient characteristics were affected by missing values ranging from 0% to 41.1%, with 22.7% of all observations missing. Multiple imputation is known to be a statistically sound method for handling incomplete data [28]. Hence, missing values were imputed ten times depending on all patient characteristics and on those observation times of HRQOL domains with a correlation of at least 0.5. Results were pooled according to Rubin's Rule [28].

Fourth, the HRQOL scores at baseline and twenty-four months after treatment of the three main treatment groups as well as the three RT subgroups were compared to German norm values for the EORTC QLQ-C30 [29] by calculating the reference score in a population with a similar age distribution and presenting the difference between the treatment groups' score and the reference value.

Post hoc statistical power analysis

A post hoc power analysis was conducted using the software package G*Power3 [30] with $\alpha = 0.05$, two-tailed. The calculation was based on a repeated measure MANOVA for the two groups with the highest and the lowest HRQOL, which had also the lowest sample sizes: nsRP (n = 127) and RP (n = 133). The expected treatment difference was the MCID, namely 10 for HRQOL and 5 for PORPUS-P. The standard deviation (SD) (between 10 and 20 for the different outcomes) and the correlation between the four repeated measures of the individuals (between 0.5 and 0.8) were estimated from the data. Power was generally far above 95%.

Results

Patients and tumour characteristics

516 of the initial 529 patients had complete or partially complete HRQOL data and were included. Approximately one of five observations for each HRQOL outcome (23.9%) and one of the ten baseline covariate values (13.3%) were missing for every patient. 256 patients received nnsRP, 127 nsRP, and 133 patients received RT, of which 44 were treated by brachyRT, 52 by externRT, and 37 by combRT. More than half of those patients treated with RT, where information on pre-baseline androgen deprivation therapy was available, additionally received androgen deprivation therapy (ADT) (52%).

Compared to patients receiving other treatment options, patients who underwent nsRP surgery were younger, were more often employed, more often living in a rural area, and had a better baseline sexual functioning (Table 1). Tumours that could not be treated nerve-sparingly during surgery had more often an advanced stage. RT patients were on average older than patients in the other treatment groups, more often not employed, living in urban areas, had a higher PSA level, more often a small tumour stage, and a lower sexual functioning. Comparison of D'Amico risk stratification revealed a much lower risk for the RT treatment groups. More than 80% of the nnsRP and nsRP patients were considered at high risk compared to less than 40% of the RT patients (data after multiple imputation, not shown). Pre-treatment PSA levels were highest in the combRT group and lowest in the nsRP group, while Gleason levels were highest in the nnsRP group and lowest in the brachyRT group.

Table 1 Sociodemographic characteristics and tumor specific data

	Radical prostatectomy		Radiotherapy				p-value[1]
	Non-nerve-sparing (reference)	Nerve-sparing	Total	Brachytherapy	Combined (External/ brachytherapy)	External	
	(n = 256)	(n = 127)	(n = 133)	(n = 44)	(n = 37)	(n = 52)	
Age [mean ± SD]	64.2 ± 6.3	59.7 ± 6.1	66.5 ± 5.5	65.0 ± 6.0	66.8 ± 5.5	67.7 ± 4.8	<0.001
Partnership [N (%)]							
Not living with a partner	14 (5.5)	6 (4.7)	10 (7.5)	4 (9.1)	3 (8.1)	3 (5.8)	0.586
Married or having a spouse	239 (93.4)	120(94.5)	121 (91.0)	39 (88.6)	33 (89.2)	49 (94.2)	
Missing	3 (1.2)	1 (0.8)	2 (1.5)	1 (2.3)	1 (2.7)	0 (0.0)	
Education [N (%)]							
without	-	-	2 (1.5)	0 (0.0)	0 (0.0)	2 (3.8)	0.113
8-9 years	127 (49.6)	50 (39.4)	65 (48.9)	20 (45.5)	21 (56.8)	24 (46.2)	
10-11 years	59 (23.0)	31 (24.4)	27 (20.3)	11 (25.0)	10 (27.0)	6 (11.5)	
>=12 years	70 (27.3)	45 (35.4)	38 (28.6)	13 (29.5)	6 (16.2)	19 (36.5)	
Missing	-	1 (0.8)	1 (0.8)	0 (0.0)	0 (0.0)	1 (1.9)	
Employment status [N (%)]							
Employed	70 (27.3)	67 (52.8)	17 (12.8)	9 (20.5)	2 (5.4)	6 (11.5)	<0.001
Non employed	180 (70.3)	59 (46.5)	114 (85.7)	33 (75.0)	35 (94.6)	46 (88.5)	
Missing	6 (2.3)	1 (0.8)	2 (1.5)	2 (4.5)	0 (0.0)	0 (0.0)	
Living area [N (%)]							
Rural	149 (58.3)	85 (66.9)	56 (42.1)	29 (65.9)	18 (48.6)	9 (17.3)	<0.001
Urban	102 (39.8)	40 (31.5)	71 (53.4)	12 (27.3)	17 (45.9)	42 (80.8)	
Missing	5 (2.0)	2 (1.6)	6 (4.5)	3 (6.8)	2 (5.4)	1 (1.9)	
Pre-therapeutic Gleason score, [mean ± SD]	6.6 ± 1.2	6.5 ± 1.0	6.0 ± 13.1	5.4 ± 1.4	6.1 ± 1.6	6.4 ± 1.1	0.110
Missing [N]	2	1	33	25	7	3	
Pre-therapeutic PSA score, [mean ± SD]	11.4 ± 21.3	8.0 ± 4.7	13.7 ± 17.0	10.8 ± 15.0	17.6 ± 14.4	13.2 ± 19.9	0.032
Missing [N]	5	1	2	1	1	-	
Pre-baseline androgen deprivation therapy [N (%)]							
Yes	10 (3.9)	1 (0.8)	51 (38.3)	20 (45.4)	13 (35.1)	18 (34.6)	<0.001
No	185 (72.2)	81 (63.8)	46 (34.6)	16 (36.4)	12 (32.4)	19 (36.5)	
Missing	61 (23.8)	45 (35.4)	36 (27.0)	8 (18.2)	12 (32.4)	16 (30.8)	
Tumour stage at diagnosis [N %)]							
T1	2 (0.8)	-	32 (24.0)	1 (2.3)	1 (2.7)	29 (55.8)	<0.001
T2	142 (55.5)	103 (81.1)	39 (29.3)	8 (18.2)	17 (45.9)	14 (26.9)	
T3	105 (41.0)	21 (16.5)	20 (15.0)	1 (2.3)	12 (32.4)	7 (13.5)	
Missing	7 (2.7)	3 (2.4)	43 (32.3)	34 (77.3)	7 (18.9)	2 (3.8)	
Risk stratification [N (%)]							
Low	13 (5.1)	7 (5.5)	25 (18.8)	6 (13.6)	0 (0.0)	19 (36.5)	<0.001
Intermediate	33 (12.9)	15 (11.8)	22 (16.5)	2 (4.5)	8 (21.6)	12 (23.1)	
High	205 (80.1)	103 (81.1)	47 (35.3)	4 (9.1)	25 (67.6)	18 (34.6)	
Missing	5 (1.9)	2 (1.6)	39 (29.3)	32 (72.7)	4 (10.8)	3 (5.8)	
Operation condition [N (%)]							
Retropubic	251 (98.0)	124 (97.6)	n.a.	n.a.	n.a.	n.a.	n.a.
Perineal	5 (2.0)	2 (1.6)					

Table 1 Sociodemographic characteristics and tumor specific data (Continued)

Missing	-	1 (0.8)					
Sexual functioning, [mean ± SD]	41.5 ± 21.2	54.7 ± 16.5	33.1 ± 22.3	26.7 ± 22.1	32.4 ± 21.6	39.7 ± 21.7	<0.001
Missing [N]	92	36	44	11	15	18	

[1]Chi-square and F- test for the three groups (non-nerve-sparing radical prostatectomy, nerve-sparing radical prostatectomy, and total radiotherapy), respectively.

Sexual functioning - IIEF

Figure 1 shows that the average sexual functioning of the RT patients remains on a similar low level over the whole observation period. Patients receiving nnsRP start off with a higher sexual functioning, but end up with the lowest scores. Patients receiving nnsRP have the highest baseline scores, but drop by more than 20 points, ending after a small recovery at a 24-month score similar to the baseline score in RT patients. Additional file 1 presents the trends for the three RT subgroups, which end with very similar scores after 24 months of follow-up.

Generic HRQOL – QLQ-C30

Several of the baseline functioning or symptom scales differed to a clinically relevant extent across the treatment groups (physical, role, emotional, and social functioning, fatigue, pain, dyspnoea, insomnia, and financial difficulties). In all cases, the RT group – especially the combRT group – had the least favourable baseline values (Figure 2 and Additional file 2). The most favourable value was generally found in the nsRP group, except for emotional functioning, social functioning, and insomnia, which was best in the externRT group. However, both the nsRP and the nnsRP group most often showed higher functioning and fewer symptoms than the total RT group.

Three months after baseline, typically a decrease in functioning scales and an increase in symptom scales were seen, followed by a recovery (Figure 2 and Additional file 2). Due to the smaller number of patients, the time trends of the individual RT groups show a larger variability and the typical time trend can be seen less clearly than in the total RT group. When comparing nnsRP, nsRP, and the total RT group, the following deviations from this pattern were observed: In contrast to the more specific functioning and symptom scales, the global health status was hardly affected by treatment: It remained nearly unchanged for the total RT group but further increased over time for the two RP groups. The increase in emotional functioning was clinically relevant in the nsRP group at six, twelve, and twenty-four months after baseline and in the nnsRP group twelve months after baseline. Physical functioning, role functioning, and cognitive functioning worsened over time for the RT group, a group of older patients compared to those in the surgery groups. Among the RT groups, the largest differences were observed for dyspnoea, insomnia, and financial difficulties.

In the multiple regression analysis, only diarrhoea was statistically significantly associated with treatment option after adjusting for baseline HRQOL, age, and other demographical and clinical data (Table 2). RT was estimated to increase the score on the diarrhoea symptom scale by 7 points, while the estimate for nsRP was –0.9. The RT effect was mostly driven by the brachyRT group (effect of 7.8 compared to 4.1 and 4.2 for combRT and externRT). The difference was not clinically relevant.

Disease-specific quality of life – PORPUS-P

At baseline, the PORPUS-P score was highest in nsRP and lowest in RT patients, in particular in patients treated with combRT (Figure 3 and Additional file 3). The difference was clinically relevant. The PORPUS-P score decreased three months after baseline, followed by a partial recovery.

In the covariate-adjusted multiple regression analysis a statistically significant but not clinically relevant association of main treatment option and HRQOL during the follow-up period was observed (Table 2), with nsRP patients having a significantly higher HRQOL and RT patients also having a (not statistically significant) higher HRQOL than nnsRP patients.

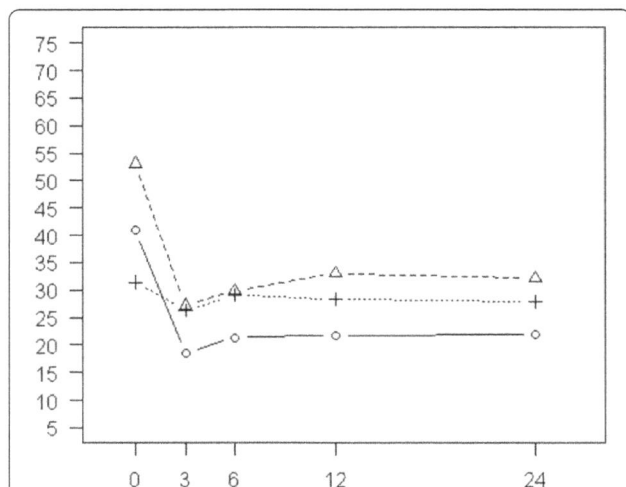

Figure 1 Sexual functioning (IIEF). Mean scores of nnsRP, nsRP, and RT cancer patients at baseline and during the 24-month follow-up period after multiple imputation of missing values (solid line: nnsRP, dashed line: nsRP, dotted line: RT).

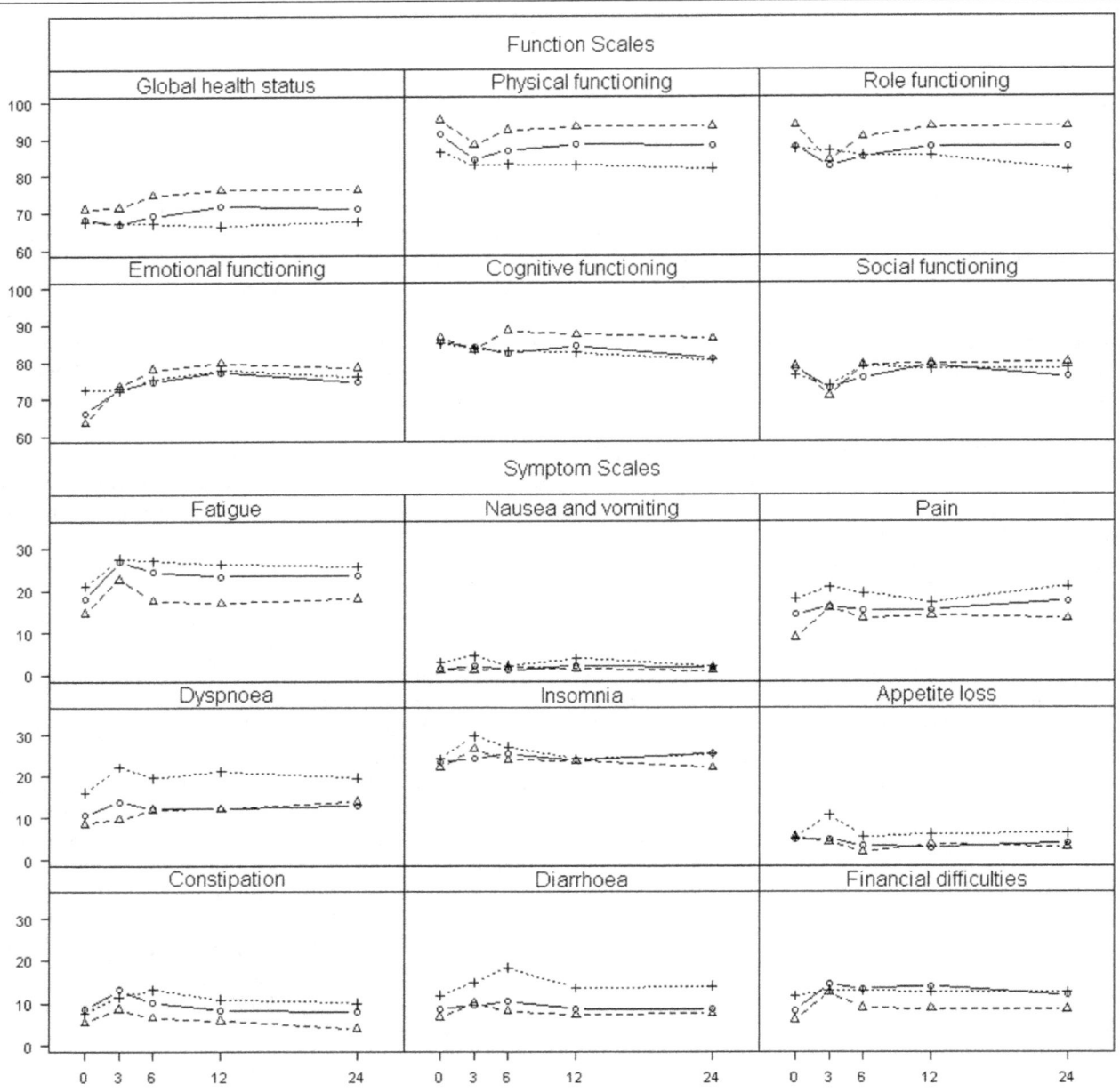

Figure 2 Health-related QoL (QLQ-C30). Mean scores of nnsRP, nsRP, and RT cancer patients at baseline and during the 24-month follow-up period after multiple imputation of missing values (solid line: nnsRP, dashed line: nsRP, dotted line: RT).

Comparison of generic HRQOL to German norm values

Overall, scores of the treatment groups at baseline and twenty-four months after treatment were mostly comparable to German norm values for the EORTC QLQ-C30 [29] (Table 3). However, patients treated with RP had clinically relevant lower scores of fatigue and pain at baseline, and the low pain score persisted for the nsRP patients for twenty-four months. The nsPR patients had a clinically relevant higher role functioning than expected at baseline and at the end of the follow-up. No clinically relevant deviations from the norm values were observed for the total group of patients treated with RT. However, the brachyRT group had a clinically relevant higher role functioning at baseline than expected. The externRT group had a higher role functioning at baseline as well, and lower symptoms of pain, which slightly decreased to a clinically non-relevant level until twenty-four months later. The combRT group had clinically relevant lower emotional and social functioning and higher insomnia scores at baseline, and less pain but more insomnia than the reference population twenty-four months after baseline.

Table 2 Estimated effect of treatment option on HRQOL in a multiple regression analysis

	Main analysis						Analysis with separation of different RT treatment groups[1]							Wald test
	Radical prostatectomy			Radiotherapy		Wald test	Radiotherapy							Wald test
	Ref.	Nerve-sparing		Total			Brachytherapy		Combined (External/ brachytherapy)		External			
	b	b	95%-CI	b	95%-CI	p-value	b	95%-CI	b	95%-CI	b	95%-CI	p-value	
QLQ-C30														
Functioning scales														
Global health status	0	2.9	(−0.6, 6.4)	−2.0	(−5.9, 2.0)	0.098	−1.0	(−6.2, 4.2)	−2.2	(−8.4, 3.9)	−4.4	(−9.9, 1.2)	0.120	
Physical functioning	0	1.7	(−0.6, 4.1)	−0.9	(−4.3, 2.4)	0.198	−0.6	(−5.4, 4.3)	−0.6	(−5.2, 3.9)	−3.5	(−8.9, 2.0)	0.224	
Role functioning	0	1.9	(−1.5, 5.3)	−0.5	(−4.8, 3.8)	0.425	−1.6	(−7.9, 4.7)	2.0	(−4.7, 8.7)	−2.5	(−8.8, 3.8)	0.314	
Emotional functioning	0	3.8	(−0.2, 7.8)	−2.7	(−7.3, 2.0)	0.074	−2.4	(−8.7, 3.9)	1.1	(−6.2, 8.3)	**−8.6**	**(−15.2, −2.0)**	0.028	
Cognitive functioning	0	2.5	(−1.1, 6.2)	−1.8	(−5.5, 1.9)	0.170	−0.7	(−6.0, 4.5)	−2.2	(−8.2, 3.8)	−2.7	(−9.5, 4.0)	0.277	
Social functioning	0	1.2	(−3.7, 6.1)	0.1	(−5.4, 5.5)	0.650	−0.7	(−7.9, 6.5)	3.0	(−5.1, 11.1)	−5.7	(−14.3, 3.0)	0.287	
Symptom scales														
Fatigue	0	−3.6	(−7.8, 0.5)	0.4	(−4.6, 5.3)	0.173	0.1	(−6.6, 6.8)	−1.6	(−9.1, 5.9)	5.4	(−2.0, 12.9)	0.174	
Nausea and vomiting	0	−0.5	(−1.6, 0.6)	1.1	(−0.5, 2.7)	0.100	**2.1**	**(0.1, 4.1)**	−0.5	(−2.2, 1.2)	0.6	(−1.8, 2.9)	0.091	
Pain	0	0.5	(−3.5, 4.5)	2.7	(−2.2, 7.5)	0.477	3.6	(−3.3, 10.5)	0.1	(−7.2, 7.3)	3.4	(−4.8, 11.6)	0.601	
Dyspnoea	0	1.4	(−2.1, 4.8)	3.5	(−0.8, 7.8)	0.177	0.1	(−5.6, 5.8)	6.8	(−0.5, 14.1)	4.8	(−1.5, 11.0)	0.122	
Insomnia	0	0.1	(−4.7, 5.0)	3.2	(−2.5, 8.9)	0.451	4.3	(−2.9, 11.5)	4.0	(−4.7, 12.7)	6.4	(−2.8, 15.6)	0.291	
Appetite loss	0	−0.1	(−2.3, 2.1)	1.5	(−1.7, 4.7)	0.317	1.5	(−1.8, 4.8)	1.0	(−3.7, 5.6)	3.1	(−1.5, 7.6)	0.276	
Constipation	0	−1.2	(−5.3, 3.0)	0.4	(−4.1, 4.9)	0.542	1.7	(−4.2, 7.5)	−0.9	(−8.4, 6.5)	3.2	(−5.5, 12.0)	0.362	
Diarrhoea	0	−0.9	(−4.4, 2.6)	**7.0**	**(2.5, 11.6)**	**0.006**	**7.8**	**(1.0, 14.5)**	4.1	(−3.3, 11.4)	4.2	(−3.6, 12.0)	**0.048**	
Financial difficulties	0	−3.1	(−7.0, 0.8)	−0.2	(−4.7, 4.3)	0.257	−2.7	(−9.1, 3.7)	−0.5	(−8.8, 7.7)	4.9	(−4.0, 13.8)	0.216	
PORPUS														
PORPUS-P	0	**2.3**	**(0.1, 4.6)**	2.2	(−0.6, 5.0)	**0.045**	2.2	(−1.6, 6.1)	3.3	(−0.6, 7.2)	1.4	(−3.0, 5.7)	0.119	

Ref = Non-nerve-sparing radical prostatectomy as reference level.
Bold values indicate significance at the 5%-level.
[1]As the regression coefficients of the radical prostatectomy group did not change much, only the regression coefficients of the radiotherapy subgroups with their confidence intervals and the Wald test p-values are reported.
Both analyses are adjusted for baseline HRQOL, age, having a partner (yes/no), highest education level (no graduation, 8–9 years ('Hauptschulabschluss'), 10–11 years ('Realschulabschluss'), >= 12 years high school ('(Fach-)Abitur')), working (yes/no), residence (rural/urban), tumour stage (T-category of the TNM-classification), pre-therapeutic Gleason score, pre-therapeutic PSA score, and sexual functioning at baseline (IIEF total scale).

Sensitivity analysis – complete case analysis

The complete case analysis was based on 248 to 254 patients, depending on the HRQOL measure. Results were mostly similar to the results after multiple imputation presented above. Global health status, emotional functioning, and appetite loss, but not diarrhoea, were additionally found to be significantly (but not clinically relevantly) related to main treatment option.

Discussion

This study analysed changes of HRQOL of prostate cancer patients over time, the effect of treatment on HRQOL, and compared HRQOL to that in a German reference population.

Changes over time

The descriptive comparison of time trends showed that a decreased sexual functioning and limited recovery is more common in RP than in RT. Although the comparison does not convey information about a treatment effect on similar/randomised groups, it describes what happens to men with prostate cancer in actual health care. The finding is in concordance with other publications [31,32]. Further, better outcomes in erectile functioning for nsRP patients compared to patients with non-nerve-sparing procedures were also found in previous studies [10,11,33]. Still, erectile functioning is a concern in RP in general [34-36].

In view of generic HRQOL, only minor changes over time were seen across groups. In several other studies

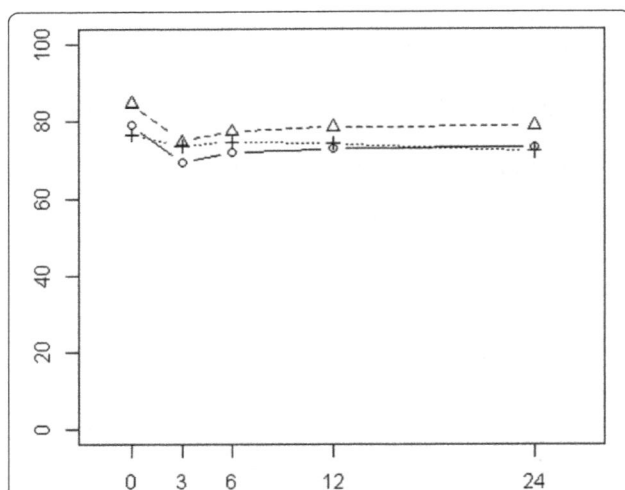

Figure 3 PORPUS-P. Mean scores of nnsRP, nsRP, and RT cancer patients at baseline and during the 24-month follow-up period after multiple imputation of missing values (solid line: nnsRP, dashed line: nsRP, dotted line: RT).

these results have been ascribed to the fact that generic instruments are not able to a) distinguish adequately between highly selected groups [26] and b) adequately measure HRQOL after diagnosis because of response shift bias [36,37]. In this analysis, the application of multiple imputation may have obscured differences; the incorporation of uncertainty due to missing values often results in conservative estimates.

A clinically relevant worsening in PORPUS-P and an increase in emotional functioning at all measurement time points after baseline were observed in the RP group (with exceptions for emotional functioning in the nnsRP group). Differences between RP patients and norm values were close to clinical relevance at baseline (−8.7 and −9.3, respectively) [29]. At the end of the follow-up differences in emotional functioning had largely disappeared, which may be ascribed to adaptation processes [38]. Our findings are in contrast to those of a Canadian study observing clinically relevant decreases of prostate-specific HRQOL after radiotherapy [39]. This is particularly interesting as over 50% of our RT patients, where information about pre-baseline androgen deprivation therapy was available, received ADT, i.e. an adjuvant

Table 3 Differences between EORTC QLQ-C30 ProCaSP data and norm data

	Baseline								24 months after baseline			
	Radical prostatectomy		Radiotherapy				Radical prostatectomy		Radiotherapy			
	nns	ns	total	brachy	comb	extern	nns	ns	total	brachy	comb	extern
Global quality of life	2.5	5.3	1.5	4.6	−1.7	1.3	5.3	10.3	2.0	3.8	2.8	0.1
Functioning scales												
Physical	7.3	9.6	3.0	3.5	2.3	3.2	5.0	8.5	0.0	1.6	−1.3	−0.5
Role	9.7	**14.0**	3.6	**11.0**	2.3	**12.2**	9.7	**14.1**	4.6	−0.5	5.9	9.6
Emotional	−8.7	−9.3	−3.8	−2.8	**−13.2**	1.5	−1.6	4.4	−0.4	2.1	−2.7	−1.6
Cognitive	1.4	2.1	1.7	3.9	−1.5	2.1	−2.4	2.0	−1.6	0.8	−6.5	−0.2
Social	−3.1	−2.9	−4.9	−6.4	**−13.1**	2.4	−5.2	−1.8	−2.2	−7.5	1.9	1.5
Symptom scales												
Fatigue	**−10.0**	**−13.5**	−6.9	−9.9	−0.4	−9.3	−4.5	−9.8	−3.4	−3.5	−1.5	−4.6
Nausea/Vomiting	−1.1	−1.7	0.4	1.8	1.9	−1.6	−0.8	−1.7	−0.6	0.8	−1.3	−1.6
Pain	**−12.9**	**−19.0**	−8.7	−8.3	−7.0	**−10.5**	−9.6	**−14.0**	−6.8	−5.4	**−10.8**	−9.4
Single items												
Dyspnoea	−9.3	−9.0	−4.9	−9.6	−1.1	−3.3	−8.1	−4.9	−2.7	−6.5	−0.5	0.7
Insomnia	−2.8	−4.8	−1.2	−4.9	**10.7**	−6.6	0.1	−4.5	0.0	−4.0	**10.6**	−1.1
Appetite loss	−2.5	−2.0	−1.6	−3.5	0.6	−1.3	−2.8	−4.3	−0.5	−2.6	−3.8	3.5
Constipation	2.8	0.3	1.7	3.5	2.6	−0.4	1.9	−1.3	2.8	5.4	0.0	3.6
Diarrhoea	0.5	−2.1	3.6	1.7	8.4	2.1	0.4	−0.9	5.8	7.7	0.4	6.5
Financial difficulties	−6.7	−8.4	−3.1	−4.3	4.5	−7.4	−2.8	−6.1	−2.3	0.0	−4.5	−2.3

Legend: positive differences = higher mean functioning or higher mean symptom score in the prostate cancer patient group than in the norm data, negative differences = lower mean functioning or higher mean symptom score in the prostate cancer patient group than in the norm data.
Bold numbers indicate clinical relevance.
nns = non-nerve-sparing, ns = nerve-sparing, brachy = brachytherapy, extern = extern radiotherapy, comb = extern radiotherapy and brachytherapy.

therapy that negatively impacts erectile functioning, social functioning, and global health/HRQOL [39]. Hence, a clinically relevant decrease of HRQOL scores in our RT patients would have been expected. In a joint analysis of the Canadian data and our data, however, we were able to show that RT patients with ADT indeed scored lower HRQOL than RT patients without ADT [40].

Treatment effects

When controlling for baseline HRQOL, sexual functioning, and other possible confounders in a GEE model, the treatment effect of nsRP compared to nnsRP was favourable for many HRQOL domains and often unfavourable for RT. The treatment effect was significant for the domain diarrhoea of the HRQOL and for the PORPUS-P. The negative effect of RT on bowel functioning is in agreement with previous research [41,42]. However, treatment effects in our analysis never reached clinical relevance.

The treatment groups differed with respect to their baseline HRQOL, sexual functioning, and sociodemographic and tumour-related characteristics. Baseline HRQOL and sexual functioning was generally highest in patients receiving nsRP and lowest in patients receiving RT, especially in the combRT group. RT patients were older than RP patients, and the combRT group had the highest risk profile. Similar results have been reported in comparable international outcome studies [12,41] which is concordant with recommendations in current therapy guidelines such as the EAU-guideline advising an estimated 10-year survival as a precondition for RP but not for RT [43]. Logistic regression indicated that the significant predictors for a successful nerve-sparing surgery (in contrast to a non-nerve-sparing surgery) were a younger age, a higher Gleason score, and a better sexual functioning of the patient, while predictors for choosing radiotherapy were a better T-category, a worse sexual functioning, and an urban living area. However, there was considerable overlap with regard to these variables between the treatment groups, and the covariate adjustment in the regression analyses allowed to derive meaningful treatment effect estimates despite the group differences.

Comparison to reference population

Patients treated with RP had clinically relevant lower scores of fatigue and pain and higher role functioning than age-matched German men of the general population. The RT group also had lower fatigue and pain scores than suggested by the reference data but the difference was not clinically relevant (except for the externRT subgroup at baseline and the combRT subgroup after 24 months for pain). It can be suspected that the high proportion of participants reporting depression in the reference population caused artificially high norm

values for fatigue and pain and low values for role functioning [29]. Even the 'low' symptom values (pain, fatigue) of the cancer patients in our study were higher than those reported by Krahn et al. (2009) for Canadian early stage prostate cancer patients [39]. The same applies to the role functioning values in the RP group.

Strengths and limitations

Important strengths of the ProCaSP Study are the multi-center design, the comparison of HRQOL outcomes in several prostate cancer treatment groups, and the application of suitable statistical methods such as GEEs and adjustments for baseline differences. The main limitation of the study is missing data due to drop-out or incomplete questionnaires, especially for IIEF questions; however, by applying multiple imputation methods we achieved a sample size sufficient for stratification of two RP and three RT groups. The exclusion of urinary measures because of insufficient psychometric properties of the Prostate Specific Module limits the scope of our study. Finally, selection bias caused by an overrepresentation of severe cases in university hospitals cannot be ruled out. Possible confounding was handled by adjustment of covariates in the GEE model, although residual confounding cannot be excluded.

Conclusions

Our results support the findings from previous research. A fundamental basis of both empirical research and evidence-based medicine is the reproducibility of findings in different settings, health care systems, and different cohorts of patients. In conclusion, RT cancer patients scored lowest on HRQOL at baseline and throughout the study. RP had a larger negative impact on sexual functioning than RT. In patients with similar baseline characteristics and similar baseline HRQOL, treatment by RT increased symptoms of diarrhoea, and nnsRP decreased prostate-specific HRQOL. In view of the relevant proportion of overdiagnosis in prostate cancer and in view of improved survival rates for prostate cancer patients, physicians should inform their patients about these differences in HRQOL outcomes and take them into account when deciding which therapy is best for an individual patient.

Additional files

Additional file 1: Sexual functioning Radiotherapy Subgroups.tiff. Sexual functioning in the radiotherapy subgroups. Mean scores of brachytherapy, external radiotherapy, and combined radiotherapy cancer patients at baseline and during the 24-month follow-up period after multiple imputation of missing values (circle: brachyRT, triangle: externRT, cross: combRT).

Additional file 2: QLQ-C30 Radiotherapy Subgroups.tiff. Health-related quality of life in the radiotherapy subgroups. Mean scores of brachytherapy, external radiotherapy, and combined radiotherapy cancer patients at baseline and during the 24-month follow-up period after multiple imputation of missing values (circle: brachyRT, triangle: externRT, cross: combRT).

Additional file 3: PorpusP Radiotherapy Subgroups.tiff. PORPUS-P in the radiotherapy subgroups. Mean scores of brachytherapy, external radiotherapy, and combined radiotherapy cancer patients at baseline and during the 24-month follow-up period after multiple imputation of missing values (circle: brachyRT, triangle: externRT, cross: combRT).

Abbreviations

brachyRT: Brachytherapy; combRT: Combined extern radiotherapy and brachytherapy; externRT: Extern radiotherapy; HRQOL: Health-related quality of life; nnsRP: Non-nerve-sparing radical prostatectomy; nsRP: Nerve-sparing radical prostatectomy; RP: Radical prostatectomy; RT: Radiotherapy; SD: Standard deviation.

Competing interests

The authors declare that they have no competing interests.

Authors' contributions

NE made substantial contributions to the design of the analysis, to the statistical analysis and interpretation, and to drafting the manuscript. SN made substantial contributions to drafting the manuscript and to revising it critically for important intellectual content. MS contributed to the statistical analysis and to drafting the manuscript. AK made substantial contributions to drafting the manuscript and to revising it critically for important intellectual content. VR planned the study and was involved in data acquisition and revised the manuscript for important intellectual content. AW contributed to the planning of the analysis, to the statistical analysis, interpretation of results, and drafting the manuscript. All authors gave final approval of the final manuscript.

Acknowledgements

We thank the German Cancer Aid for funding the ProCaSP Study.

Author details

[1]Institute of Cancer Epidemiology, University of Luebeck, Ratzeburger Allee 160, 23562 Luebeck, Germany. [2]Medical Clinic, Department of Psychosomatic Medicine, Charité - Universitätsmedizin Berlin, Charitéplatz 1, 10117 Berlin, Germany. [3]Deakin University, 221 Burwood Highway, Burwood, VIC 3125, Australia. [4]Institute of Social Medicine and Epidemiology, University Hospital Schleswig-Holstein, Campus Luebeck, Ratzeburger Allee 160, 23562 Luebeck, Germany. [5]Medical Practice of Urology, Auguststr. 4, 23611 Bad Schwartau, Germany. [6]Department of Urology, Pediatric Urology and Andrology, Justus Liebig University of Giessen, Rudolf-Buchheim-Str. 7, 35392 Giessen, Germany.

References

1. Haas GP, Delongchamps N, Brawley OW, Wang CY, de la Roza G. The worldwide epidemiology of prostate cancer: perspectives from autopsy studies. Can J Urol. 2008;15(1):3866–71.
2. Zlotta AR, Egawa S, Pushkar D, Govorov A, Kimura T, Kido M, et al. Prevalence of prostate cancer on autopsy: cross-sectional study on unscreened Caucasian and Asian men. J Natl Cancer Inst. 2013;105(14):1050–8.
3. Andriole GL, Crawford ED, Grubb 3rd RL, Buys SS, Chia D, Church TR, et al. Mortality results from a randomized prostate-cancer screening trial. N Engl J Med. 2009;360(13):1310–9.
4. Andriole GL, Crawford ED, Grubb 3rd RL, Buys SS, Chia D, Church TR, et al. Prostate cancer screening in the randomized Prostate, Lung, Colorectal, and Ovarian Cancer Screening Trial: mortality results after 13 years of follow-up. J Natl Cancer Inst. 2012;104(2):125–32.
5. Starker A, Saß A. Participation in cancer screening in Germany. Results of the German Health Interview and Examination Survey for Adults (DEGS1). Bundesgesundheitsblatt. 2013;56(5–6):858–67.
6. Robert Koch-Institute, Association of population-based cancer registries in Germany. Cancer in Germany 2009/2010. 9th edition. Robert Koch Institute (ed.) and the Association of Population-based Cancer

Registries in Germany (ed.). . Incidence and Trends. Berlin, 2014. (http://www.rki.de/Krebs/EN/Home/homepage_node.html)
7. Hayes JH, Barry MJ. Screening for prostate cancer with the prostate-specific antigen test: a review of current evidence. JAMA. 2014;311(11):1143–9.
8. Heidenreich A, Aus G, Bolla M, Joniau S, Matveev VB, Schmid HP, et al. EAU guidelines on prostate cancer. Eur Urol. 2008;53(1):68–80.
9. Penson DF. Quality of life after therapy for localized prostate cancer. Cancer J. 2007;13(5):318–26.
10. Kessler TM, Burkhard FC, Studer UE. Nerve-sparing open radical retropubic prostatectomy. Eur Urol. 2007;51(1):90–7.
11. Litwin MS, Flanders SC, Pasta DJ, Stoddard ML, Lubeck DP, Henning JM. Sexual function and bother after radical prostatectomy or radiation for prostate cancer: multivariate quality-of-life analysis from CaPSURE. Cancer Prostate Strategic Urol Res Endeavor Urol. 1999;54(3):503–8.
12. Litwin MS, Gore JL, Kwan L, Brandeis JM, Lee SP, Withers HR, et al. Quality of life after surgery, external beam irradiation, or brachytherapy for early-stage prostate cancer. Cancer. 2007;109(11):2239–47.
13. Sanda MG, Dunn RL, Michalski J, Sandler HM, Northouse L, Hembroff L, et al. Quality of life and satisfaction with outcome among prostate-cancer survivors. N Engl J Med. 2008;358(12):1250–61.
14. Potosky AL, Davis WW, Hoffman RM, Stanford JL, Stephenson RA, Penson DF, et al. Five-year outcomes after prostatectomy or radiotherapy for prostate cancer: the prostate cancer outcomes study. J Natl Cancer Inst. 2004;96(18):1358–67.
15. Gulati R, Inoue LY, Gore JL, Katcher J, Etzioni R. Individualized estimates of overdiagnosis in screen-detected prostate cancer. J Natl Cancer Inst. 2014;106(2):djt367.
16. Hugosson J, Carlsson S. Overdetection in screening for prostate cancer. Curr Opin Urol. 2014;24(3):256–63.
17. Vickers AJ, Sjoberg DD, Ulmert D, Vertosick E, Roobol MJ, Thompson I, et al. Empirical estimates of prostate cancer overdiagnosis by age and prostate-specific antigen. BMC Med. 2014;12:26.
18. Singh J, Trabulsi EJ, Gomella LG. Is there an optimal management for localized prostate cancer? Clin Interv Aging. 2010;5:187–97.
19. Eisemann N, Waldmann A, Rohde V, Katalinic A. Quality of life in partners of patients with localised prostate cancer. Qual Life Res. 2013;23(5):1557–68.
20. Wittekind C, Meyer H-J, Bootz F. TNM Klassifikation maligner Tumoren, vol. 6. Berlin Heidelberg New York: Springer; 2002.
21. D'Amico AV, Whittington R, Malkowicz SB, Schultz D, Blank K, Broderick GA, et al. Biochemical outcome after radical prostatectomy, external beam radiation therapy, or interstitial radiation therapy for clinically localized prostate cancer. JAMA. 1998;280(11):969–74.
22. Bestmann B, Rohde V, Siebmann JU, Galalae R, Weidner W, Kuchler T. Validation of the German prostate-specific module. World J Urol. 2006;24(1):94–100.
23. Fayers P, Aaronson N, Bjordal K, Groenvold M, Curran D, Bottomley A, et al. The EORTC QLQ-C30 scoring manual. 3rd ed. Brussels: European Organization for Research and Treatment of Cancer; 2001.
24. Osoba D, Rodrigues G, Myles J, Zee B, Pater J. Interpreting the significance of changes in health-related quality-of-life scores. J Clin Oncol. 1998;16(1):139–44.
25. Krahn M, Ritvo P, Irvine J, Tomlinson G, Bezjak A, Trachtenberg J, et al. Construction of the Patient-Oriented Prostate Utility Scale (PORPUS): a multiattribute health state classification system for prostate cancer. J Clin Epidemiol. 2000;53(9):920–30.
26. Ritvo P, Irvine J, Naglie G, Tomlinson G, Bezjak A, Matthew A, et al. Reliability and validity of the PORPUS, a combined psychometric and utility-based quality-of-life instrument for prostate cancer. J Clin Epidemiol. 2005;58(5):466–74.
27. R Development Core Team. R: A language and environment for statistical computing. Vienna, Austria: R Foundation for Statistical Computing; 2013.
28. Schafer J. Analysis of Incomplete Multivariate Data. London: Chapman & Hall; 1997.
29. Waldmann A, Schubert D, Katalinic A. Normative data of the EORTC qlq-c30 for the german population: a population-based survey. PLoS One. 2013;8(9):e74149.
30. Faul F, Erdfelder E, Buchner A, Lang AG. Statistical power analyses using G*Power 3.1: tests for correlation and regression analyses. Behav Res Methods. 2009;41(4):1149–60.
31. Miwa S, Mizokami A, Konaka H, Ueno S, Kitagawa Y, Koh E, et al. Prospective longitudinal comparative study of health-related quality of life and treatment satisfaction in patients treated with hormone therapy, radical retropubic prostatectomy, and high or low dose rate brachytherapy for prostate cancer. Rrostate Int. 2013;1(3):117–24.

32. van Tol-Geerdink JJ, Leer JW, van Oort IM, van Lin EJ, Weijerman PC, Vergunst H, et al. Quality of life after prostate cancer treatments in patients comparable at baseline. Br J Cancer. 2013;108(9):1784–9.

33. Hashine K, Kusuhara Y, Miura N, Shirato A, Sumiyoshi Y, Kataoka M. A prospective longitudinal study comparing a radical retropubic prostatectomy and permanent prostate brachytherapy regarding the health-related quality of life for localized prostate cancer. Jpn J Clin Oncol. 2008;38(7):480–5.

34. Marien TP, Lepor H. Does a nerve-sparing technique or potency affect continence after open radical retropubic prostatectomy? BJU Int. 2008;102(11):1581–4.

35. Dubbelman Y, Wildhagen M, Schroder F, Bangma C, Dohle G. Orgasmic dysfunction after open radical prostatectomy: clinical correlates and prognostic factors. J Sex Med. 2010;7(3):1216–23.

36. Noldus J, Michl U, Graefen M, Haese A, Hammerer P, Fernandez S, et al. Die nerverhaltende radikale retropubische Prostatektomie. Ergebnisse nach Patientenbefragung. [Nerve-sparing radical retropubic prostatectomy. Results of a patient survey]. Urol A. 2001;40(2):102–6.

37. Sprangers MA, Schwartz CE. The challenge of response shift for quality-of-life-based clinical oncology research. Ann Oncol. 1999;10(7):747–9.

38. Wyler SF, Engeler DS, Seelentag W, Ries G, Schmid HP. Health-related quality of life after radical prostatectomy and low-dose-rate brachytherapy for localized prostate cancer. Urol Int. 2009;82(1):17–23.

39. Krahn MD, Bremner KE, Tomlinson G, Naglie G. Utility and health-related quality of life in prostate cancer patients 12 months after radical prostatectomy or radiation therapy. Prostate Cancer Prostatic Dis. 2009;12(4):361–8.

40. Waldmann A, Rohde V, Bremner K, Krahn M, Kuechler T, Katalinic A. Measuring prostate-specific quality of life in prostate cancer patients scheduled for radiotherapy or radical prostatectomy and reference men in Germany and Canada using the Patient Oriented Prostate Utility Scale-Psychometric (PORPUS-P). BMC Cancer. 2009;9:295.

41. Ferrer M, Suarez JF, Guedea F, Fernandez P, Macias V, Marino A, et al. Health-related quality of life 2 years after treatment with radical prostatectomy, prostate brachytherapy, or external beam radiotherapy in patients with clinically localized prostate cancer. Int J Radiat Oncol Biol Phys. 2008;72(2):421–32.

42. Katz A, Ferrer M, Suarez JF, Multicentric Spanish Group of Clinically Localized Prostate C. Comparison of quality of life after stereotactic body radiotherapy and surgery for early-stage prostate cancer. Radiat Oncol (London, England. 2012;7:194.

43. Heidenreich A, Bellmunt J, Bolla M, Joniau S, Mason M, Matveev V, et al. EAU guidelines on prostate cancer. Part 1: screening, diagnosis, and treatment of clinically localised disease. Eur Urol. 2011;59(1):61–71.

4

Primary melanoma of the prostate

Georgi Tosev[1]*, Timur H. Kuru[1], Johannes Huber[1], Gerald Freier[1], Frank Bergmann[2], Jessica C. Hassel[3], Sascha A. Pahernik[1], Markus Hohenfellner[1] and Boris A. Hadaschik[1]

Abstract

Background: Primary melanoma of the prostate has an extremely rare incidence. Only five cases have been reported in the literature and prognosis is poor. The most likely origin of prostatic melanoma is the transitional epithelium of the prostatic urethra. Surgical care for primary melanoma of mucosal sites is less well established than for primary cutaneous melanoma, but excision of the primary is recommended if the patient has no systemic disease.

Case presentation: Here, we describe a case of primary malignant melanoma of the prostate. A 37-year-old male patient with history of both chemo- and radiation therapy for Hodgkin's disease was admitted to the University Hospital Heidelberg on suspicion of pleomorphic sarcoma of the bladder. In-house diagnostic work-up revealed a malignant melanoma of the prostate. We then performed radical prostatectomy with extended lymphadenectomy. Despite presumably curative surgery, the patient suffered from early relapse of disease with pulmonary metastasis. Systemic chemotherapy and subsequent immuno-oncologic treatment was thereafter initiated.

Conclusion: Since prostatic melanoma is a rare disease and a melanoma metastasis of unknown primary is the differential diagnosis, a multidisciplinary approach including early imaging to rule out possible metastases and to search for another potentially existing primary is advisable. To prevent complications related to local tumor progression and to receive tissue for mutational analysis, we recommend complete surgical resection to reduce the tumor mass. Novel immune and targeted oncologic therapies can lead to an improved survival in some cases and support of clinical trials is needed.

Keywords: Prostate, Prostatic neoplasm, Prostatectomy, Ipilimumab, Nivolumab

Background

Primary melanoma of the prostate has an extremely rare incidence. The first report of this disease was in 1980. Since then only five cases have been reported worldwide [1–5]. We report on one case including diagnosis, surgical management, and subsequent therapy with darcabazine, ipilimumab and nivolumab.

Case presentation

A 37-year old man was admitted to the University Hospital Heidelberg for a second opinion after diagnosis of a pleomorphic sarcoma of the bladder in April 2012. His medical history included Hodgkin's disease stage IIb

which was first diagnosed in August 2004 in supraclavicular and mediastinal lymph nodes. In 2004 he received two cycles each of BEACOPP and ABVD chemotherapy, resulting in complete remission. Consolidating treatment consisted of involved-field radiotherapy with 30 Gy in 2005.

The patient reported that one month before his first consultation at our Clinic he suffered from macrohaematuria and urinary retention. He was admitted to an outside urology unit and a transurethral resection was performed. Histopathology reported a pleomorphic sarcoma of the bladder neck with malignant melanoma as a possible differential diagnosis.

Neither digital rectal examination, nor a serum prostate antigen of 1.57 ng/ml, were indicative of primary prostate cancer, but in-house cystoscopy showed an asymmetric prostate enlargement with purple discoloration. Thus,

* Correspondence: georgi.tosev@med.uni-heidelberg.de
[1]Department of Urology, University of Heidelberg, Im Neuenheimer Feld 110, D-69120 Heidelberg, Germany
Full list of author information is available at the end of the article

transrectal prostate biopsy was performed with inconclusive results, followed by a diagnostic TUR-P yielding two specimens from the dubious area of the left prostate lobe above the level of the verumontanum. Final histopathology and immunohistochemical staining showed positive expression of Vimentin, Melan A, CD56, and HMB 45 and negative expression of CD30, Desmin, PSMA, S100, AE 1/3, CD34, LCA, PLAP, BerEp4, EMA, CD68, Inhibin and Calretinin, which confirmed the diagnosis of a melanoma [6]. Clear cell sarcoma was excluded via the lack of EWSR-ATF-1 translocation in the areas of the lesion analyzed.

No evidence for primary melanoma at other sites, particulary skin and mucosal by dermatologic, ophthalmologic and otolaryngologic examinations, as well as colonoscopy and gastroscopy, or distant metastases were found on imaging (CT with contrast of chest and abdomen and pelvic MRI with contrast in April 2012; Fig. 1, Ia and Ib). Therefore, open retropubic radical prostatectomy with extended lymph-node dissection was performed with curative intention in June 2012. Histopathologic examination (Fig.1, IIa, IIb, IIc) revealed a primary melanoma of the prostate with clear surgical margins (pR0) and tumour-free lymph nodes (pN0 0/22). One year after surgery the patient was completely continent and reported normal erectile function. Additionally, follow-up imaging did not show any local recurrence in the small pelvis. However CT imaging of the chest and, abdomen, and an MRI of the head with contrast in October 2012 and January 2013 (Fig. 1, IIIa) detected multiple small pulmonary lesions of up to 24 mm in size, suspicious for pulmonary metastases. Bronchoscopy was performed and biopsies from the pulmonary nodules were taken. Histopathology showed metastases of the melanoma confirming systemic relapse. According to the results of subsequent molecular analyses, no BRAF, cKIT, NRAS or GNAQ mutations and again no EWSR-1-translocation were identified. Systemic therapy with DTIC (Dacarbazine) 1000mg/m^2 for three cycles was initiated. Due to disease progression (Fig. 1, IIIb), therapy was switched to Ipilimumab (3 mg/kg). Staging after four cycles of Ipilimumab again revealed a massive disease progression and the patient was subsequently included in a phase three study of an anti-PD1 antibody receiving five cycles (NCT 01721746). As before, the patient experienced a pronounced progression of lung and hilar lymph node metastases (Fig. 1, IIIc). Another treatment regimen consisting of chemotherapy with carboplatin and paclitaxel was offered to the patient, but was declined. The patient died 16 months after initial diagnosis in palliative care.

Consent

Written informed consent was obtained from the parents of the patient for publication of this Case report and any accompanying images. A copy of the written consent is available for review by the Editor of this journal.

Discussion

Primary melanoma of the prostate is exceedingly rare. In the present case our patient suffered from melanoma of the prostate as a secondary malignancy.

The patient's history of Hodgkin disease (HD) and prior treatment with chemotherapy and radiochemotherapy (RT) may play a pathogenetic role in the development of the secondary malignancy. HD often involves cervical and mediastinal lymph nodes, and RT is known to target these nodal regions resulting in the irradiation of adjacent mammary tissue and lung. The risk of secondary lung cancer, breast, bladder, gastric and oesophageal cancer has been associated with radiation dose and with field size, but it is mostly described > 10 years after treatment [7, 8]. Similarly, secondary malignancy rates after BEACOPP-chemotherapy are 5.7–6 %, respectively [9]. Among adult survivors of childhood cancer, the prevalence of adverse health outcomes is high and an ongoing health monitoring for this group of patients is very important [10]. Due to the uncommon localization, no previous staging CT or MRI included the prostate in the present case. Only symptoms of locally advanced disease such as hematuria and urinary retention lead to further diagnostic work-up and to the final diagnosis. As seen on upon MRI analysis, the location of the tumor was in the transition zone of the prostate. Thus, the most likely origin of the prostatic melanoma was the transitional epithelium of the prostatic urethra. However, we cannot completely exclude that the patient had a stage IV melanoma with unknown primary where the prostate was the first location of metastases. In disseminated metastatic melanoma it has been reported that the prostate may be involved in 3 % of autopsies.

Initial management of cutaneous melanoma after biopsy is directed by depth of tumor, presence of ulceration, and dermal mitoses and may involve wide local excision with margins ranging from 1 to 2 cm plus/minus sentinel lymph node biopsy, and adjuvant interferon or immuno-oncologic therapy depending on final staging [11]. Surgical care for primary melanoma of mucosal sites is less well established than for primary cutaneous melanoma, but excision of the primary is always the goal if the patient has no systemic disease.

Despite low chances of a cure, we performed radical prostatectomy (RP) with extended lymph node dissection due to clinical lower urinary tract symptoms and to prevent further local complications. RP is a strong independent predictor of survival benefit in patients with prostate cancer [12]. However, radical prostatectomy can

Ia April 2012 pelvic MRT

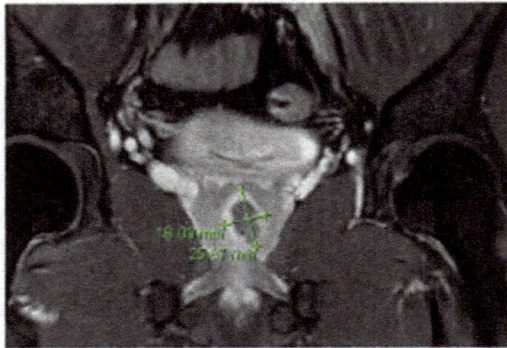

preoperative pelvic T1-weighted image MRI with suspicious lesion in the left prostate

Ib April 2012 CT Thorax

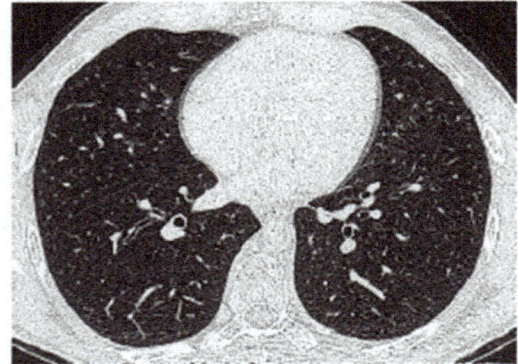

no suspicion of pulmonary lesions

II June 2012 histology of radical prostatectomy specimen

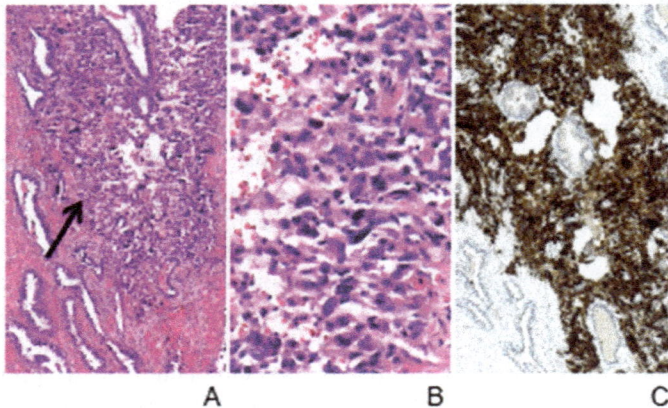

A   B   C

Microscopic aspect of the melanoma within the prostate. A: Ill-defined tumour nodules (arrow) are found within the glandular prostatic parenchyma. B: The tumor consists of highly pleomorphic cells with ovaloid irregular shaped nuclei with frequent nucleoli and pale basophilic cytoplasm. C: The tumor cells show immunohistochemical expression of melan A Stainings: H&E (A, B), immunohistochemical melan A staining (C). Original magnification: x100 (A, C), x400 (B)

IIIa January 2013
Follow up stagings

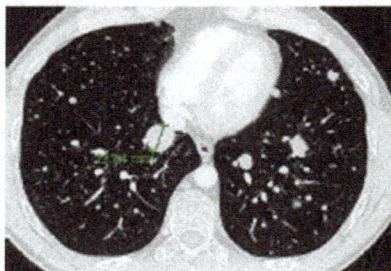

IIIb May 2013

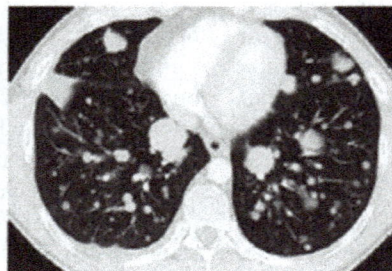

IIIc August 2013

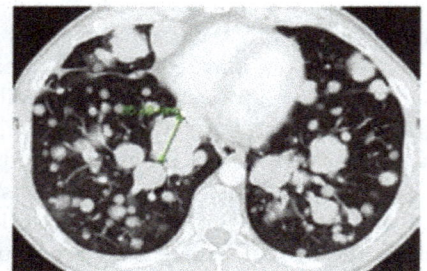

Fig. 1 Case time-line

also have detrimental side effects, especially if performed at low volume hospitals [13]. Thus, the decision of dissection of the tumor was an individual approach, based on the current knowledge of the treatment of prostate carcinoma and melanoma and based on the fact that macrohaematuria and lower urinary tract symptoms significantly impair quality of life. In the present case, the patient fully recovered lower urinary tract function after surgery.

Unfortunately, the patient suffered from systemic relapse with pulmonary metastases shortly afterwards. Systemic therapy was initiated, and 16 months after initial diagnosis the patient died due to multi-organ failure. Advanced imaging such as PET/CT may have detected systemic disease earlier than the staging we had performed. However, first metastases occurred in the lungs for which PET scanning is not clearly superior to CT. In addition, the management of the patient would not have changed significantly since one of the main indications for surgery was to improve micturition and to prevent local complications.

Systemic therapeutic options for advanced melanoma have substantially increased over the last several years. They can be divided into targeted therapies such as BRAF, MEK, cKIT inhibitors or immuno-oncologic treatments such as CTLA4 and PD-(L)-1 antibodies which manipulate the immune system. At present, trials are addressing various combination therapies to improve overall survival.

Melanomas arising in visceral organs are less likely to be BRAF or NRAS positive. While mucosal melanomas are more likely to have cKIT mutations and if positive can benefit from targeted therapy such as tyrosine kinase inhibition, this was not the case in our patient. In the case report of Ma et al. before novel immunotherapeutic drugs were available, the patient survived three months on systemic treatment. Although our patient showed disease progression under therapy with novel immunotherapeutics, the overall survival was better than the case stated above. Whether this means that tumor growth was slowed down under treatment with checkpoint inhibitors is at this point speculative.

Interestingly, the anti-cytotoxic T lymphocyte-associated receptor 4 (CTLA4) antibody Ipilimumab is also under investigation for patients with metastatic, castration-resistant prostate cancer (mCRPC) [14].

Conclusion

Due to the extreme rarity of prostatic melanoma, only very few cases have been reported. This increases the scientific importance of each individual case report. A multidisciplinary team approach to search for another potentially existing primary and early imaging to rule out possible metastases are advisable. In case of prostatic melanoma we recommend complete surgical resection with extended lymphadenectomy by experienced surgeons to prevent complications related to local tumor progression.

Advanced melanoma shows a wide heterogeneity and testing for different mutations of the tumor is needed to choose drug regimens individually for the patient. Novel immuno-oncologic therapy may lead to an improved survival in some cases.

Abbreviations
BEACOPP: Bleomycin Etoposide, Adriamycin (doxorubicin), Cyclophosphamide, Oncovin = Vincristine, Procarbazine, Prednisone; ABVD: Adriamycin Bleomycin, Vinblastine, Dacarbazine; DTIC: Dacarbazine; RT: Radiotherapy; HD: Hodgkin disease; TUR-B: Transurethral resection of the bladder; TUR-P: Transurethral resection of the prostate.

Competing interest
The authors declare that they have no competing interest.

Authors' contributions
Conception and design: GT, SP, MH and BH. Administrative support: SP, MH, BH. Acquisition of data: GT, GF, TK, JH, JH, FB. Analysis and interpretation of data: GT, TK, JH, GF, JH, SP, MH, BH. Manuscript writing: All authors read and approved the final manuscript.

Acknowledgements
All authors have made significant contributions by making diagnosis, treatment and intellectual input in the case and writing the manuscript. All authors have contributed to this paper and consent the publication. The authors would like to thank Nina Korzeniewski for providing editing services in English.

Author details
[1]Department of Urology, University of Heidelberg, Im Neuenheimer Feld 110, D-69120 Heidelberg, Germany. [2]Institute of Pathology, University of Heidelberg, Heidelberg, Germany. [3]Department of Dermatology, University of Heidelberg, Heidelberg, Germany.

References
1. Doublali M, Chouaib A, Khallouk A, Tazi MF, Fassi MJEI, Farih MyH, et al. Primary malignant melanoma of prostate. Urol Ann. 2010;2(2):76–7.
2. Hubler J, Pajor L, Kincses I. Primary malignant melanoma of the prostate. Acta Chir Acad Sci Hung. 1980;21(3):239–43.
3. Ma L. Primary malignant melanoma of the prostate. Int J Urol. 2010;17:94–5.
4. Wang CJ. Followup of primary malignant melanoma of the prostate. J Urol. 2001;166(1):214.
5. Wong JA, Bell DG. Primary malignant melanoma of the prostate: case report and review of the literature. Can J Urol. 2006;13(2):3053–6.
6. Garbe C, Peris K, Hauschild A, Saiag P, Middleton M, Spatz A, et al. Diagnosis and treatment of melanoma. European consensus-based interdisciplinary guideline–Update 2012. Eur J Cancer. 2012;48(15):2375–90.
7. Dores GM, Metayer C, Curtis RE, Lynch CF, Clarke EA, Glimelius B, et al. Second malignant neoplasms among long-term survivors of Hodgkin's disease: a population-based evaluation over 25 years. J Clin Oncol. 2002;20(16):3484–94.
8. Castellino SM, Geiger AM, Mertens AC, Leisenring WM, Tooze JA, Goodman P, et al. Morbidity and mortality in long-term survivors of Hodgkin lymphoma: a report from the Childhood Cancer Survivor Study. Blood. 2011;117(6):1806–16.
9. Engert A, Diehl V, Franklin J, Lohri A, Dörken B, Ludwig WD, et al. Escalated-dose BEACOPP in the treatment of patients with advanced-stage Hodgkin's lymphoma: 10 years of follow-up of the GHSG HD9 study. J Clin Oncol. 2009;27(27):4548–54.
10. Hudson MM, Ness KK, Gurney JG, Mulrooney DA, Chemaitilly W, Krull KR, et al. Clinical ascertainment of health outcomes among adults treated for childhood cancer. JAMA. 2013;309(22):2371–81.
11. Balch CM, Gershenwald JE, Soong SJ, Thompson JF, Atkins MB, Byrd DR, et al. Final version of 2009 AJCC melanoma staging and classification. J Clin Oncol. 2009;27(36):6199–206.
12. Engel J, Bastian PJ, Baur H, Beer V, Chaussy C, Gschwend JE, et al. Survival benefit of radical prostatectomy in lymph node-positive patients with prostate cancer. Eur Urol. 2010;57(5):754–61.
13. Hu JC, Gold KF, Pashos CL, Mehta SS, Litwin MS. Role of surgeon volume in radical prostatectomy outcomes. J Clin Oncol. 2003;21(3):401–5.
14. Agarwal N, Sonpavde G, Sternberg CN. Novel molecular targets for the therapy of castration-resistant prostate cancer. Eur Urol. 2012;61(5):950–60.

5

External validation of risk classification in patients with docetaxel-treated castration-resistant prostate cancer

Kazuhiko Nakano*, Kenji Komatsu, Taro Kubo, Shinsuke Natsui, Akinori Nukui, Shinsuke Kurokawa, Minoru Kobayashi and Tatsuo Morita

Abstract

Background: Castration-resistant prostate cancer (CRPC) patients have poor prognoses, and docetaxel (DTX) is among the few treatment options. An accurate risk classification to identify CRPC patient groups for which DTX would be effective is urgently warranted. The Armstrong risk classification (ARC), which classifies CRPC patients into 3 groups, is superior; however, its usefulness remains unclear, and further external validation is required before clinical use. This study aimed to examine the clinical significance of the ARC through external validation in DTX-treated Japanese CRPC patients.

Methods: CRPC patients who received 2 or more DTX cycles were selected for this study. Patients were classified into good-, intermediate-, and poor-risk groups according to the ARC. Prostate-specific antigen (PSA) responses and overall survival (OS) were calculated and compared between the risk groups. A multivariate analysis was performed to clarify the relationship between the ARC and major patient characteristics.

Results: Seventy-eight CRPC patients met the inclusion criteria. Median PSA levels at DTX initiation was 20 ng/mL. Good-, intermediate-, and poor-risk groups comprised 51 (65%), 17 (22%), and 10 (13%) patients, respectively. PSA response rates ≥30% and ≥50% were 33%, 41%, and 30%, and 18%, 41%, and 20% in the good-, intermediate-, and poor-risk groups, respectivcixely, with no significant differences (p = 0.133 and 0.797, respectively). The median OS in the good-, intermediate-, and poor-risk groups were statistically significant (p < 0.001) at 30.1, 14.2, and 5.7 months, respectively. A multivariate analysis revealed that the ARC and PSA doubling time were independent prognostic factors.

Conclusions: Most of CRPC patients were classified into good-risk group according to the ARC and the ARC could predict prognosis in DTX-treated CRPC patients.

Keywords: Castration-resistant prostate cancer, Docetaxel, Risk classification, Validation study

Background

Castration-resistant prostate cancer (CRPC) patients have poor prognoses. Although many treatment options have been developed, truly effective ones remain limited [1-6]. In Japan, the currently available drugs are limited even further. Predictions and classifications of CRPC patients' clinical outcomes and prognoses for the effective use of the limited treatment options offer prolonged

survival to the patients. In particular, docetaxel (DTX) [1,2] has been established as effective and has become widely used in CRPC treatment; however, in some patients, DTX is ineffective and induces a high incidence of adverse events. Thus, the development of an accurate risk classification that can identify the CRPC patient group in which DTX would be effective is urgently warranted. Although some reports have demonstrated the usefulness of superior nomograms for predicting prognosis in CRPC patients [7-9], these nomograms include many investigation items and are therefore somewhat difficult to implement

* Correspondence: nknkzhk@jichi.ac.jp
Department of Urology, Jichi Medical University, Yakushiji 3311-1, Shimotsuke, Tochigi 329-0498, Japan

in clinical practice. The Armstrong risk classification (ARC), which classifies CRPC patients into 3 groups according to 4 risk factors, including visceral metastases, bone scan progression, significant pain, and anemia (hemoglobin [Hb] level < 13 g/dL), is also a superior risk classification because it can be easily used in clinical practice without reducing the predictive abilities of nomograms and can predict not only survival but also post-chemotherapy prostate-specific antigen (PSA) declines and tumor responses [10]. ARC is highly reliable because it was developed from 656 CRPC patients who were administered DTX and was also internally validated in 333 CRPC patients who were administered mitoxantrone among the 1006 CRPC patients in the TAX327 study [1]. Furthermore, ARC was demonstrated to significantly classify the clinical outcomes of estramustine phosphate (EMP) treatment in CRPC patients [11].

However, few reports have externally validated ARC in CRPC patients who were administered DTX. Under external validation, risk classifications and nomograms might be found to have positive [12] or negative [13] effects and, sometimes, to clarify characteristics at the time of clinical use [14]. Kawahara et al. [15] reported that CRPC patients who were administered DTX in 10 or more cycles had favorable prognosis; in this study, the authors examined whether ARC would be useful when selecting CRPC patients who could continue a DTX regimen for 10 or more cycles. However, the Hb criteria were changed to 10 g/dL from 13 g/dL, the bone scan progression risk factor was replaced with alkaline phosphatase (ALP) levels, and the association between PSA response and ARC was not referenced. Armstrong, the developer of the ARC, externally validated ARC and the above-mentioned nomograms in CRPC patients who were administered DTX [16] and indicated the superior but insufficient discriminatory abilities and necessary improvements of these tools. Thus, the usefulness of ARC remains unclear and needs further external validation before clinical use.

The objective of this study was to examine the clinical significance of ARC through external validation in DTX-treated Japanese CRPC patients.

Methods

Patients and treatment

This study was approved by the institutional review board of Jichi Medical University. The clinical trial was registered in the University Hospital Medical Information Network Clinical Trials Registry (UMIN-CTR) UMIN000011969. Written informed consent to participate in this study was obtained from all patients. At our institution, patients with metastatic and/or first treatment-refractory prostate cancer (PCa) are treated with androgen deprivation therapy (ADT). After progressing to CRPC, the patients are principally treated in the following order: 1) combined androgen blockade (CAB), 2) anti-androgen withdrawal, 3) anti-

androgen substitution, 4) EMP, 5) DTX, 6) dexamethasone, and 7) best supportive care. These treatments are continued until disease progression and/or unacceptable toxicity occurs. Of the CRPC patients who received DTX in our institution between July 2003 and September 2012, those who met the following inclusion criteria were eligible for this study: 1) confirmed histological PCa diagnosis, 2) refractory to ADT with CAB, anti-androgen withdrawal, and anti-androgen substitution, 3) refractory to EMP, and 4) received 2 or more cycles of DTX.

A modified version of the regimen used in the SWOG9916 study [2] was used as the DTX treatment protocol [17]. Briefly, DTX (60 mg/m^2) was administered by intravenous drip infusion for 1 hour on day 1, once every 3–4 weeks. Twice-daily EMP (280 mg) was orally administered in combination with DTX. EMP could be reduced to 280 mg/day according to the degree of adverse events and, if already administered before DTX initiation, continued at the same dose that was administered before DTX treatment. As a premedication, 8 mg of dexamethasone was administered by intravenous drip infusion before and after the DTX treatment. The DTX treatment was continued until disease progression, unacceptable toxicity, or a patient's request for its cessation. Disease progression was defined as increases in the number of evaluable lesions observed on imaging tests and/or biological progression characterised by an elevated serum PSA level of 25% and an absolute increase of 2 ng/mL or higher than the nadir in at least 3 consecutive measurements.

Armstrong risk classification

The patients were classified as good-, intermediate-, and poor-risk according to the ARC, which included the following 4 risk factors: visceral metastases, bone scan progression, significant pain, and anemia (Hb level < 13 g/dL) [10]. Patients with 0 or 1, 2, and 3 or 4 risk factors were classified as good-, intermediate-, and poor-risk, respectively. The risk factor of visceral metastases was defined as "presence" if computed tomography (CT) and/or magnetic resonance imaging (MRI) were performed at DTX initiation and revealed visible visceral metastases. The risk factor of bone scan progression was subject to satisfaction that a bone scan had been performed at DTX initiation, comparable prior bone scans had also been performed, and progression or increases in the numbers of hot spots were demonstrated by these scans. Although significant pain was defined as a Present Pain Intensity score (PPI) ≥ 2 and/or an analgesic score (AS) ≥ 10 in the ARC [10], we defined the use of some types of analgesic at DTX initiation as a surrogate measurement of significant pain because the PPI and AS of the patients in this study were not measured. The risk factor of anemia was defined as "presence" if the patient met the criteria of Hb levels < 13 g/dL at DTX initiation.

Assessment

According to the recommendations of the Prostate Cancer Clinical Trial Working Group [18], PSA responses were demonstrated in waterfall plot of decreasing PSA rates for each patient. Decreasing PSA rates were obtained from the values determined just before DTX initiation and the lowest PSA values during DTX treatment. Overall survival (OS) was defined as the period from DTX initiation to death. When patients were lost to follow-up, OS was considered up to the last day of confirmed patient survival. Adverse events were determined according to the National Cancer Institute Common Toxicity Criteria (NCI-CTC) version 3.

Statistical analysis

PSA responses were compared with a chi-square test. OS was determined according to the Kaplan-Meier method and compared with the log-rank test. A multivariate analysis of OS was performed to compare the prognostic factors in a Cox proportional hazard analysis. Continuous data were divided into 2 groups according to median value. A concordance index (c-index) was estimated as a measure of the ARC discriminatory index. A c-index of 0.50 represents random prediction, whereas a c-index of 1.0 represents a perfect discriminatory ability [9,10,19]. $P < 0.05$ was considered statistically significant.

Results

Patients

During the study period, 102 CRPC patients received DTX at our institution, among whom, 78 met the inclusion criteria. The patient characteristics are shown in Table 1. The median observation period was 24 months (range, 3–74 months). The median number of administered DTX cycles was 5 (range, 2–46 cycles), and the median DTX administration period was 9 months (range, 1–66 months). In addition, 0, 1, 2, 3, and 4 ARC risk factors were observed in 9, 42, 17, 9, and 1 patients, respectively. The good-, intermediate-, and poor-risk groups according to the ARC included 51 (65%), 17 (22%), and 10 (13%) patients, respectively. CRPC patients with a history of EMP use were 47/51 (92%), 14/17 (82%), and 8/10 (80%) patients in the good-, intermediate-, and poor-risk groups, respectively, with no statistically significant difference (p = 0.367). A total of 67 patients (86%) discontinued DTX treatment during the observation period, of whom 51, 8, 2, 4, and 2 patients discontinued DTX treatment because of disease progression, adverse events, death, patient request, and other reasons, respectively. The remaining 11 patients (14%) were still undergoing DTX treatment during the course of the study.

Armstrong risk classification assessment

Waterfall plots of PSA response according to each ARC risk group are shown in Figure 1. PSA responses ≥0%, ≥30%,

Table 1 Patient characteristics

	(n = 78)
Age (years)	70 (50–88)
PSA at PCa diagnosis (ng/mL)	124.6 (4.7-19523.1)
PSA at DTX initiation (ng/mL)	19.7 (0.6-1053.0)
Time from PCa diagnosis to DTX initiation (months)	37 (4–189)
PSADT (months)	2.4 (0.6-33.9)
ECOG performance status, n (%)	
0	40 (51)
1	28 (36)
2	10 (13)
Gleason score, n (%)	
<6	5 (6)
7	16 (21)
>8	50 (64)
Unknown	7 (9)
Metastatic site, n (%)	
Bone	42 (54)
Lymph nodes	19 (24)
Liver	3 (4)
Lung	1 (1)
None	28 (36)
Bone scan progression, n (%)	
Yes	15 (19)
No	63 (81)
Pain at baseline, n (%)	
Yes	24 (31)
No	54 (69)
Haemoglobin (g/dL)	11.8 (8.4-14.1)
ALP (IU/L)	290 (59-8689)
Prior treatment, n (%)	
Combined androgen blockade	78 (100)
Prostatectomy	3 (4)
Radiotherapy	10 (13)
Estramustine	69 (88)
No. of DTX cycles	5 (2–46)

Abbreviations: PSA, prostate-specific antigen; PCa, prostate cancer; DTX, docetaxel; PSADT, prostate-specific antigen doubling time; ECOG, Eastern Cooperative Oncology Group; ALP, alkaline phosphatase. All continuous data are described in median (range).

and ≥50% were observed in 48 (62%), 27 (35%), and 18 (23%) of the total patients, respectively. PSA response rates ≥30% and ≥50% were observed in 33%, 41%, and 30%, and 18%, 41%, and 20% of the good-, intermediate-, and poor-risk groups, respectively, with no statistically significant differences between the groups (p = 0.133 and 0.797, respectively).

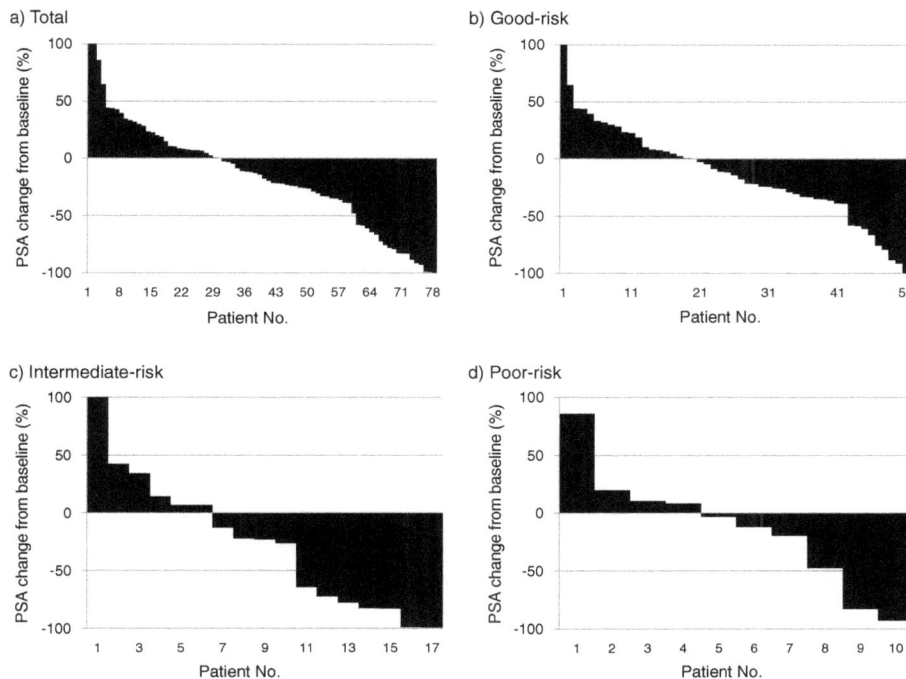

Figure 1 Waterfall plots of prostate-specific antigen (PSA) responses according to total (a), good-(b), intermediate-(c), and poor-(d) risk group of Armstrong risk classification.

The OS according to each ARC risk factor is shown in Table 2. Regarding the risk factor of anemia, which was divided into 2 groups according to the relatively high Hb value of 13 g/dL, the group with Hb levels ≤ 13 g/dL dominated with 64 patients (82%). There were significant associations between OS and the risk factors of visceral metastases (p < 0.001), bone scan progression (p < 0.001), and significant pain (p < 0.001), but not anemia (p = 0.442).

Patient distributions and OS curves according to the ARC risk groups are shown in Figure 2. The CRPC patients at our institution were mostly classified as good-risk (65%). The median OS durations in the good-, intermediate-, and poor-risk groups were 30.1 months (95% confidence interval [CI]: 17.8–42.5 months), 14.2 months (95% CI: 3.7–

24.7 months), and 5.7 months (95% CI: 3.1–8.2 months), respectively, with statistically significant differences between the groups (p < 0.001). During the observation period, death occurred in 39 patients (46%), of whom 18, 14, and 7 were in the good-, intermediate-, and poor-risk groups, respectively. The c-index was 0.60 for OS, indicating that the ARC had a modest discriminatory ability in our cohort.

Subgroup analysis

A multivariate analysis was performed to clarify the relationship between the ARC and the major patient characteristics that are often evaluated in clinical practice. The following 6 factors at DTX initiation were covariates of interest: age, PSA level, PSA doubling time (PSADT),

Table 2 Univariate analysis for overall survival according to each risk factor of Armstrong risk classification [10]

Risk factor	Category	n	Median (months)	Hazard ratio	95% CI	p value*
Visceral metastases	no	74	20.3	1.00		<0.001
	yes	4	3.9	19.47	5.51 - 68.83	
Bone scan progression	no	63	25.8	1.00		<0.001
	yes	15	9.1	3.78	2.00 - 7.14	
Significant pain	no	54	25.8	1.00		<0.001
	yes	24	8.7	2.98	1.72 - 5.17	
Hemoglobin (g/dL)	>13.0	14	22.9	1.00		0.442
	≦ 13.0	64	19.5	1.31	0.66 - 2.60	

Abbreviations: CI, confidence interval. *log rank test.

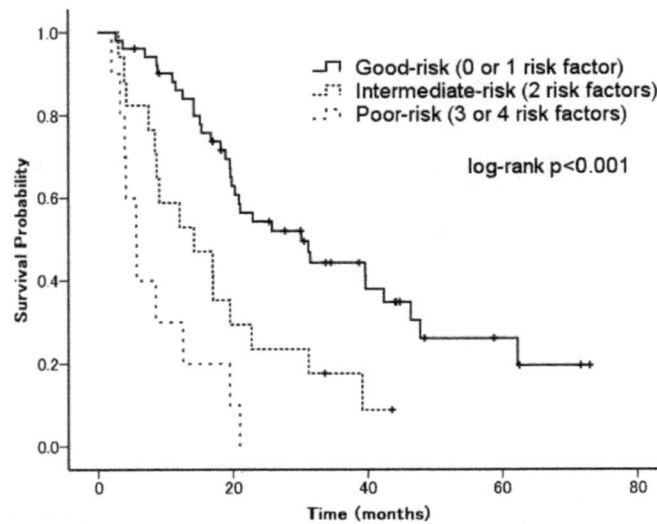

risk	n	median OS (mo)	95% CI
Good	51	30.1	17.8 - 42.5
Intermediate	17	14.2	3.7 - 24.7
Poor	10	5.7	3.1 - 8.2

p=0.003
p=0.034
p=0.001

Figure 2 Overall survival curves according to Armstrong risk classification [10].

Eastern Cooperative Oncology Group (ECOG) performance status, Gleason score, and ARC. A univariate analysis conducted with the log-rank test revealed significant associations between OS and 4 factors (PSA at DTX initiation, PSADT, ECOG performance status, and ARC). A multivariate analysis with these 4 factors revealed that the ARC and PSADT were independent prognostic factors (Table 3).

Discussion

We externally validated the ARC in CRPC patients who were administered DTX in 2 or more cycles and showed that there were statistically significant differences in OS among the ARC risk groups. The median OS and 95% CI for each ARC risk group were similar between the CRPC patients used for validation in this study (the

Table 3 Univariate and multivariate analysis for overall survival of major prognostic factors

Prognostic factor	Category	n	Median (months)	Univariate			Multivariate		
				Hazard ratio	95% CI	p value*	Hazard ratio	95% CI	p value**
Age (years)	$\leq$ 70	43	17.0	1.00		0.062			
	>70	35	22.7	0.60	0.35 - 1.03				
PSA at DTX initiation (ng/ml)	$\leq$ 20	39	39.6	1.00		<0.001	1.00		0.058
	>20	39	12.6	3.44	1.94 - 6.11		2.07	0.98 - 4.37	
PSADT (months)	>2.4	38	31.4	1.00		0.001	1.00		0.033
	$\leq$ 2.4	40	16.7	2.56	1.48 - 4.41		1.88	1.05 - 3.36	
ECOG performance status	$\leq$ 1	68	20.3	1.00		0.001	1.00		0.740
	2	10	4.1	3.11	1.55 - 6.26		1.16	0.49 - 2.74	
Gleason score	$\leq$ 7	21	31.2	1.00		0.113			
	>8	57	18.2	1.63	0.89 - 3.00				
Armstrong risk classification	Good	51	30.1	1.00		<0.001	1.00		0.060
	Intermediate	17	14.2	2.48	1.32 - 4.66		1.33	0.60 - 2.97	0.487
	Poor	10	5.7	6.58	3.07 - 14.11		3.21	1.17 - 8.80	0.024

Abbreviations: CI, confidence interval; PSA, prostate-specific antigen; PSADT, prostate-specific antigen doubling time; ECOG, Eastern Cooperative Oncology Group; ALP, alkaline phosphatase. *log rank test. **Cox proportional hazards model.

validation group) and the CRPC patients used to develop the ARC [10] (the development group). The c-index for OS was 0.60, indicating that the ARC had a modest discriminatory ability in the validation group. A multivariate analysis revealed that the ARC was an independent prognostic factor. Thus, the ability of the ARC to classify and approximately predict the OS of CRPC patients with certain reproducibility was confirmed, suggesting that the ARC is useful when predicting prognosis in DTX-treated CRPC patients. This means that CRPC patients who are classified into good- and intermediate-risk groups are recommended for aggressive DTX administration, because these patients would be expected to experience prolonged OS in response to DTX. However, CRPC patients who are classified as poor-risk should be recommended for clinical trial participation or other treatments because given the poor outcomes, these patients would be expected to experience a limited prognosis despite the use of DTX.

ARC was also reported to be able to classify PSA response in CRPC patients, although this system was principally aimed at classifying OS [10]. We also externally validated the usefulness of ARC in classifying the PSA response of CRPC patients. However, there were no statistically significant differences in PSA response between the ARC risk groups. This result was considered to be caused by the reason that most of CRPC patients in the validation group had a history of EMP use; the frequency of a history of EMP use was high in good-risk group (92%) compared to intermediate-risk (82%) and poor-risk (80%) groups. The CRPC patients with a history of EMP use showed significantly lower PSA response during DTX treatment than those without a history of EMP use [10]. Thus, considering that PSA response during DTX treatment are likely to be low in the CRPC patients with a history of EMP use, our cohort might not be suitable for validating the usefulness of ARC in classifying the PSA response of CRPC patients.

This validation study exhibited the following characteristics with respect to the ARC: the development group presented with median PSA levels of 110 ng/mL at DTX initiation. From this group, symptoms and imaging test items that are often observed after some disease progression, including bone scan progression [9], significant pain [20], and visceral metastases [8,21], were identified as risk factors. However, as the efficacy of DTX was established in CRPC patients and DTX initiation in patients with low PSA levels was found to confer better prognosis [9,15,17,21], the likelihood of initiating DTX at lower PSA levels has increased to a level higher than those reported in the TAX327 and SWOG9916 trials. The validation group presented median PSA levels of 20 ng/mL at DTX initiation, a lower value than that of the development group, and possessed few ARC risk factors; this led to a disproportionate distribution in which 65% of CRPC patients in the validation group were classified as good-risk. Thus, the ARC tends to classify

many CRPC patients with low PSA levels as good-risk. At the comparison of the prognoses and/or treatment responses of CRPC patients, the ARC would ensure more accurate outcomes while considering the above-mentioned ARC characteristics.

This study had the following limitations: a retrospective study design; a small sample size; different patient backgrounds in the validation and development groups in terms of EMP exposure, lower PSA levels, lack of visceral spread, and lower numbers of DTX cycles; and a different definition of significant pain as a risk factor. Although these major limitations could have possibly deteriorated the quality of this external validation study of ARC, it was noteworthy that the ARC indicated good discriminatory ability for OS even in this validation group.

Conclusions
Most of CRPC patients were classified into good-risk group according to the ARC and the ARC could predict prognosis in DTX-treated CRPC patients.

Competing interests
The authors declare that they have no competing interests.

Authors' contributions
This study has been designed by KN and TM. The clinical database of the patients have been acquired by KN, KK, TK, SN, AN, SK, MK and TM. Manuscript has been written by KN and TM. KN is responsible for the statistical analyses. Conclusions have been drawn mainly by KN and TM. TM has given final approval of the version to be published. All authors read and approved the final manuscript.

Acknowledgement
We thank Mayumi Takasawa for the assistance with manuscript preparation.

References
1. Tannock IF, de Wit R, Berry WR, Horti J, Pluzanska A, Chi KN, Oudard S, Theodore C, James ND, Turesson I, Rosenthal MA, Eisenberger MA, TAX Investigators: **Docetaxel plus prednisone or mitoxantrone plus prednisone for advanced prostate cancer.** *N Engl J Med* 2004, 351:1502–1512.
2. Petrylak DP, Tangen CM, Hussain MHA, Lara PJ, Jones JA, Taplin ME, Burch PA, Berry D, Moinpour C, Kohli M, Benson MC, Small EJ, Raghavan D, Crawford ED: **Docetaxel and estramustine compared with mitoxantrone and prednisone for advanced refractory prostate cancer.** *N Engl J Med* 2004, 351:1513–1520.
3. de Bono JS, Oudard S, Ozguroglu M, Hansen S, Machiels JP, Kocak I, Gravis G, Bodrogi I, Mackenzie MJ, Shen L, Roessner M, Gupta S, Sartor AO: **Prednisone plus cabazitaxel or mitoxantrone for metastatic castration-resistant prostate cancer progressing after docetaxel treatment: a randomised open-label trial.** *Lancet* 2010, 364:1147–1154.
4. de Bono JS, Logothetis CJ, Molina A, Fizazi K, North S, Chu L, Chi KN, Jones RJ, Goodman OB Jr, Saad F, Staffurth JN, Mainwaring P, Harland S, Flaig TW, Hutson TE, Cheng T, Patterson H, Hainsworth JD, Ryan CJ, Sternberg CN, Ellard SL, Flechon A, Saleh M, Scholz M, Efstathiou E, Zivi A, Bianchini D, Loriot Y, Chieffo N, Kheoh T, *et al*: **Abiraterone and increased survival in metastatic prostate cancer.** *N Engl J Med* 2011, 364:1995–2005.
5. Scher HI, Fizazi K, Saad F, Taplin ME, Sternberg CN, Miller K, de Wit R, Mulders P, Chi KN, Shore ND, Armstrong AJ, Flaig TW, Flechon A, Mainwaring P, Fleming M, Hainsworth JD, Hirmand M, Selby B, Seely L, de Bono JS: **Increased survival with enzalutamide in prostate cancer after chemotherapy.** *N Engl J Med* 2012, 367:1187–1197.
6. Kantoff PW, Higano CS, Shore ND, Berger ER, Small EJ, Penson DF, Redfern CH, Ferrari AC, Dreicer R, Sims RB, Xu Y, Frohlich MW, Schellhammer PF, Impact

Study Investigators : Sipuleucel-T immunotherapy for castration-resistant prostate cancer. *N Engl J Med* 2010, **363**:411–422.

7. Smaletz O, Scher HI, Small EJ, Verbel DA, McMillan A, Regan K, Kelly WK, Kattan MW: Nomogram for overall survival of patients with progressive metastatic prostate cancer after castration. *J Clin Oncol* 2002, **20**:3972–3982.

8. Halabi S, Small EJ, Kantoff PW, Kattan MW, Kaplan EB, Dawson NA, Levine EG, Blumenstein BA, Vogelzang NJ: Prognostic model for predicting survival in men with hormone-refractory metastatic prostate cancer. *J Clin Oncol* 2003, **21**:1232–1237.

9. Armstrong AJ, Garrett-Mayer ES, Yang YCO, de Wit R, Tannock IF, Eisenberger M: A contemporary prognostic nomogram for men with hormone-refractory metastatic prostate cancer: a TAX327 study analysis. *Clin Cancer Res* 2007, **13**:6396–6403.

10. Armstrong AJ, Tannock IF, de Wit R, George DJ, Eisenberger M, Halabi S: The development of risk groups in men with metastatic castration-resistant prostate cancer based on risk factors for PSA decline and survival. *Eur J Cancer* 2010, **46**:517–525.

11. Minato A, Fujimoto N, Kubo T, Harada S, Akasaka S, Matsumoto T: Efficacy of estramustine phosphate according to risk classification of castration-resistant prostate cancer. *Med Oncol* 2012, **29**:2895–2900.

12. Yu JB, Makarov DV, Sharma R, Peschel RE, Partin AW, Gross CP: Validation of the partin nomogram for prostate cancer in a national sample. *J Urol* 2010, **183**:105–111.

13. Bhojani N, Ahyai S, Graefen M, Capitanio U, Suardi N, Shariat SF, Jeldres C, Erbersdobler A, Schlomm T, Haese A, Steuber T, Heinzer H, Montorsi F, Huland H, Karakiewicz PI: Partin Tables cannot accurately predict the pathological stage at radical prostatectomy. *Eur J Surg Oncol* 2009, **35**:123–128.

14. Naito S, Kuroiwa K, Kinukawa N, Goto K, Koga H, Ogawa O, Murai M, Shiraishi T: Validation of partin tables and development of a preoperative nomogram for Japanese patients with clinically localized prostate cancer using 2005 international society of urological pathology consensus on gleason grading: data from the clinicopathological research group for localized prostate cancer. *J Urol* 2008, **180**:904–909.

15. Kawahara T, Miyoshi Y, Sekiguchi Z, Sano F, Hayashi N, Teranishi J, Misaki H, Noguchi K, Kubota Y, Uemura H: Risk factors for metastatic castration-resistant prostate cancer (CRPC) predict long-term treatment with docetaxel. *PLoS One* 2012, **7**:e48186.

16. Pond GR, Armstrong AJ, Wood BA, Leopold L, Galsky MD, Sonpavde G: Ability of C-reactive protein to complement multiple prognostic classifiers in men with metastatic castration resistant prostate cancer receiving docetaxel-based chemotherapy. *BJU Int* 2012, **110**:E461–468.

17. Nakano K, Ohta S, Komatsu K, Kubo T, Nukui A, Suzuki K, Kurokawa S, Kobayashi M, Morita T: Docetaxel with or without estramustine for estramustine refractory castration-resistant prostate cancer: a single institution experience. *BMC Urol* 2012, **12**:3.

18. Scher HI, Halabi S, Tannock I, Morris M, Sternberg CN, Carducci MA, Eisenberger MA, Higano C, Bubley GJ, Dreicer R, Petrylak D, Kantoff P, Basch E, Kelly WK, Figg WD, Small EJ, Beer TM, Wilding G, Martin A, Hussain M: Design and end points of clinical trials for patients with progressive prostate cancer and castrate levels of testosterone: recommendations of the prostate cancer clinical trials working group. *J Clin Oncol* 2008, **26**:1148–1159.

19. Armstrong AJ, Garrett-Mayer E, de Wit R, Tannock I, Eisenberger M: Prediction of survival following first-line chemotherapy in men with castration-resistant metastatic prostate cancer. *Clin Cancer Res* 2010, **16**:203–211.

20. Oudard S, Banu E, Medioni J, Scotte F, Banu A, Levy E, Wasserman J, Kacso G, Andrieu JM: What is the real impact of bone pain on survival in patients with metastatic hormone-refractory prostate cancer treated with docetaxel? *BJU Int* 2009, **103**:1641–1646.

21. Bamias A, Bozas G, Antoniou N, Poulias I, Katsifotis H, Skolarikos A, Mitropoulos D, Alamanis C, Alivizatos G, Deliveliotis H, Dimopoulos MA: Prognostic and predictive factors in patients with androgen-independent prostate cancer treated with docetaxel and estramustine: a single institution experience. *Eur Urol* 2008, **53**:323–332.

6

Erectile function in men with end-stage liver disease improves after living donor liver transplantation

You-Chiuan Chien[1†], Heng-Chieh Chiang[1†], Ping-Yi Lin[2] and Yao-Li Chen[3,4*]

Abstract

Background: Impaired liver function in men can result in erectile dysfunction or hypogonadism or both. We investigated whether living donor liver transplantation (LDLT) results in improvement in male sexual function.

Methods: A total of 58 patients with end-stage liver disease (ESLD) were included in this prospective, cross-sectional study. Erectile function was measured before and after LDLT using a five-item modified version of the International Index of Erectile Function scale (IIEF-5) and hypogonadism was evaluated before and after LDLT using the Androgen Deficiency in the Aging Male (ADAM) questionnaire. Differences in mean values from the questionnaires before and after the operation were than evaluated to determine whether there is an association between LDLT and improvement in sexual function.

Results: We found that mean IIEF-5 scores significantly increased after LDLT (from 11.7 ± 7.7 before LDLT to 14.7 ± 7.5 after LDLT, $p < 0.01$), indicating that the operation played a role in improving erectile function. In addition, the prevalence of hypogonadism among the patients with ESLD decreased markedly after liver transplantation (hypogonadism before LDLT, n = 41 versus hypogonadism after LDLT, n = 31, $p = 0.03$). Patients with hypogonadism reported a higher prevalence of erectile dysfunction after LDLT than patients without hypogonadism ($p < 0.01$).

Conclusions: LDLT results in improvement in erectile function. In addition, improvement in erectile function is associated with self-reported absence of hypogonadism.

Background

Liver transplantation is considered standard curative therapy for patients with advanced hepatocellular carcinoma and for patients with alcohol-related end-stage liver disease (ESLD). Improvements in surgical techniques as well as medical therapy have resulted in better long-term survival outcomes for patients who require liver transplantation. However, patients with chronic disease tend to care more about quality of life than about the duration of life. Sexual function, a component of quality of life, is a major concern for men with ESLD and for those who have received liver transplantation [1, 2]. Damage to the hypothalamic-pituitary-gonadal axis and impaired

liver function are the main causes of sexual dysfunction in patients with cirrhosis [1, 3]. Studies have shown that orthotopic liver transplantation (OLT) can result in restoration of the hypothalamic-pituitary-gonadal axis [4, 5].

Religious beliefs, cultural values, educational systems and differences in legislation associated with brain death help to explain why OLT is not as common in Asian countries as in Western countries [6]. Increased need for liver transplantation and a shortage of deceased donors led to the development of living donor liver transplantation (LDLT) as an alternative to OLT. Although long-term survival rates, organ rejection rates, and rates of hepatitis C virus (HCV) recurrence have been shown to be more or less equal between LDLT and OLT, studies have shown that LDLT is associated with a shorter ischemic time, a lower mortality rate, and greater perioperative benefits than OLT [7].

The prevalence of erectile dysfunction is high in patients with ESLD [8]. Although the gold standard for

* Correspondence: 31560@cch.org.tw

[†]Equal contributors

[3]School of Medicine, Kaohsiung Medical University, Kaohsiung, Taiwan

[4]Department of General Surgery, Changhua Christian Hospital, No.135 Nan-Hsiao Street, Changhua county 50006, Taiwan

Full list of author information is available at the end of the article

determining the presence of hypogonadism in men is measuring free testosterone level, that test is not widely performed in clinical laboratories. An alternative to measuring free testosterone in serum is to administer the self-report Androgen Deficiency in the Aging Male (ADAM) questionnaire, which is designed to assess symptoms associated with androgen deficiency and, therefore, can be used as a tool to detect and measure the degree of hypogonadism. The ADAM questionnaire is a simple, non-invasive measure that has been shown to have a high sensitivity and a relatively acceptable specificity [9, 10].

Erectile dysfunction (ED) is defined as the inability to develop or maintain an erection during sexual intercourse and is the main domain of sexual dysfunction in men [8]. Although ED is an important quality-of-life issue, it is often underestimated by patients and physicians. The five-item International Index of Erection Function (IIEF-5) questionnaire provides a measurable scale with which to estimate the true prevalence of ED [11]. To the best of our knowledge, no studies have evaluated the effect of LDLT on sexual function in men. Thus, in this study, we measured the differences in pre- and post-surgical IIEF-5 and ADAM questionnaire scores to investigate whether LDLT affects sexual function in men.

Methods

Patients

The patients in this prospective cohort study comprised 68 men with end-stage liver disease who were scheduled to undergo LDLT at the Changhua Christian hospital (Changhua, Taiwan) during the period 2006–2012. Written informed consents were obtained from the patients. The five-item International Index of Erection Function (IIEF-5) questionnaire, designed to evaluate erectile dysfunction,

and the Androgen Deficiency in the Aging Male (ADAM) questionnaire, designed to measure the degree of hypogonadism, were administered to the patients before LDLT and six months after the operation. Patients were required to complete the IIEF-5 questionnaire in the outpatient department about six to seven months after transplantation. At the end of the study period, 10 men were excluded from the study because of because of working abroad (n = 2), because they refused to complete the questionnaires (n = 6), or because of self-reported inability to understand the questionnaire during the post-operative period (n = 2). Therefore, data on 58 patients were evaluated (Fig. 1).

The Institutional Review Board of the Changhua Christian hospital approved the study.

Inclusion and exclusion criteria

Adult (≥18 years) male recipients of living donor liver transplant who had completed a 6-month follow-up assessment were considered eligible for inclusion. Exclusion criteria included female gender, age < 18 years, liver graft failure, refusal to complete the post-LDLT questionnaires, and loss to follow-up for any reason.

Survey

An introductory letter comprising a detailed description of the methodology of the study, the future consequences of the study, the name of the contact person of the study, and associated information was presented to each participant before LDLT. Data collection was completed by two doctors in the urology division of the surgery department via telephone or face-to-face interview. Etiology of liver disease (hepatitis B virus, hepatitis C virus, or alcoholism),

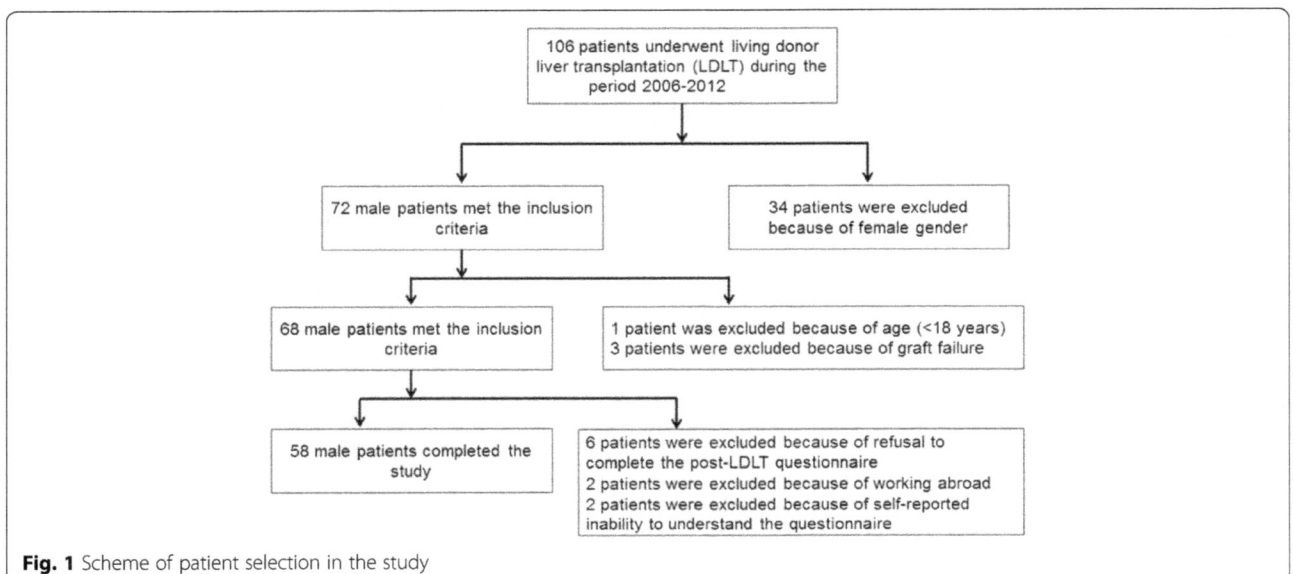

Fig. 1 Scheme of patient selection in the study

alcohol intake history, the presence of diabetes and demographic data were obtained through chart review.

Main outcome measures
Measures
The International Index of Erectile Function (IIEF), also known as the Sexual Health Inventory for Men (SHIM), is a widely used questionnaire for the evaluation of male sexual function and is recommended as a primary endpoint for diagnostic evaluation of ED severity by the National Institutes of Health Consensus Panel on Impotence [12]. The IIEF-5 is a modified version of the IIEF comprising five items instead of 15 items and was designed to shorten the time needed to complete the survey. The IIEF-5 questionnaire shows the presence and severity of ED over the past six months [13]. Studies have shown that the validity and sensitivity of the IIEF-5 are similar to those of the original IIEF scale [11, 14]. The IIEF-5 is graded on a scale from 1 to 5 points for each of the five items. The total score therefore ranges from 5 to 25. The primary score is classified into five categories of severity, namely severe (score 5–7), moderate (score 8–11), mild-to-moderate (score 12–16), mild (score 17–21), and no ED (score 22–25). The Androgen Deficiency in the Aging Male (ADAM) questionnaire is a self-report, ten-item scale designed to evaluate the degree of androgen deficiency [10]. ADAM consists of 10 questions and answering "yes" to question 1 or 7 or to 3 or more of the questions is regard as an indication of possible hypogonadal status. ADAM has been shown to be a highly sensitive but poorly specific measure for determining androgen deficiency [15]. Nonetheless, Tancredi et al. found that hormone analysis of blood samples correlated with ADAM scores [9]. Patients who reported decreased libido or inadequate erectile "strength" and patients who provided positive answers to 3 of the other questions listed in the questionnaire were considered to have androgen deficiency. Both questionnaires were given to patients before LDLT and at least six months after the operation to evaluate whether LDLT had an effect on erectile dysfunction and hypogonadism.

Statistical analysis
Categorical data were compared by the McNemar's test or the Chi-square test. Differences in continuous variables were compared by the Wilcoxon signed-rank test. A *p* value of less than 0.05 was considered to indicate statistical significance. All statistical analyses were performed on a personal computer with the statistical package SPSS for Windows (Version 18.0, SPSS, Chicago, Il).

Results
During the period November 2012 to May 2013, 58 of the 68 (85 %) adult men who were eligible to participate in the study completed both questionnaires before and after LDLT. Reasons for not completing the questionnaires during the post-operative period included refusal to participate (n = 6), working abroad (n = 2), and self-reported inability to understand the questionnaire (n = 2). Table 1 summarizes the general characteristics of the patients who participated in the study. The mean age at the time of LDLT was 53.86 ± 7.53 years. Alcohol abuse was self-reported in 17 patients before LDLT and in 4 after the operation. In addition, 15 of the patients had diabetes mellitus before surgery and 27 had the disorder after LDLT (Table 1).

Change in erectile dysfunction
We found that mean IIEF-5 scores significantly increased after LDLT (from 11.7 ± 7.7 before LDLT to 14.7 ± 7.5 after LDLT, *p* <0.01), indicating that the operation played a role in improving erectile function. Overall, 28 patients reported improvement in erectile function, 23 patients reported no change in erectile function and 7 patients reported worse erectile function. We also found that the degrees of ED changed among the study population after surgery (Table 2). The percentage of patients with IIEF-5 scores indicative of severe ED or mild-to-moderate ED was markedly lower after LDLT (24.1 % vs. 37.9 % and 17.2 % vs. 31.0 % respectively) and the percentage of patients with IIEF-5 scores indicating no ED was noticibly higher after LDLT (13.8 % vs. 6.9 %). Interestingly, however, the percentage of patients with scores indicative of moderate ED or mild ED was higher

Table 1 Characteristics of the population before and after transplantation

	Before transplantationN (%)	After transplantationN (%)	p value
Age (years; mean ± SD)	53.86 ± 7.53	55.02 ± 7.33	< 0.001
Alcohol abuse	17 (29.3)	4 (6.9)	< 0.001
HBV	34 (58.6)	1 (1.7)	< 0.001
HCV	17 (29.3)	6 (10.3)	0.001
Diabetes	15 (25.9)	27 (46.6)	< 0.001
IIEF5 score (mean ± SD)	11.7 ± 7.7	14.7 ± 7.5	0.001
Suspected hypogonadism via ADAM questionnaire	41 (70.6)	31 (53.4)	0.031

Table 2 Changes of erectile dysfunction prior to and after liver transplantation

		Before transplantationN (%)	After transplantationN (%)	p value
Categories of IIEF5 score	Severe ED	22 (37.9)	14 (24.1)	< 0.001
	Moderate ED	2 (3.4)	3 (5.2)	
	Mild to moderate ED	18 (31.0)	10 (17.2)	
	Mild ED	12 (20.7)	23 (39.7)	
	No ED	4 (6.9)	8 (13.8)	

after LDLT (5.2 % vs. 3.4 % and 39.7 % vs. 20.7 %, respectively) (Table 2) (Fig. 2).

Change in hypogonadism

The prevalence of hypogonadism among the patients with ESLD decreased markedly after liver transplantation based on the scores from the ADAM questionnaires administered before and after surgery (hypogonadism before LDLT, n = 41 vs. hypogonadism after LDLT, n = 31, $p = 0.031$).

Association of erectile dysfunction and hypogonadism

We found that hypogonadism before LDLT was associated with improvement in erectile function after LDLT. There was a significant correlation between hypogonadism before LDLT and IIEF-5 score prior to LDLT (Fig. 3). In patients with ADAM questionnaire scores indicating no hypogonadism, the mean IIEF-5 score was 15.35 ± 6.89 prior to LDLT and 19.92 ± 4.92 after LDLT (p <0.01) (Table 3). In patients with ADAM scores indicative of hypogonadism, the mean IIEF-5 score was 8.75 ± 7.07 before surgery and 10.53 ± 6.65 after LDLT ($p = 0.107$).

Factors associated with post-LDLT erectile dysfunction

The existence of HCV infection was significantly associated with lower IIEF-5 scores (mean IIEF-5 score in patients with HCV = 11.06 ± 7.81 vs. mean IIEF-5 score in patients without HCV = 16.27 ± 6.97, $p = 0.015$). Patients with clinical evidence of DM had lower IIEF-5 scores than those without diabetes (IIEF-5 of patients with DM = 12.15 ± 7.40 vs. IIEF-5 of patients without DM = 17.00 ±

7.02, $p = 0.013$). Other parameters such as alcohol-related origin of liver disease, development of post-transplantation DM, and gender of donor were not associated with the development of post-LDLT erectile dysfunction or hypogonadism.

Discussion

Determination of sexual health is challenging, especially in Asian men who are often reluctant to undergo evaluation of sexual function. The response rate among participants to questionnaires designed to survey sexual function has been reported to range from 22.5 % to 81 % [8, 11, 16]. In our study, however, the response rate was 85 %. The introductory letters written by the surgeon who performed the LDLT procedures most likely contributed to the relatively high compliance rate in our study. The etiology of sexual dysfunction is multi-factorial and ESLD is one of many factors associated with the disorder. Liver transplantation restores liver function and should, theoretically, result in improvements in sexual function [8]. However, immunosuppressive drugs, which are key to survival after liver transplantation, are known to impair sexual function [17]. Alterations in the hypothalamic-pituitary-gonadal axis, changes in estrogen-over-androgen ratio, and altered sex hormone transport have been shown to cause hypogonadism in patients with impaired liver function [16, 18, 19]. Decreased testosterone level, libido, testis size and even infertility have been reported in patients with cirrhosis [3, 20]. Foresta et al. reported decreased sex hormone binding protein levels and higher free testosterone in serum in patients after OLT, which may explain the

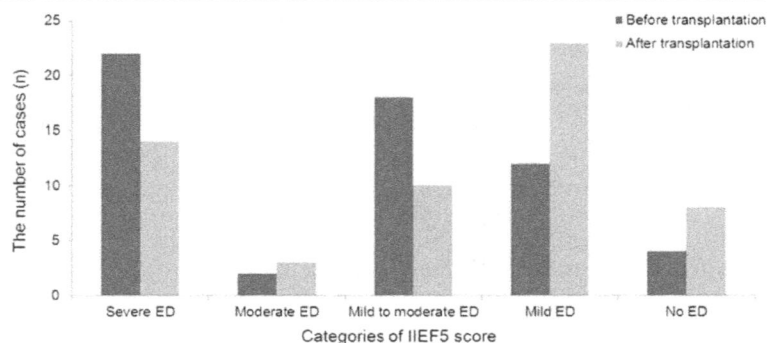

Fig. 2 Prevalence of erectile dysfunction prior to and after liver transplantation

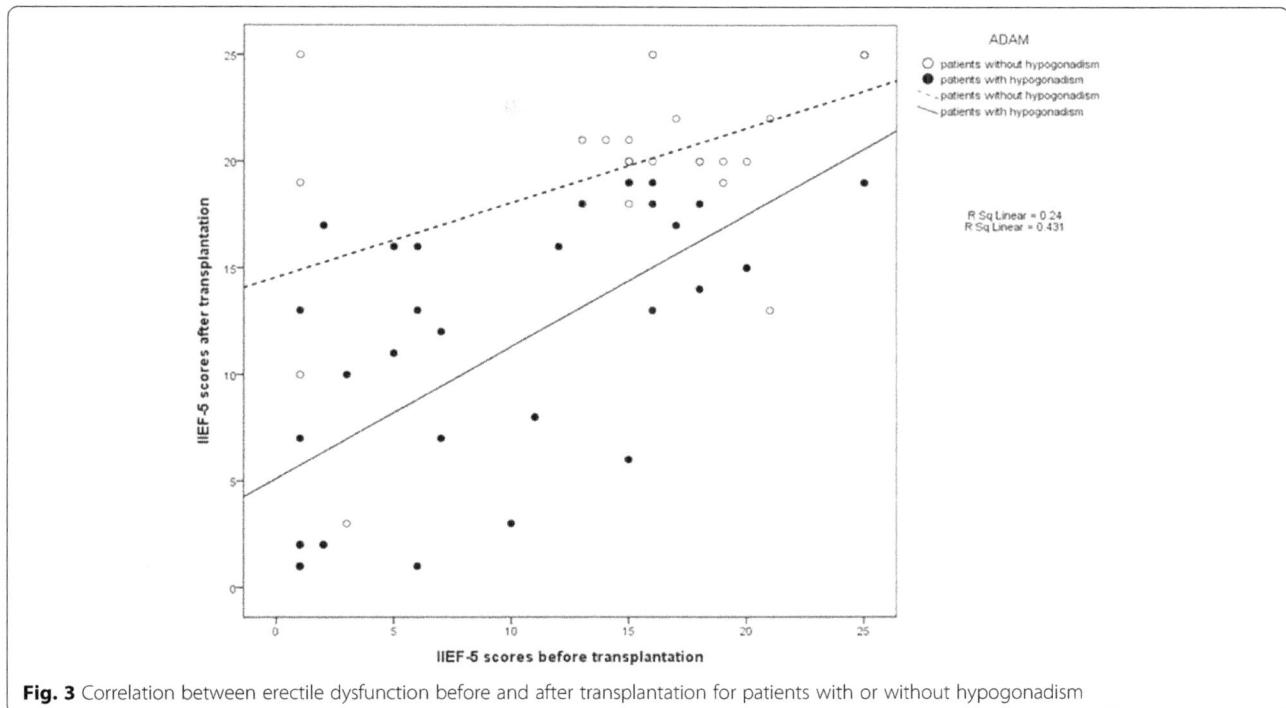

Fig. 3 Correlation between erectile dysfunction before and after transplantation for patients with or without hypogonadism

improvement in physiological function after the operation, even under immunosuppressive therapy [4]. Park et al. reported that up to 60 % of men reported no improvement in erectile function after OLT [10]. Klein and colleagues reported improvement in sexual function including erectile function, sexual satisfaction and sexual desire and a statistical trend in improvement in IIEF scores after liver transplant [21]. In our study, we found that nearly half of the patients reported improvement in erectile function. Many factors contribute to ED, including drugs, neurogenic disorders, cavernosal disorders, hormones, psychological causes, surgery, aging, and diabetes [22]. In our study, higher IIEF-5 scores were associated with absence of hypogonadism after the operation. That is, improvement in erectile function after liver transplantation is mainly hormone related. Theoretically, irreversible damage of the hypothalamic-pituitary-gonadal axis by

long-term consumption of alcohol implies the low possibility of improvement in sexual function after LDLT [23]. However, Huyghe E et al. reported no higher risk of erectile dysfunction in patients with end-stage liver disease secondary to alcohol consumption [8]. Burra et al. also reported that there was no significantly lower trend in IIEF score in patients with alcohol-induced ESLD [3]. Sorrell and Brown found that 40 % of patients developed erectile dysfunction and 25 % reported having a lower level of sexual satisfaction after liver transplantation [16]. Ho et al. reported that 32 % of patients developed de novo sexual dysfunction after OLT [24]. Cardiovascular disease, post-transplantation diabetes, alcohol abuse, antidepressants and angiotensin II receptor blockers have been shown to be associated with new onset erectile dysfunction after liver transplantation [8]. In our study, 12 % (n = 7) of our patients reported a decrease in erectile function

Table 3 IIEF-5 scores before and after transplantation for each group

| | IIEF-5 score | | |
	Before transplantation(mean ± SD)	After transplantation(mean ± SD)	p value
With hypogonadism	8.75 ± 7.07	10.53 ± 6.65	0.109
Without hypogonadism	15.35 ± 6.89	19.92 ± 4.92	0.001
HCV positive	9.24 ± 6.98	11.06 ± 7.81	0.247
HCV negative	12.73 ± 7.80	16.27 ± 6.97	0.001
With DM	10.48 ± 6.51	12.15 ± 7.40	0.094
Without DM	12.77 ± 8.53	17.00 ± 7.02	0.002

after LDLT. The low incidence of de novo erectile dysfunction might be due to the relatively short follow-up period in our study.

There are several limitations in this study. First, immunosuppressive regimens after transplantation were not consistent throughout the study population. Therefore, we were not able to take pharmacologic factors into account. Second, our findings are limited by the relatively small sample size and short follow-up period. Third, we did not measure serum testosterone levels and therefore we do not have laboratory data to support the change in prevalence of hypogonadism. Nonetheless, to the best of our knowledge, this is the first study to compare changes in sexual function before and after LDLT. Large-scale studies with longer follow-up periods are needed to clarify the role liver transplantation plays in sexual function.

Conclusions
LDLT results in improvement in erectile function. In addition, improvement in erectile function is associated with absence of hypogonadism before LDLT.

Competing interests
The authors declare that they have no competing interests.

Authors' contributions
YCC, HCC and YLC conceptualised and planned the study. YCC writing of the manuscript, collection and analysis of data and writing of the manuscript drafts. HCC, PYL and YLC advised on study design and manuscript drafts. All authors read and approved the final manuscript.

Funding
None declared.

Author details
[1]Division of urology, Department of Surgery, Changhua Christian Hospital, No.135, Nansiao St. Changhua city, Changhua county 50006, Taiwan. [2]Transplant Medicine & Surgery Research Centre, Changhua Christian Hospital, Changhua, Taiwan. [3]School of Medicine, Kaohsiung Medical University, Kaohsiung, Taiwan. [4]Department of General Surgery, Changhua Christian Hospital, No.135 Nan-Hsiao Street, Changhua county 50006, Taiwan.

References
1. Bravata DM, Olkin I, Barnato AE, Keeffe EB, Owens DK. Health-related quality of life after liver transplantation: a meta-analysis. Liver transplantation and surgery : official publication of the American Association for the Study of Liver Diseases and the International Liver Transplantation Society. 1999;5:318–31.
2. Durazzo M, Premoli A, Di Bisceglie C, Bo S, Ghigo E, Manieri C. Male sexual disturbances in liver diseases: what do we know? J Endocrinol Invest. 2010;33:501–5.
3. Burra P, Germani G, Masier A, De Martin E, Gambato M, Salonia A, et al. Sexual dysfunction in chronic liver disease: is liver transplantation an effective cure? Transplantation. 2010;89:1425–9.
4. Foresta C, Schipilliti M, Ciarleglio FA, Lenzi A, D'Amico D. Male hypogonadism in cirrhosis and after liver transplantation. J Endocrinol Invest. 2008;31:470–8.
5. Madersbacher S, Ludvik G, Stulnig T, Grunberger T, Maier U. The impact of liver transplantation on endocrine status in men. Clin Endocrinol (Oxf). 1996;44:461–6.
6. Chen CL, Kabiling CS, Concejero AM. Why does living donor liver transplantation flourish in Asia? Nat Rev Gastroenterol Hepatol. 2013;10:746–51.
7. Akamatsu N, Sugawara Y, Kokudo N. Living-donor vs deceased-donor liver transplantation for patients with hepatocellular carcinoma. World j hepatol. 2014;6:626–31.
8. Huyghe E, Kamar N, Wagner F, Yeung SJ, Capietto AH, El-Kahwaji L, et al. Erectile dysfunction in liver transplant patients. Am j transplant : official journal of the American Society of Transplantation and the American Society of Transplant Surgeons. 2008;8:2580–9.
9. Tancredi A, Reginster JY, Schleich F, Pire G, Maassen P, Luyckx F, et al. Interest of the androgen deficiency in aging males (ADAM) questionnaire for the identification of hypogonadism in elderly community-dwelling male volunteers. Eur j endocrinol / European Federation of Endocrine Societies. 2004;151:355–60.
10. Morley JE, Charlton E, Patrick P, Kaiser FE, Cadeau P, McCready D, et al. Validation of a screening questionnaire for androgen deficiency in aging males. Metab: clin exp. 2000;49:1239–42.
11. Wu CJ, Hsieh JT, Lin JS, Hwang TI, Jiann BP, Huang ST, et al. Comparison of prevalence between self-reported erectile dysfunction and erectile dysfunction as defined by five-item International Index of Erectile Function in Taiwanese men older than 40 years. Urology. 2007;69:743–7.
12. Rosen RC, Cappelleri JC, Gendrano 3rd N. The International Index of Erectile Function (IIEF): a state-of-the-science review. Int J Impot Res. 2002;14:226–44.
13. Rosen RC, Cappelleri JC, Smith MD, Lipsky J, Pena BM. Development and evaluation of an abridged, 5-item version of the International Index of Erectile Function (IIEF-5) as a diagnostic tool for erectile dysfunction. Int J Impot Res. 1999;11:319–26.
14. Heidelbaugh JJ. Management of erectile dysfunction. Am Fam Physician. 2010;81:305–12.
15. Morley JE, Perry 3rd HM, Kevorkian RT, Patrick P. Comparison of screening questionnaires for the diagnosis of hypogonadism. Maturitas. 2006;53:424–9.
16. Sorrell JH, Brown JR. Sexual functioning in patients with end-stage liver disease before and after transplantation. Liver transpl : official publication of the American Association for the Study of Liver Diseases and the International Liver Transplantation Society. 2006;12:1473–7.
17. Rovira J, Diekmann F, Ramirez-Bajo MJ, Banon-Maneus E, Moya-Rull D, Campistol JM. Sirolimus-associated testicular toxicity: detrimental but reversible. Transplantation. 2012;93:874–9.
18. Gavaler JS, Van Thiel DH. Gonadal dysfunction and inadequate sexual performance in alcoholic cirrhotic men. Gastroenterology. 1988;95:1680–3.
19. Wang G, Yang J, Li M, Liu B, Jiang N, Fu B, et al. Liver transplant may improve erectile function in patients with benign end-stage liver disease: single-center Chinese experience. Exp clin transplant : official journal of the Middle East Society for Organ Transplantation. 2013;11:332–8.
20. Karagiannis A, Harsoulis F. Gonadal dysfunction in systemic diseases. Eur j endocrinol / European Federation of Endocrine Societies. 2005;152:501–13.
21. Klein J, Tran SN, Mentha-Dugerdil A, Giostra E, Majno P, Morard I, et al. Assessment of sexual function and conjugal satisfaction prior to and after liver transplantation. Ann transplant : quarterly of the Polish Transplantation Society. 2013;18:136–45.
22. McMahon CG, Jannini E, Waldinger M, Rowland D. Standard operating procedures in the disorders of orgasm and ejaculation. J Sex Med. 2013;10:204–29.
23. Burra P. Liver abnormalities and endocrine diseases. Best Pract Res Clin Gastroenterol. 2013;27:553–63.
24. Ho JK, Ko HH, Schaeffer DF, Erb SR, Wong C, Buczkowski AK, et al. Sexual health after orthotopic liver transplantation. Liver transpl: official publication of the American Association for the Study of Liver Diseases and the International Liver Transplantation Society. 2006;12:1478–84.

7

Active surveillance of prostate cancer: a questionnaire survey of urologists, clinical oncologists and urology nurse specialists across three cancer networks in the United Kingdom

Yiannis Philippou[1], Hary Raja[2] and Vincent J. Gnanapragasam[2]*

Abstract

Background: Active surveillance is considered a mainstream strategy in the management of patients with low-risk prostate cancer. A mission-critical step in implementing a robust active surveillance program and plan its resource and service requirements, is to gauge its current practice across the United Kingdom. Furthermore it is imperative to determine the existing practices in the context of the recommendations suggested by the recent National Institute for Health and Clinical Excellence guidance on active surveillance of prostate cancer.

Methods: An internet questionnaire was circulated to urologists, clinical oncologists and urology nurse specialists across three geographically distinct cancer networks. Twenty five questions across four domains were assessed. (i) hospital resources (staff and clinical areas) utilised for active surveillance (ii) enrolment criteria (iii) follow up (iv) criteria that trigger conversion to active treatment.

Results: We received 35 responses, 20 of which were from urologists. The survey data suggests that there is marked heterogeneity in enrolment criteria with patients having features of intermediate-risk prostate cancer often recruited into Active Surveillance programs. Only 60 % of our respondents use multiparametric MRI routinely to assess patient suitability for active surveillance. In addition, marked variation exists in how patients are followed up with regard to PSA testing intervals and timing of repeat biopsies. Only 40 % undertake a repeat biopsy at 12 months. Tumour upgrading on repeat biopsy, an increase in tumour volume or percentage of core biopsies involved would prompt a recommendation for treatment amongst most survey respondents. In addition allocation of resources and services for active surveillance is poor. Currently there are no dedicated active surveillance clinics, which are well-structured, -resourced and -supported for regular patient counselling and follow up.

Conclusion: This variability in enrolment criteria and follow up is also demonstrated in international and national series of active surveillance. Resources are not currently in place across the UK to support an active surveillance program and a national discussion and debate to plan resources is much required so that it can become a mainstream therapeutic strategy.

Keywords: Prostate cancer, Active surveillance, Questionnaire survey

* Correspondence: vjg29@cam.ac.uk
[2]Academic Urology Group, Department of Surgery & Oncology, University of Cambridge, Cambridge Biomedical Campus, Cambridge CB2 0QQ, UK
Full list of author information is available at the end of the article

Background

There is a clear trend, both in the UK and worldwide, towards managing patients diagnosed as having low-risk prostate cancer (LRPC) with active surveillance (AS) [1, 2]. The recent publication of the Prostate Cancer Intervention Versus Observation Trial (PIVOT) has further added to the growing evidence which supports that LRPC can be safely managed by AS and without the treatment-related side effects [3]. There are however major caveats in considering widespread adoption of AS for LRPC in the UK and indeed in other health-care systems. Firstly, there is an increasing concern that the current diagnostic method of an elevated prostate specific antigen (PSA), digital rectal examination (DRE) and a single 10–12 core trans-rectal biopsy, carries a significant potential of missing higher risk disease. Secondly there remain no universally accepted inclusion criteria for AS and there is a lack of consensus on what an AS regime should consist of. Whereas there are national and international guidelines on standards of surgery and radiotherapy for prostate cancer these are lacking for AS [4]. Thirdly, the timing of PSA checks, repeat examination, place and role of imaging, repeat biopsies and triggers for intervention vary considerably from centre to centre and even from clinician to clinician. Finally, AS requires structured, well-resourced and supported clinics for regular patient reviews, and these will be needed for many years. It is therefore clear that an expansion of AS will be a significant resource implication for any health service let alone an already overstretched National Health Service (NHS).

A move to a wider implementation of AS will require in addition to a uniform protocol, a national consensus on the resource and service requirements in setting this up and on the likely cost-implications of a long-term AS programme. As an initial step in this process the recent publication of the updated National Institute for Health and Clinical Excellence (NICE) guidance (CG175) has proposed a guideline for how men on AS may be managed (Table 1) [5]. A mission-critical step however in any attempt to adopt this guideline, is to gauge how AS is currently practiced in the UK.

Methods

We conducted an online survey of urologists, clinical oncologists (these were both medical and radiation oncologists with a special interest in uro-oncology) and urology nurse specialists with regard to the practice of AS within the East of England (EoE) cancer network. Data was collected during the year 2012–2013. The EoE cancer network delivers cancer care to 2.63 million people and is comprised mainly of two university hospitals and six district general hospitals. It employs approximately 50 consultant urologists. An internet questionnaire was circulated by email to urological departments of the

Table 1 Protocol for Active Surveillance as outlined by NICE: prostate cancer: diagnosis and treatment (CG175)

Timing	Tests
At enrolment in active surveillance	Multiparametric MRI if not previously performed
Year 1 of active surveillance	Every 3–4 months: measure PSA
	Throughout active surveillance: monitor PSA kinetics
	Every 6–12 months: DRE
	At 12 months prostate rebiopsy
Years 2–4 of active surveillance	Every 3–6 months: measure PSA
	Throughout active surveillance: monitor PSA kinetics
	Every 6–12 months: DRE
Year 5 and every year thereafter until active surveillance ends	Every 6 months: measure PSA
	Throughout active surveillance: monitor PSA kinetics
	Every 12 months: DRE

eight hospitals within the network. The email address of each urological department within each hospital was available on the hospital website. After receiving the email secretarial staff within each hospital were able to forward the questionnaire to all urological consultants, oncologists and urology nurse specialists working within each hospital. A further email was sent 1 month after in order to remind non-responders to complete the questionnaire. We also distributed the survey to two other cancer networks in geographically distinct areas of the UK. These were the North of England Cancer network and the Avon Somerset and Wiltshire cancer network. The reason behind the inclusion of a further two geographically distinct cancer networks was that we felt that this would allow us to form a more comprehensive opinion on the practice of AS across the UK and also allow comparison of our practice with other networks. Twenty five questions across four domains were assessed with associated multiple-choice answers (Additional file 1). Where more than one answer was possible respondents were able to select more options. The four domains were: (i) what hospital resources are currently utilised (staff and clinical areas) to counsel and follow up patients on AS (ii) enrolment criteria for AS (iii) how patients on AS are followed up (iv) respondents opinions on criteria that would trigger conversion to active treatment. Results were collated and rounded up to the closest percentage and represent the frequency of the answer selected for a particular question against the number of respondents answering the question.

Ethics approval

The above study is registered as an audit at Addenbrooke's hospital NHS trust. Ref: 3631.

Table 2 Distribution of responses according to specialty

Specialty	Response percent (%)	Response count
Urology	57	20
Medical oncology	0	0
Clinical oncology	20	7
Urology specialist nurse	20	7
Oncology specialist nurse	3	1
Total		35
Skipped question		0

Results

Completed questionnaires were received from 15 urologists, six clinical oncologists and four specialist nurses within our cancer network with all invited trusts taking part. We received a further 10 responses from the other two cancer networks we surveyed (Table 2). From the 35 respondents, 31 were directly involved in managing patients on AS with most centres reported managing more than 30 men a year by AS.

Current setting of AS

Resources allocated to AS counselling were first assessed (Fig. 1). Dedicated urology prostate cancer clinics were used in 74 % of cases but counselling and reviews also occurred in general urology clinics, oncology clinics, joint oncology and urology clinics as well as nurse led

clinics. AS counselling was primarily done by urologists in 75 % of cases. However oncologists and nurse specialists were also actively involved in this process. Respondents were then asked about the existence of an AS policy used in their unit. Of all respondents 68 % reported the use of a policy to guide selection of men suitable for AS. The rest however stated of not being aware of any agreed policy. These results suggest that currently there is little evidence of a dedicated service for men managed by AS within current NHS resource provisions.

Enrolment criteria for AS

Respondents were then asked about different enrolment criteria used in enlisting patients to their AS programme (Fig. 2a). With regards to age, there was a strong agreement that AS would not be considered in men of 55 years or younger. A sizeable proportion (46 %) would not consider it in men over 75 years either with the preference here being for watchful waiting. There was a strong agreement also that a classical definition of low risk (Gleason score of 6, a PSA level of ≤10 ng/ml and a TNM stage of ≤ T2) were necessary for enrolment into an AS programme. Some would also consider a PSA level between 10 and 20 ng/ml as long as other characteristics such as Gleason score and TNM stage were favourable. 64.5 % and 29 % of respondents would consider patients for AS if the TNM stage was T2b or T2c respectively. A significant majority considered the number of cores involved as well as the

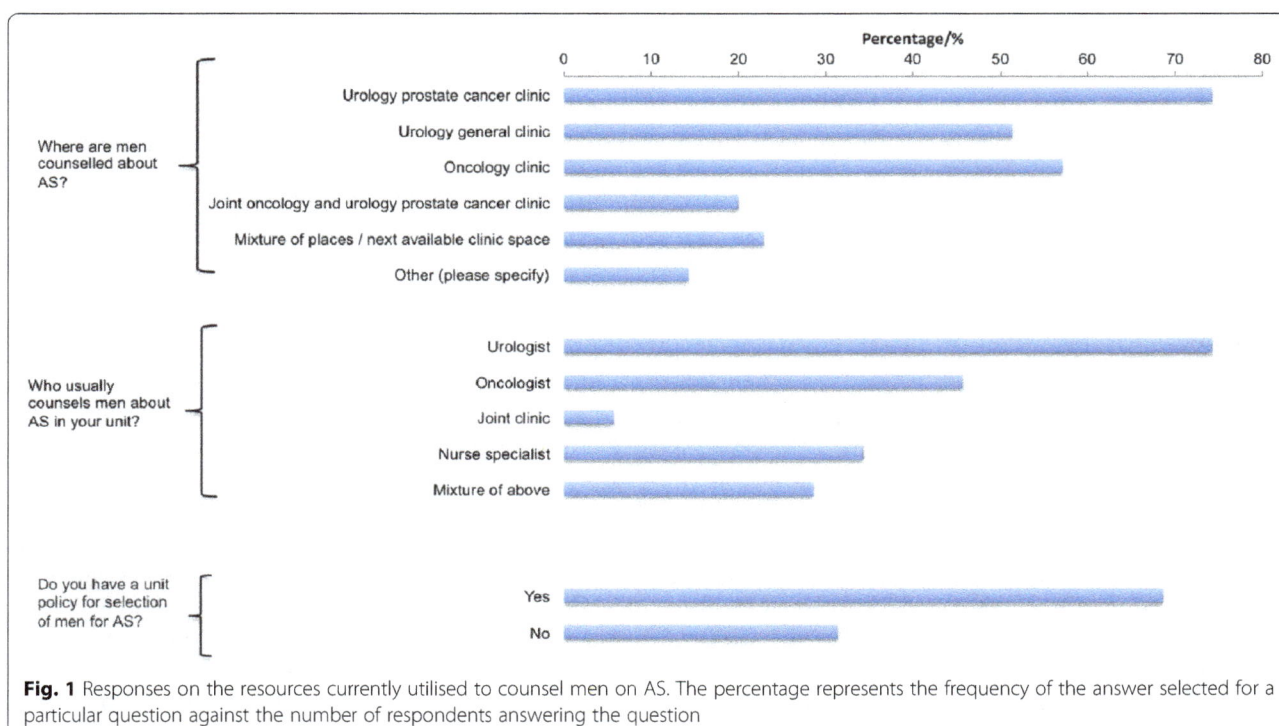

Fig. 1 Responses on the resources currently utilised to counsel men on AS. The percentage represents the frequency of the answer selected for a particular question against the number of respondents answering the question

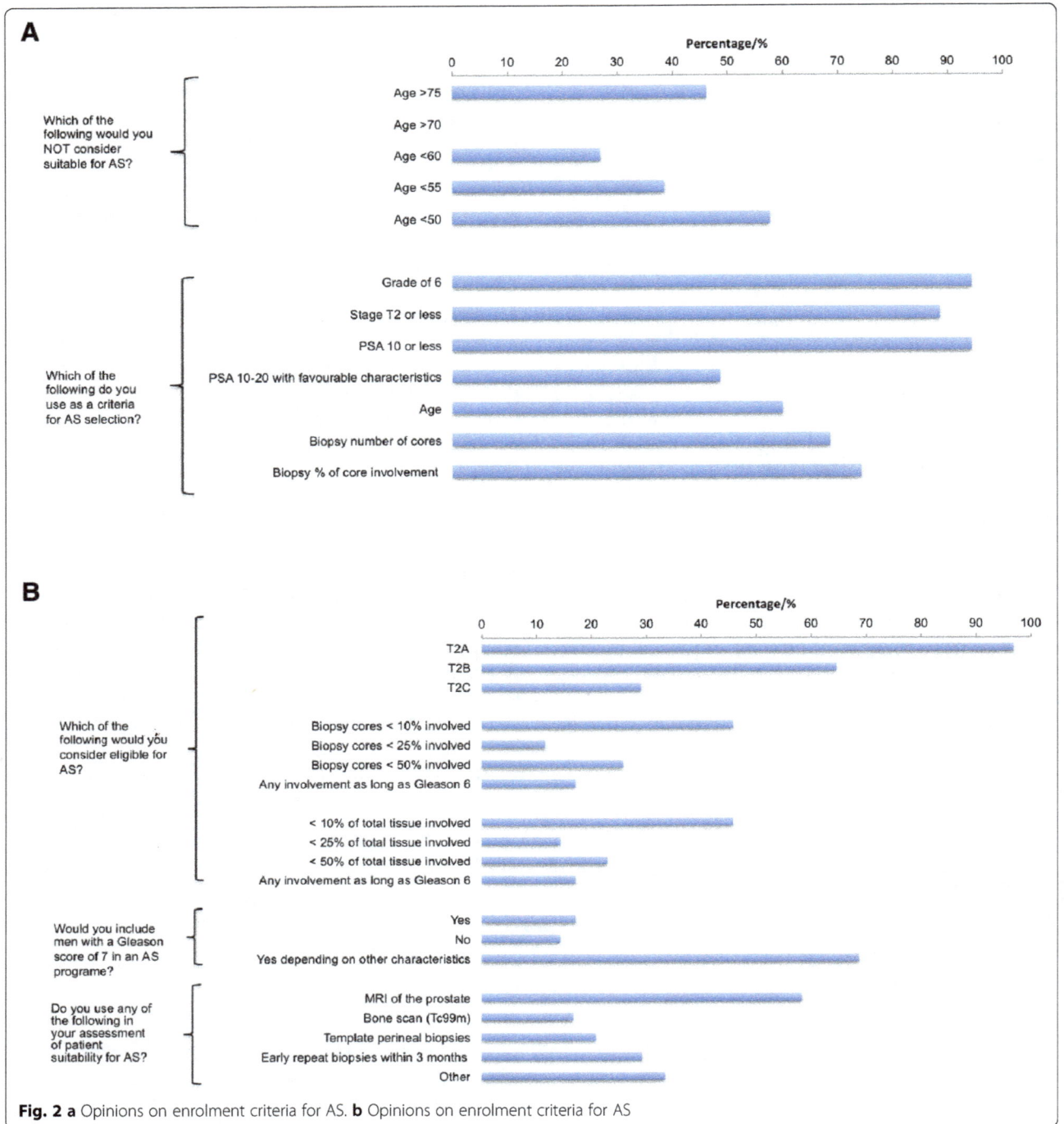

Fig. 2 a Opinions on enrolment criteria for AS. **b** Opinions on enrolment criteria for AS

percentage of the core involved as important points in decision making for AS enrolment. Specifically, 17 % would not be deterred from AS if more than 50 % of total number of cores biopsied were involved as long as the Gleason score is 6. We also observed that patients were being enrolled in programs with characteristics of intermediate risk prostate cancer (Fig. 2b). Interestingly, nearly 70 % would

consider AS in patients with a Gleason score of 7 if other tumour characteristics such as TNM stage, age, PSA level and information on biopsy core involvement were favourable. 58.3 % routinely use multiparametric MRI (mp MRI) and 29.2 % perform an early repeat biopsy (TRUS or template) within 3 months to aid in the selection of patients suitable for AS. These findings highlight the current significant variability and lack of standardisation in the inclusion criteria for men on AS across hospitals even within a single network.

Follow up of patients on AS

Respondents were asked about how they followed up patients on AS (Fig. 3a). The majority of respondents (62 %) indicated that they followed patients up with 3 monthly PSA at least in the first 2 years on AS and nearly 40 % would carry out the first repeat biopsy within 12 months. A significant minority however would only re-biopsy if there was evidence of change in the serum PSA or other clinical changes. Most respondents (60 %) used DRE as an integral part of AS monitoring. The vast majority did not use MRI as a tool to monitor men on AS. Follow up was undertaken in a multidisciplinary setting with

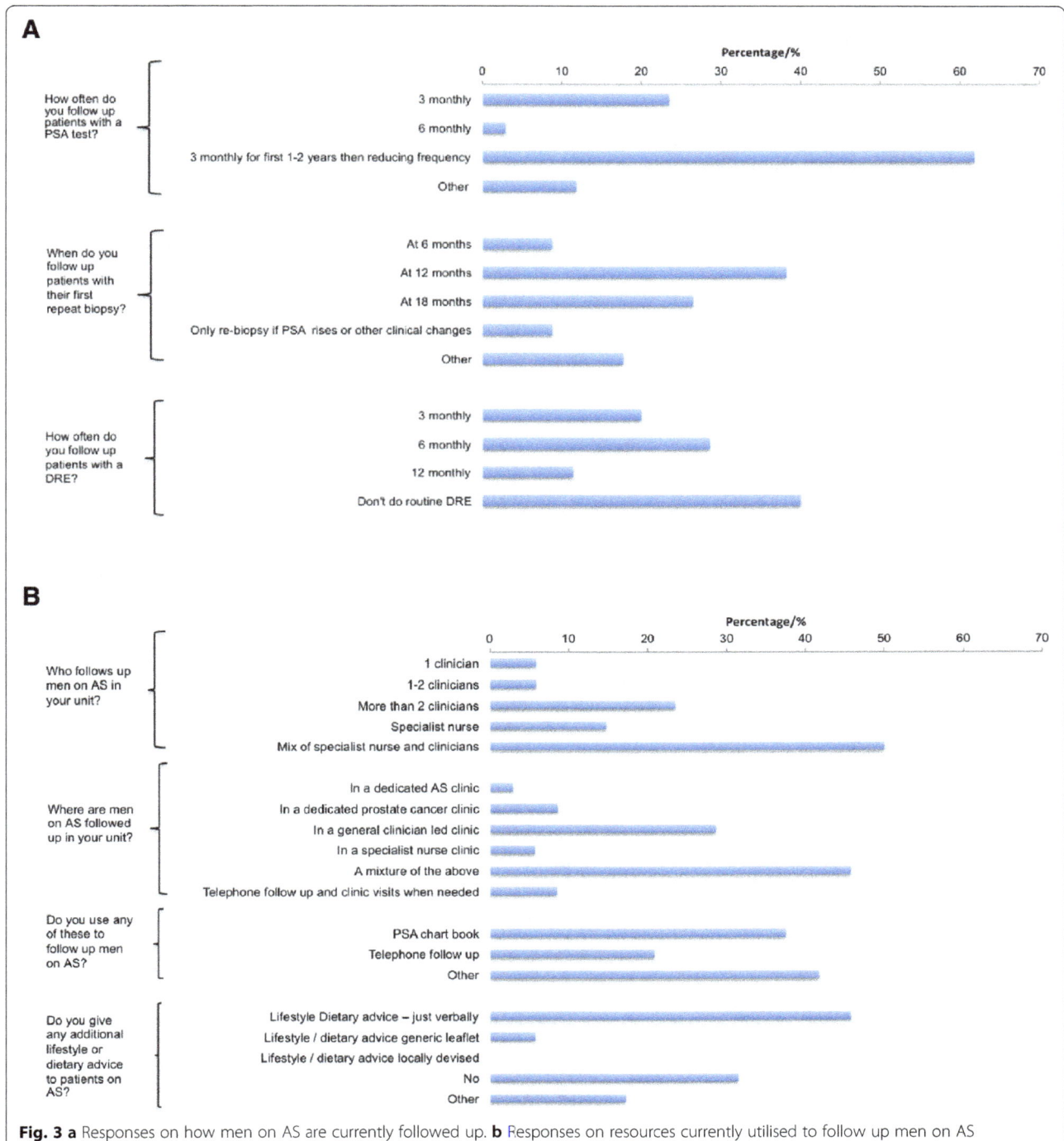

Fig. 3 a Responses on how men on AS are currently followed up. **b** Responses on resources currently utilised to follow up men on AS

at least two clinicians or a mixture of clinicians and nurse specialists involved in patient care (Fig. 3b). This however did not often occur in dedicated AS prostate cancer clinics but mainly in clinician led general urology clinics. There was also a mixture of follow up methods including PSA chart books and telephone checks. A majority of respondents also stated that they felt it was important to give patients on AS certain life-style and dietary advice either verbally or in the form of a patient information leaflet. Finally, we asked what would trigger a recommendation for active treatment. Here there was broad agreement that tumour upgrading on repeat biopsy or an increase in tumour volume or percentage of core biopsies involved would prompt a recommendation for treatment. Half of our respondents however would recommend active treatment based on evidence of a rising PSA alone or an increase in PSA velocity. Finally changes in DRE findings as well as evidence of radiological progression of the tumour would prompt radical treatment in more than 50 % of cases (Fig. 4).

Comparison with other network trusts

The same questionnaire was sent out to members of trusts part of two other UK cancer networks. We received a total of 10 responses, five from each cancer network. The findings were very comparable to our own network. There was broad agreement that men under 50 years would not be suitable for AS. In both networks surveyed, there was significant variation in respondent's views on inclusion criteria for AS (Fig. 5a). Similar to our data, most respondents would include Gleason grade 7 patients in an active surveillance programme but dependent on other clinical characteristics. In one of the two networks studied, a significant number of respondents advocated MRI and transperineal repeat biopsies as part of their assessment of patients suitability for AS. However only a minority

of respondents in the other network used any additional biopsy or imaging in evaluating patients suitability. On the question of timing of repeat biopsies there was again variability in the responses (Fig. 5b). The majority advocated re-biopsy at 12 or 18 months after entry onto an AS programme. Finally, we compared triggers to initiate a change in management. Here there was broad consistency in terms of what would initiate a change and included an increase in grade and/or tumour volume. This comparison demonstrated that the lack of dedicated resources and variability in inclusion and follow up in AS is likely to be a universal issue across the NHS.

Discussion

In contemporary UK practice LRPC accounts for 20 % of all new prostate cancer diagnoses [6]. The perception that LRPC is over-treated has gained the ascendancy among the urological community following results from randomised studies such as the European Randomised Study of Screening for Prostate Cancer (ERSPC) trial [7] and Prostate Cancer Intervention vs Observation Trial (PIVOT) [8]. It is therefore easy to foresee that AS will most likely become the preferred option of managing patients with LRPC. The UK NICE guidelines define men suitable for AS as having the following characteristics: clinical stage T1c; a Gleason score of 3 + 3; a PSA density of < 0.15 ng/mL/mL; and cancer in < 50 % of their total number of biopsy cores with < 10 mm of any core involved (http://guidance.nice.org.uk/CG175) [5]. These recommendations are very similar to the European, American and Canadian urological guidelines which universally recommend that AS is suitable for patients with Gleason score of 6 or less [1, 2, 9]. Our survey demonstrated that the NICE guidelines regarding AS enrolment are generally followed. However, in certain cases patients are being recruited into AS programmes with characteristics of intermediate-risk

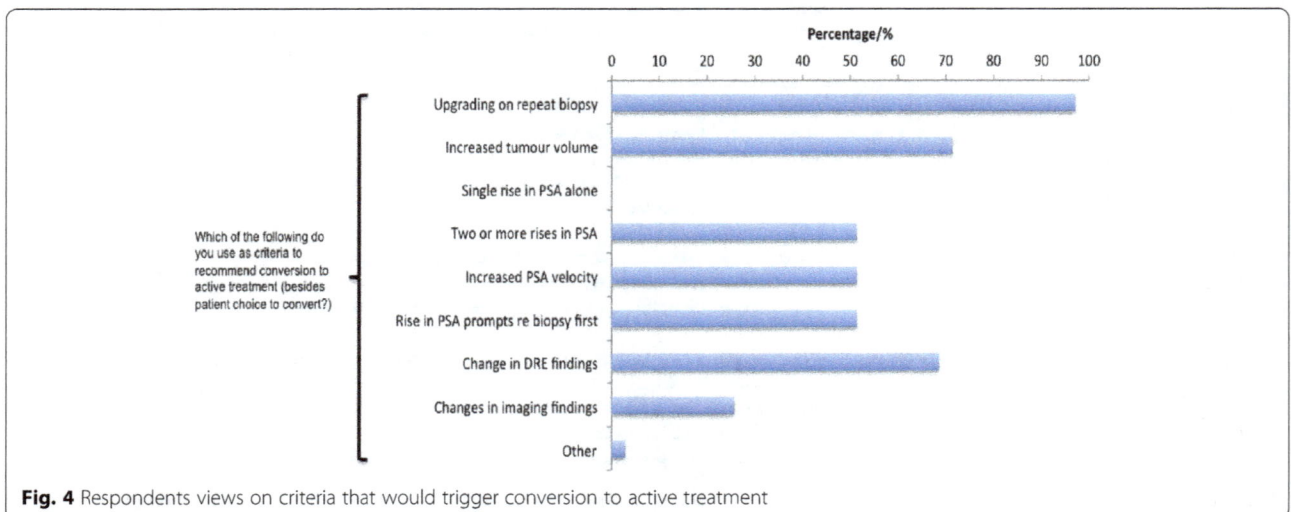

Fig. 4 Respondents views on criteria that would trigger conversion to active treatment

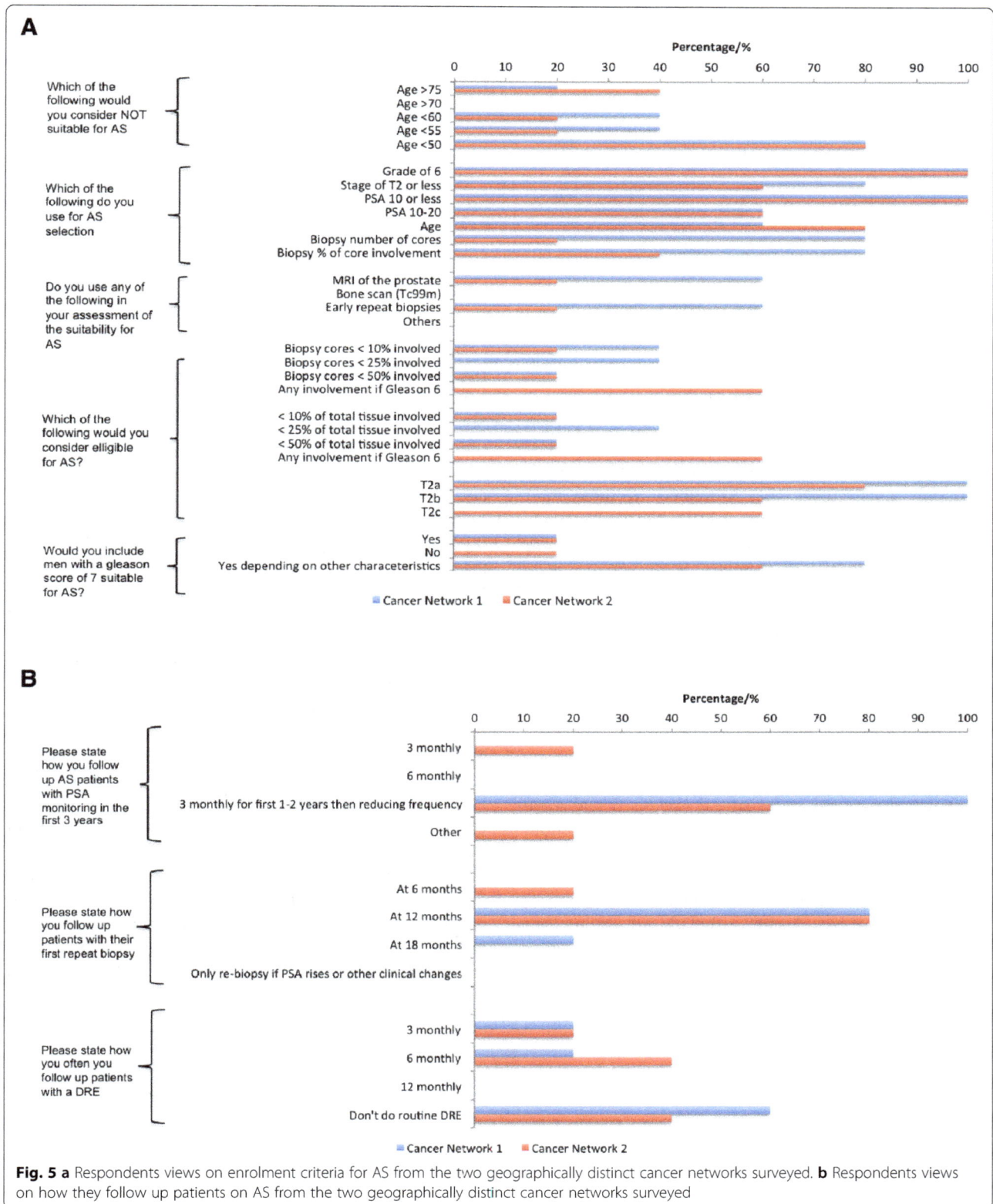

Fig. 5 a Respondents views on enrolment criteria for AS from the two geographically distinct cancer networks surveyed. **b** Respondents views on how they follow up patients on AS from the two geographically distinct cancer networks surveyed

Table 3 Selection criteria for Active Surveillance in international published series

Publication	Gleason Score	PSA (ng/ml)	Positive cores	% positive biopsy cores	% cancer involvement per core	cT
Dall' Era [11]	≤6	<10	-	<33	-	≤2a
Bul [10]	≤7	<20	≤3	-	-	-
Soloway [12]	≤6	≤10	≤2	-	<20	≤2
Tosoian [18]	≤6	≤10	≤2	-	<50	1c
Ercole [13]	≤6	<10	≤2	-	<50	≤2a
Klotz [14]	≤6	≤10	-	-	-	≤2b
Ischia [15]	≤6	<10	-	-	-	≤2a
Thomsen [16]	≤6	≤10	≤3	-	<50	≤2a
Selvadurai [17]	≤6	<15	-	≤50	-	≤2

cT clinical tumour category, *PSA* prostate specific antigen

prostate cancer. A significant proportion of our respondents considered men for AS who had T2b or T2c disease, a PSA of 10–20 ng/ml, a Gleason score of 7 and patients with tumour involvement of more than 50 % of their total biopsy cores. This reflects that routine UK practice of AS commonly outstretches that described in most international published series of AS and also the recommendations of European, American and Canadian urological guidelines. Encouragingly however, there was a general agreement between our respondents as to the criteria that would trigger conversion to radical treatment.

Our survey demonstrated the marked heterogeneity which exists in the practice of AS across our cancer network. This variability is not unique to our cancer network alone but also evident in other cancer networks too in geographically distinct areas of the UK. This striking variability in AS enrolment criteria, follow up and triggers for intervention is also demonstrated in international and national series of AS (Tables 3 and 4). In these studies, patients were followed up with a combination of repeat biopsies, serial PSA measurements and clinical examination. The frequency of repeat biopsies varied widely analogous to our own cancer network. Some carried out biopsies annually [10–12], while others every 2 or 3 years [13–16], and in some depending on clinical characteristics [17, 18]. Almost unanimously in

the studies we reviewed tumour upgrading on repeat biopsy would prompt a recommendation for treatment. Some studies also considered an increase in tumour volume or percentage of core biopsies involved as a trigger to radical treatment. PSA doubling time or velocity was also sometimes a trigger to proceed to radical treatment.

The updated NICE guidance has advocated the use of mpMRI at the time of AS enrolment followed by a repeat biopsy at year one and has put in place a follow up regime as its key suggestions. To understand what the impact of these recommendations would be on routine clinical practice, our survey assessed the current reported patterns of practice. Amongst our respondents only 40 % of respondents performed a repeat biopsy at 12 months and only 60 % use mpMRI routinely as a tool for selecting patients suitable for AS. It should be noted however that although the NICE guidelines have clearly stated that mpMRI should occur at the time of AS enrolment, the EUA and AUA guidelines are not so prescriptive. Similarly Canadian urological guidelines from Ontario recommend that mpMRI may be included in AS protocols but is not currently a necessity [1, 2, 9]. In contrast, the recommendation on 3–4 monthly PSA checks is consistent with current routine practice in our survey. Even so there will need to be a method to monitor and track the PSA. Similarly recommendations for DRE every 6–12 months is

Table 4 Triggers to treatment used in patients under Active Surveillance

Publication	Gleason Score on repeat biopsy	Positive cores	% cancer involvement per single core	% positive biopsy cores	PSAdt cT (years)	PSAv (ng/ml/year)	cT
Dall'Era [11]	Progression	-	-	-	-	>0.75	-
Tosoian [18]	>6	>2	>50	-	-	-	-
Ercole [13]	Progression	Increase	Increase	-	-	-	Upstage
Klotz [14]	≥4	-	-	-	3	-	-
Ischia [15]	Progression	-	-	-	-	-	Upstage
Thomsen [16]	≥3 + 4	>3	-	-	3	-	Upstage
Selvadurai [17]	≥4 + 3	-	-	>50	-	>1	-

cT clinical tumour category, *PSAdt* prostate-specific antigen doubling time, *PSAv* PSA velocity

Active surveillance of prostate cancer: a questionnaire survey of urologists, clinical oncologists...

49

probably best combined with clinic reviews. Of note, in our survey there was great variability in who did the AS follow up including DRE. Moreover 40 % of respondents did not routinely perform a DRE during the follow up appointment. Again adherence to the NICE guidelines will require a significant change in practice and ideally necessitate consistency in AS follow up providers.

From the results of this survey it is quite clear that the implementation of a robust and consistent AS program according to the recommendations of the NICE guidelines will prove challenging due to the current variation in its practice. In addition the burden of follow-up with clinical examinations and serum PSA testing on both men and healthcare systems is far from cost-neutral. Even more so the use of novel strategies such as mpMRI at the time of AS enrollment will further put a strain on radiology providers. It is clear that in addition to reducing the variability in the practice of AS there is also the need for robust cost-effectiveness studies to ensure that such novel strategies are both clinically and cost-effective.

This study however does not come without its limitations. Firstly the methodology of this study is a questionnaire survey study with a total of 35 respondents which is a low number of participants and may not accurately depict the practice of AS within the EoE cancer network. Also this study was UK specific and may not mirror the trends in the world-wide practice of AS though our review of other international published series of AS did demonstrate variability in its practice. Furthermore the majority of our respondents were from primarily academic institutions therefore it is likely that the practice of AS is even more heterogeneous outside the academic setting.

Conclusions

Despite its limitations, the present survey has demonstrated the marked heterogeneity in which AS is practiced across a cancer network in the UK. This is also mirrored across other hospitals in the UK. It is clear that if the NICE guidelines are adopted then the resource requirements are likely to be very significant and not currently in place across the UK. These issues need urgent resolution and now is the time for a national discussion and planning. This would provide the much needed reassurance to clinicians and patients of the robustness of an AS programme on a par with current standard therapeutic options.

Abbreviations
LRPC: Low-risk prostate cancer; AS: Active Surveillance; EoE: East of England; PIVOT: Prostate Cancer Intervention Versus Observation Trial; PSA: Prostate specific antigen; DRE: Digital Rectal Examination; NICE: National Institute for Health and Clinical Excellence; NHS: National Health Service; mp MRI: Multiparametric MRI.

Competing interest
The authors declare that they have no competing interests.

Authors' contributions
YP contributed to the data analysis and manuscript writing. HR contributed to data collection and analysis. VJG conceived the project and contributed to data collection, data analysis and final manuscript approval. All authors read and approved the final manuscript.

Author details
[1]Department of Surgery, Basildon & Thurrock University Hospital, Essex SS16 5NL, UK. [2]Academic Urology Group, Department of Surgery & Oncology, University of Cambridge, Cambridge Biomedical Campus, Cambridge CB2 0QQ, UK.

References
1. Thompson I, Trasher JB, Aus G, Burnett AL, Canby-Hagino ED, Cookson MS, et al. AUA Prostate Cancer Clinical Guideline Update Panel. Guideline for the management of clinically localised prostate cancer: 2007 update. J Urol. 2007;177:2106–31.
2. Heidenreich A, Bellmunt J, Bolla M, Joniau S, Mason M, Matveev V, et al. EUA guidelines on prostate cancer. Part 1: screening, diagnosis and treatment of clinically localised disease. Eur Urol. 2011;59:61–71.
3. Wilt TJ, Brawer MK, Jones KM, Barry MJ, Aronson WJ, Fox S, et al. Radical prostatectomy versus observation for localized prostate cancer. N Engl J Med. 2012;367:203–13.
4. Dall'Era MA, Albertsen PC, Bangma C, Caroll PR, Carter HB, Cooperberg MR, et al. Active surveillance for prostate cancer: a systematic review of the literature. Eur Urol. 2012;62:976–83.
5. NICE guideline on prostate cancer: diagnosis and treatment. February 2014 (CG175). Available at http://www.nice.org.uk/guidance/cg175. Accessed October 2014
6. National Institute for Health and Clinical Excellence. Costing statement: prostate cancer: diagnosis and treatment. Implementing the NICE guidance on prostate treatment(CG175). Available at: https://www.nice.org.uk/guidance/cg175/resources/cg175-prostate-cancer-costing-statement2. Accessed August 2014
7. Schröder FH, Hugosson J, Roobol MJ, Tammela TL, Ciatto S, Nelen V, et al. Screening and prostate-cancer mortality in a randomized European study. N Engl J Med. 2009;360:1320–8.
8. Bill-Axelson A, Holmberg L, Ruutu M, Garmo H, Stark JR, Busch C, et al. Radical prostatectomy versus watchful waiting in early prostate cancer. N Engl J Med. 2011;364:1708–17.
9. Cancer Care Ontario. Active surveillance for the management of localized prostate cancer. Available at www.cancercare.on.ca. Accessed March 2015
10. Bul M, van den Bergh RC, Zhu X, Rannikko A, Vasarainen H, Bangma CH, et al. Outcomes of initially expectantly managed patients with low or intermediate risk screen-detected localized prostate cancer. BJU Int. 2012;110:1672–7.
11. Dall'Era MA, Konety BR, Cowan JE, Shinohara K, Stauf F, Cooperberg MR, et al. Active surveillance for the management of prostate cancer in a contemporary cohort. Cancer. 2008;112:2664–70.
12. Soloway MS, Soloway CT, Eldefrawy A, Soloway MS, Soloway CT, Eldefrawy A, et al. Careful selection and close monitoring of low-risk prostate cancer patients on active surveillance minimizes the need for treatment. Eur Urol. 2010;58:831–5.
13. Ercole B, Marietti SR, Fine J, Albertsen PC. Outcomes following active surveillance of men with localized prostate cancer diagnosed in the prostate specific antigen era. J Urol. 2008;180:1336–9.
14. Klotz L, Zhang L, Lam A, Nam R, Mamedov A, Loblaw A. Clinical results of long-term follow-up of a large, active surveillance cohort with localized prostate cancer. J Clin Oncol. 2010;28:126–31.

15. Ischia JJ, Pang CY, Tay YK, Suen CF, Aw HC, Frydenberg M. Active surveillance for prostate cancer: an Australian experience. BJU Int. 2012;109:40–3.

16. Thomsen FB, Roder MA, Hvarness H, Iversen P, Brasso K. Active surveillance can reduce overtreatment in patients with low-risk prostate cancer. Dan Med J. 2013;60:A4575.

17. Selvadurai ED, Singhera M, Thomas K, Mohammed K, Woode-Amissah R, Horwich A, et al. Medium-term outcomes of active surveillance for localised prostate cancer. Eur Urol. 2013;64:981–7.

18. Tosoian JJ, Trock BJ, Landis P, Feng Z, Epstein JI, Partin AW, et al. Active surveillance program for prostate cancer: an update of the Johns Hopkins experience. J Clin Oncol. 2011;29:2185–90.

8

Association between plasma fluorescent oxidation products and erectile dysfunction

Shuman Yang[1], Edward Giovannucci[5,6], Bruce Bracken[2], Shuk-Mei Ho[3,4] and Tianying Wu[1*]

Abstract

Background: Existing epidemiological studies of the association between oxidative stress and erectile dysfunction (ED) are sparse and inconclusive, which is likely due to cross-sectional design and small sample size. Therefore, we investigated the association between biomarkers of oxidative stress and ED in prospective setting among a relatively large sample size of men.

Methods: We conducted the prospective study among 917 men ages between 47 and 80 years at the time of blood draw, which is a part of nested prospective case–control study of prostate cancer in the Health Professionals Follow-up Study. Plasma fluorescent oxidation products (FlOPs), a global biomarker for oxidative stress, were measured at three excitation/emission wavelengths (360/420 nm named as FlOP_360; 320/420 nm named as FlOP_320 and 400/475 nm named as FlOP_400).

Results: Approximately 35 % of men developed ED during follow-up. We did not find an independent association between FlOP_360, FlOP_320, FlOP_400 and risk of ED in the multivariable adjusted model (Tertile 3 vs. tertile 1: odds ratio [OR] = 0.90, 95 % confidence interval [CI] = 0.61-1.34, P_{trend} = 0.54 for FlOP_360; OR = 0.73, 95 % CI = 0.49-1.07, P_{trend} = 0.27 for FlOP_320; and OR = 0.98, 95 % CI = 0.66-1.45, P_{trend} = 0.72 for FlOP_400). Further analysis of the association between FlOPs and ED in the fasting samples or controls only (free of prostate cancer incidence) did not change the results appreciably.

Conclusions: Plasma FlOPs were not associated with the risk of ED, suggesting oxidative stress may not be an independent risk factor for ED.

Background

Oxidative stress reflects an imbalance between systemic levels of reactive oxygen species (ROSs) and host antioxidant defense systems that are able to counteract (detoxify) these ROSs. Insufficient antioxidant defense systems against ROSs can result in damage to proteins, lipids and DNA in cells and organs in humans. High level of oxidative stress is an important risk factor for many prevalent diseases including cardiovascular disease, breast cancer and reduced renal function [1–3].

The level of plasma fluorescent oxidation products (FlOPs) is a reliable and convenient approach to assess circulating oxidative stress in large epidemiological studies. One advantage of this marker as compared to other traditional specific oxidation markers (i.e., F2-isoprostanes and malondialdehyde) is that FLOP assay reflects oxidation pathways from multiple sources including lipid, protein and DNA [4, 5], whereas traditional specific oxidation markers reflect only a portion of oxidative stress. In large observational studies, we found that the level of plasma FlOPs is increased with hypertension, smoking and reduced renal function as defined by reduced levels of glomerular filtration rate [1, 3, 5, 6]. Furthermore, we have documented that the FlOP assay is robust in epidemiologic and clinical setting in which the collection and processing of blood samples cannot be well-controlled. We have found that FlOPs are stable in the blood samples with delayed processing up to 48 h at 4 °C, stable for more than 10 years in plasma samples in liquid-nitrogen freezers, and

* Correspondence: tianying.wu@uc.edu
[1]Division of Epidemiology and Biostatistics, Department of Environmental Health, University of Cincinnati Medical Center, Kettering Complex, 3223 Eden Ave, Cincinnati, OH, USA, 45267-0056
Full list of author information is available at the end of the article

highly reproducible over 1–2 year among the same individuals [5, 7].

The association between oxidative stress and erectile dysfunction (ED) is sparse and inconclusive, which is likely due to cross-sectional design and small sample size. It is well known that oxidative stress plays an important role in the development of atherosclerotic diseases [8, 9]. Atherosclerosis reduces cavernosal blood flow, leading to vasculogenic ED [10, 11]. However, existing epidemiological studies of the association between oxidative stress and ED either had small sample size (N ≤ 60) or were cross-sectional [12–14]. Further, none of above studies adjusted for important potential confounders such as diabetes, hypertension and cigarette smoking which are the risk factors for ED and are important determinants of oxidative stress [5, 15, 16]. Large and prospective studies are warranted to examine the independent relationship between oxidative stress and ED. Therefore, we investigated the association between plasma FlOPs and ED in prospective settings among a relatively large sample size of men.

Methods
Study participants and blood collection
The Health Professionals Follow-up Study (HPFS) initiated in 1986 is an ongoing prospective study of 51,529 men. Between 1993 and 1995, blood collection kits were sent to participants and 18,140 men returned specimens on ice by using an overnight courier. All returned blood samples were processed within 36 h after blood draw and stored in liquid nitrogen freezers. Based on the participants who donated blood samples, a 1:1 matched nested prospective case–control study of prostate cancer was performed from the time of blood draw [17]. All participants were free of diagnosed cardiovascular diseases and cancers at the time of blood draw. After excluding the ineligible participants (Fig. 1), we finally included 917 men ages between 47 and 80 years (median = 62 years) at the time of blood draw in the prospective study. Among 917 men, 457 and 460 men were subsequent incident prostate cancer cases and controls, respectively. Written informed consent was obtained from all participants. This investigation was approved by Institutional Review Board of the Brigham and Women's Hospital, the Harvard School of Public Health and the University of Cincinnati.

Measurement of FlOPs
Assay procedure
We measured plasma FlOPs using previously described procedures [5]. In brief, plasma was extracted with ethanol/ether (3:1, v/v) and centrifuged to obtain supernatant. We measured fluorescence of the supernatant at three wavelengths (360/420 nm [excitation/emission] named as FlOP_360, 320/420 nm named as FlOP_320 and 400/475 nm named as FlOP_400). FlOP_360 represents the interaction between lipid oxidation products and proteins, DNA and carbohydrates. FlOP_320 can be produced when oxidation products such as lipid hydroperoxides, aldehydes, and ketones react with DNA in the presence of metals, and FlOP_360 reflects the interaction between malondialdehyde, proteins and phospholipids [18]. The

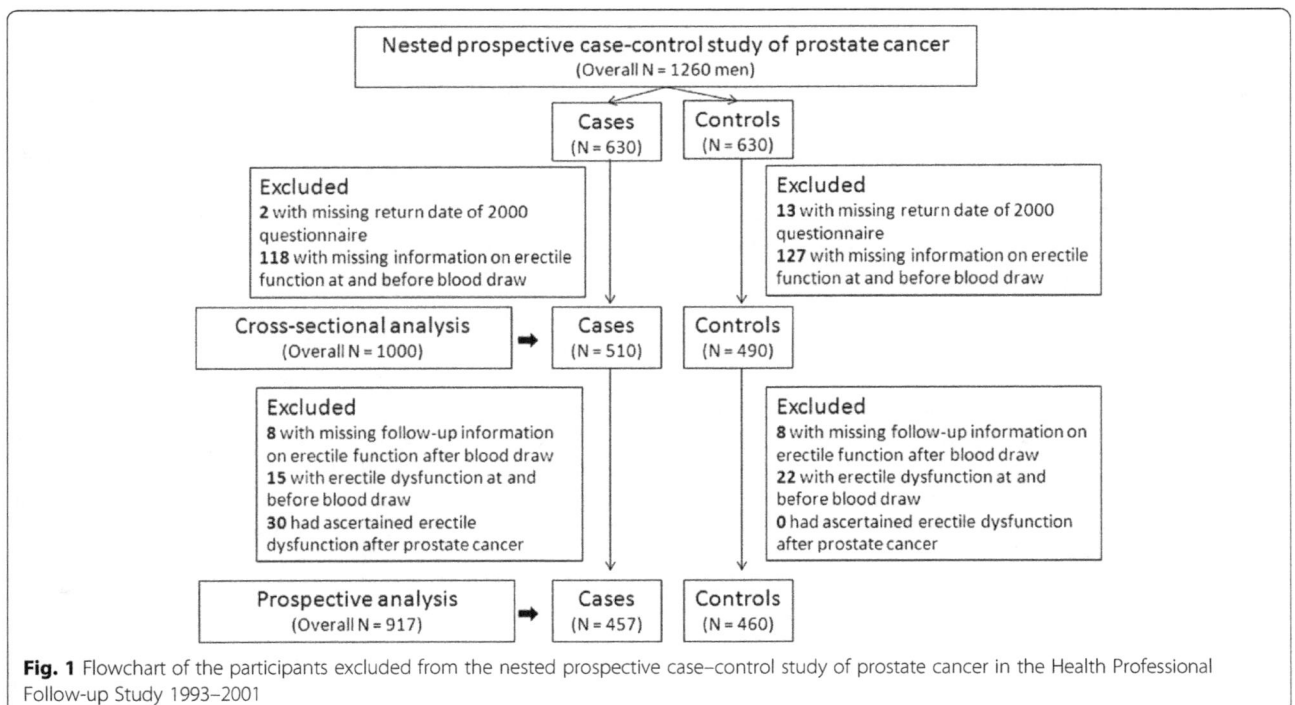

Fig. 1 Flowchart of the participants excluded from the nested prospective case–control study of prostate cancer in the Health Professional Follow-up Study 1993–2001

within-run average coefficient of variations for FlOP measurements were < 13 %.

Assay stability in blood samples with delayed processing

All blood samples were processed within 36 h after receiving the samples. The delay in processing blood samples up to 36 h appeared to have minimal influence on the measurement of FlOPs. The overall intraclass correlation coefficients (ICCs) of FlOPs were all greater than 0.95 in the shorter- (0 to 24 h) and longer-delayed processing (0 to 36 h) [7].

Assay between- and within- person reproducibility

We conducted a pilot study in 40 participants who donated two blood samples from the Nurse Health Study. After adjusting for fasting status, the ICC of the between- and within- person variations of the FlOPs for repeated measurements over 1.4 year apart (range: 0.8-2.2 years) was 0.44 for FlOP_360, 0.55 for FlOP_320, and 0.70 for FlOP_400 [3].

ED Ascertainment

Between 2000 and 2001, a recall questionnaire in HPFS participants was initiated to rate their ability to have and maintain an erection sufficient for sexual intercourse. The question was "Please rate your ability (without treatment) to have and maintain an erection good enough for intercourse for the following time periods:". Time periods included "before 1986", "1986-1989", "1990-1994", "1995 or later" and "in the last 3 months". Responses of the questionnaire included "very poor", "poor", "fair", "good" and "very good". ED was defined if participants answered "very poor" or "poor". Any ED cases ascertained clearly after blood draw (1993–1995) were considered incident ED. If year of blood draw and year of ED ascertainment may be overlapping (i.e., year of blood draw was 1995 and period of ED ascertainment was '1995 or later'), these ED cases were not defined as incident ED. If the ED cases were not defined as incidence above, these ED cases were used in the cross-sectional analysis only (Fig. 1). Regardless ED cases recovered at a later time or not, they were defined as ED cases in the current study. Whether these cases were included in the cross-sectional or prospective analysis was dependent on the time period of ED ascertainment.

Statistical analyses

To make a comprehensive understanding on relationship between plasma FlOPs and ED, we performed both prospective and cross-sectional analysis (Fig. 1). In the prospective analysis, we analyzed the association between plasma FlOPs and incidence of ED with logistic regression model, but not with Cox proportional hazard model as we were not exactly sure the year of incident EDThe risk of incident ED in lowest tertile of FlOPs was compared with

that in the second and third tertile of FlOPs. The covariates included in the prospective analysis were age (continuous), body mass index (BMI, continuous), alcohol intake (in quartiles: < 0.9, ≥ 0.9 and < 6.6, ≥ 6.6 and < 17.2, ≥ 17.2 g/day), physical activity (in quartiles: < 13.85, ≥ 13.85 and < 28.9, ≥ 28.9 and < 51.95, ≥ 51.95 MET-hours/ week), Caucasian (yes/no), fasting hours (continuous), benign prostatic hyperplasia with surgery (yes/no), history of hypertension (yes/no), history of diabetes (yes/no), smoking status (current smokers, past smokers and non-smokers), month of blood draw (in seasons: Spring [March, April and May], Summer [June, July and August], Fall [September, October and November], Winter [December, January and February]) and year of blood draw (1993, 1994 and 1995). To further rule out the potential confounding by fasting status and subclinical factors of prostate cancer incidence, we also examined the association between FlOPs and ED in fasting samples and controls only (free of prostate cancer incidence), respectively. In the cross-sectional analysis, we examined the association between plasma FlOPs and ED at baseline with logistic regression model. The covariates included in the cross-sectional analysis were same as the prospective analysis. All analyses were performed with Statistical Analysis System (Version 9, SAS Institute Inc., Cary, NC).

Results

Baseline characteristics according to plasma FlOP levels

In the prospective analysis, higher levels of plasma FlOP_360, FlOP_320 and FlOP_400 were associated with older age, greater alcohol intake, lower proportion of men who had fasted ≥ 8 h before blood draw and great proportion of current and past smokers (Table 1). Higher levels of FlOP_360 were correlated with greater proportion of history of hypertension. Higher levels of FlOP_400 were correlated with greater BMI. When similar analysis was performed in prostate cancer cases and controls separately, the relationship between baseline characteristics and FlOPs in either group was similar to that in the overall samples (Additional file 1: Table S1 and Additional file 2: Table S2). Moreover, the relationship between baseline characteristics in propective analysis (Table 1) was comparable to that in cross-sectional analysis (Additional file 3: Table S3).

Association between plasma FlOPs and ED

In the prospective analysis, 35 % (N = 323) of men were identified having incident ED after blood draw. Although the proportion of incident ED appeared to be higher among men with higher levels of FlOPs (Table 2), we did not find an independent association between FlOP_360, FlOP_320, FlOP_400 and risk of ED in the multivariable adjusted model (Tertile 3 vs. tertile 1: OR = 0.90, 95 % CI = 0.61-1.34, P_{trend} = 0.54 for FlOP_360; OR = 0.73,

Table 1 Baseline characteristics according to tertiles of plasma fluorescent oxidation products (FlOPs) (N = 917): prospective analysis in the Health Professional Follow-up Study, 1993-1995

Variables	FlOP_360			FlOP_320			FlOP_400		
Tertile	1	2	3	1	2	3	1	2	3
Range (Fl/ml)	< 184	≥ 184; < 233	≥ 233	< 356	≥ 356; < 524	≥ 524	< 49.1	≥ 49.1; < 62.6	≥ 62.6
N	305	306	306	305	306	306	305	306	306
Age (years)	**61.1**	**61.9**	**62.3**	**60.4**	**62.2**	**62.6**	**60.7**	**62.3**	**62.2**
Body mass index (kg/m²)	25.8	25.8	25.7	25.5	25.9	25.9	**25.4**	**25.9**	**26.0**
Alcohol intake (g/day)[a]	**2.9**	**8.2**	**10.0**	**3.5**	**8.8**	**8.6**	**2.4**	**8.2**	**10.4**
Physical activity (MET-hours/week)[a]	26.0	33.6	29.1	27.9	34.2	26.5	28.3	29.8	28.1
Caucasians (%)	92	92	95	91	95	93	93	91	95
Fasting status (≥ 8 h; %)	**76.4**	**56.2**	**50.3**	**75.7**	**56.5**	**50.7**	**71.2**	**59.5**	**52.3**
History of BPH with surgery (%)	1.6	3.6	3.3	1.3	3.3	3.9	2.0	3.6	2.9
History of hypertension (%)	**23.3**	**23.9**	**31.4**	20.3	30.4	27.8	21.3	31.1	26.1
History of diabetes (%)	3.6	2.6	2.9	2.6	3.3	3.3	2.3	3.9	2.9
Current smokers (%)	**1.1**	**6.7**	**13.0**	**1.1**	**9.6**	**9.4**	**1.1**	**4.2**	**16.5**
Past smokers (%)	**37.8**	**49.8**	**60.8**	**38.6**	**55.4**	**54.4**	**35.1**	**50.9**	**62.7**

Variables with normal distribution are shown in mean, unless otherwise specified
[a]Variables with skew distribution are shown in median
Abbreviations: FlOP = Fluorescent oxidation products, Fl = Fluorescent intensity unites, MET = Metabolic equivalent, BPH = Benign prostatic hyperplasia
Bold-faced values indicate statistically significance at P < 0.05 across tertiles of FlOPs

95 % CI = 0.49-1.07, P_{trend} = 0.27 for FlOP_320; and OR = 0.98, 95 % CI = 0.66-1.45, P_{trend} = 0.72 for FlOP_400).

Further analysis of the association between FlOPs and ED in the fasting samples (≥ 8 h) did not change the results appreciably (Tertile 3 vs. tertile 1: OR = 0.91, 95 % CI = 0.56-1.47, P_{trend} = 0.69 for FlOP_360; OR = 0.75, 95 % CI = 0.46-1.21, P_{trend} = 0.52 for FlOP_320; and OR = 0.83, 95 % CI = 0.51-1.35, P_{trend} = 0.53 for FlOP_400).

When we analyzed the relationship between plasma FlOPs and risk of ED in controls only (free of prostate cancer incidence), levels of FlOP_360, FlOP_320 and FlOP_400 were again not associated with increased risk of ED (Table 3).

In the cross-sectional analysis, we found 3.7 % (N = 37) of men with ED at the time of blood draw. Higher levels of FlOP_360 were associated with increased risk of baseline ED (Tertile 3 vs. tertile 1: odds ratio [OR] = 2.68, 95 % confidence interval [CI] = 1.01-7.12), and the relationship had a significant trend (P_{trend} = 0.03). However, higher levels of FlOP_320 and FlOP_400 were not associated with baseline ED (Additional file 4: Table S4).

Discussion

To our knowledge, this is the first study that comprehensively assessed the association between oxidative stress and ED in both prospective and cross-sectional designs. Although higher levels of FlOP_360 were associated with increased risk of ED in the cross-sectional design, none of FlOP_360, FlOP_320 or FlOP_400 was associated with incidence of ED in the prospective design. Since the relationship between biomarkers of oxidative stress and ED is largely derived from animal models [10], the results of our study have challenged the traditional understandings on the independent detrimental effects of oxidative stress on ED in human.

We only found FlOP_360, but not FlOP_320 or FlOP_400, was positively associated with ED in cross-sectional design. Several reasons may be responsible: First, we cannot fully exclude a possibility of false-positive findings due to the fact that cross-sectional analysis had a small number of ED cases (N = 37) and only one type of FlOPs (FlOP_360 only) was associated with ED. Second, because of the cross-sectional design, the positive relationship between FlOP_360 and ED in cross-sectional design may be due to ED-related diseases that are correlated with oxidative stress. Certainly, further studies are warranted to confirm this.

In contrast to the positive association between FlOP_360 and ED in the cross-sectional study, we did not show consistent evidence of a positive association between oxidative stress and risk of ED in the prospective design, which had approximately 9 times as many cases as cross-sectional analysis. Besides the much larger number of cases, the prospective design limited reverse causation. However, it is possible that the underlying mechanism of oxidative stress on ED was not due to a global oxidative burden but a specific type of ROSs. There is animal and tissue evidence suggesting that superoxide with nitric oxide can result in acute impairment of cavernosal relaxation but also long-term penile vasculopathy [19–21].

Table 2 Association between plasma fluorescent oxidation products (FlOPs) and erectile dysfunction in prostate cancer cases (N =457) and controls (N = 460): prospective analysis in the Health Professional Follow-up Study, 1993-2001

Tertile	1	2	3	P for trend
Variables	FlOP_360			
Range (Fl/ml)	< 184	≥ 184; < 233	≥ 233	—
N	305	306	306	—
Median (Fl/ml)	160	207	280	—
Erectile dysfunction incidence (n, %)	100 (33 %)	112 (37 %)	111 (36 %)	—
Age adjusted	1 (ref)	1.13 (0.79, 1.61)	1.07 (0.75, 1.52)	0.84
Multivariable adjusted[a]	1 (ref)	1.03 (0.71, 1.51)	0.90 (0.61, 1.34)	0.54
	FlOP_320			
Range (Fl/ml)	< 356	≥ 356; < 524	≥ 524	—
N	305	306	306	—
Median (Fl/ml)	302	410	1837	—
Erectile dysfunction incidence (n, %)	102 (33 %)	114 (37 %)	107 (35 %)	—
Age adjusted	1 (ref)	1.00 (0.70, 1.42)	0.86 (0.60, 1.23)	0.30
Multivariable adjusted[a]	1 (ref)	0.75 (0.51, 1.11)	0.73 (0.49, 1.07)	0.27
	FlOP_400			
Range (Fl/ml)	< 49.1	≥ 49.1; < 62.6	≥ 62.6	—
N	305	306	306	—
Median (Fl/ml)	44.0	55.1	72.6	—
Erectile dysfunction incidence (n, %)	100 (33 %)	99 (32 %)	124 (41 %)	—
Age adjusted	1 (ref)	0.82 (0.57, 1.17)	1.24 (0.87, 1.77)	0.14
Multivariable adjusted[a]	1 (ref)	0.67 (0.45, 0.99)	0.98 (0.66, 1.45)	0.72

Values are odds ratio (95 % confidence interval), unless otherwise specified. Fl = Fluorescent intensity units

[a]Risk factors include age (continuous), body mass index (continuous), alcohol intake (in quartiles: < 0.88, ≥ 0.88 and < 5.58, ≥ 5.58 and < 16.38, ≥ 16.38 g/day), physical activity (in quartiles: < 15.6, ≥ 15.6and < 30.6, ≥ 30.6 and < 56.9, ≥ 56.9 MET-hours/week), Caucasian (yes/no), fasting hours (continuous), benign prostatic hyperplasia with surgery (yes/no), history of hypertension (yes/no), history of diabetes (yes/no), smoking status (current smokers, past smokers and non-smokers), month of blood draw (in seasons: Spring [March, April and May], Summer [June, July and August], Fall [September, October and November], Winter [December, January and February]) and year of blood draw (1993, 1994 and 1995)

The study has several limitations. First, a single measurement of FlOPs may not accurately reflect the average levels of the biomarker over a prolonged period of time. However, we have assessed their reproducibility over approximately a one-year period, and high ICCs suggest that this marker can be used as a marker for chronic exposure. Second, since we only ascertained ED via a single self-reported questionnaire on ED onset during approximately 7 years after blood draw, we cannot exclude the recall bias as a possible explanation of our results. Furthermore, our assessment of ED has not been validated; however, we note that a prior report using these data [22] were consistent with what has been found in other studies [15, 23]. Nonetheless, these two methodological weaknesses regarding the ascertainment of ED may lead to misclassification between incident ED and healthy controls. Third, our study is limited because the specific oxidative stress level at penile site was not available. Fourth, as our study only included history of BPH with surgery, some BPH cases with less severe clinical conditions might not be included. Fifth, the bias due to other known (i.e., duration of hypertension and smoking) or unknown residual confounding factors that are related to plasma FlOPs and ED is likely present. Sixth, our study was derived from another study designed to study prostate cancer but not ED. The sampling of that nested case–control study may introduce biases that affected our study and may limit the generation of our results. All the above limitations may cause the null association between plasma FlOPs and incident ED.

The strength of the study is that it contained relatively large sample size of men and incident EDs. In addition, as mentioned above, the prospective study design is a better design than cross-sectional design to reduce the possibility of the reverse causation between oxidative stress and ED, although an effect of subclinical disease on biomarkers cannot be excluded.

Table 3 Association between plasma fluorescent oxidation products (FlOPs) and erectile dysfunction in controls only (N = 460): prospective analysis in the Health Professional Follow-up Study, 1993-2001

Tertile	1	2	3	P for trend
Variables	FIOP_360			
Range (Fl/ml)	< 184	≥ 184; < 233	≥ 233	—
N	164	144	152	—
Median (Fl/ml)	159	206	279	—
Erectile dysfunction incidence (n, %)	55 (34 %)	51 (35 %)	51 (32 %)	—
Age adjusted	1 (ref)	1.06 (0.64, 1.75)	0.90 (0.54, 1.48)	0.59
Multivariable adjusted[a]	1 (ref)	1.02 (0.58, 1.79)	0.83 (0.47, 1.47)	0.46
	FIOP_320			
Range (Fl/ml)	< 356	≥ 356; < 524	≥ 524	—
N	160	142	158	—
Median (Fl/ml)	297	411	1858	—
Erectile dysfunction incidence (n, %)	52 (33 %)	53 (37 %)	52 (33 %)	—
Age adjusted	1 (ref)	0.96 (0.57, 1.60)	0.73 (0.44, 1.22)	0.17
Multivariable adjusted[a]	1 (ref)	0.75 (0.42, 1.35)	0.55 (0.31, 0.99)	0.10
	FIOP_400			
Range (Fl/ml)	< 49.1	≥ 49.1; < 62.6	≥ 62.6	—
N	150	160	150	—
Median (Fl/ml)	43.4	54.9	73.3	—
Erectile dysfunction incidence (n, %)	50 (33 %)	48 (31 %)	59 (39 %)	—
Age adjusted	1 (ref)	0.77 (0.46, 1.28)	1.23 (0.74, 2.03)	0.29
Multivariable adjusted[a]	1 (ref)	0.72 (0.41, 1.28)	1.07 (0.60, 1.88)	0.68

Values are odds ratio (95 % confidence interval), unless otherwise specified. Fl = Fluorescent intensity units
[a]Risk factors include age (continuous), body mass index (continuous), alcohol intake (in quartiles: < 0.88, ≥ 0.88 and < 5.58, ≥ 5.58 and < 16.38, ≥ 16.38 g/day), physical activity (in quartiles: < 15.6, ≥ 15.6and < 30.6, ≥ 30.6 and < 56.9, ≥ 56.9 MET-hours/week), Caucasian (yes/no), fasting hours (continuous), benign prostatic hyperplasia with surgery (yes/no), history of hypertension (yes/no), history of diabetes (yes/no), smoking status (current smokers, past smokers and non-smokers), month of blood draw (in seasons: Spring [March, April and May], Summer [June, July and August], Fall [September, October and November], Winter [December, January and February]) and year of blood draw (1993, 1994 and 1995)

Conclusions

In conclusion, we found no overall association between plasma FlOPs and risk of ED. This has raised an important message that systemic oxidative stress markers overall may not be a relevant measure for assessing the risk of incident ED. Therefore, the necessity of oxidative stress measurement in the risk of ED assessment is questionable. Since this is the first prospective study on biomarkers of global oxidation only, further investigation of other biomarkers of oxidative stress in relation to ED is warranted.

Additional files

Additional file 1: Table S1. Baseline characteristics according to tertiles of plasma fluorescent oxidation products in the Health Professional Follow-up Study in prostate cancer cases (N = 457), 1993–1995.

Additional file 2: Table S2. Baseline characteristics according to tertiles of plasma fluorescent oxidation products in the Health Professional Follow-up Study in controls (N = 460), 1993–1995. (DOCX 15 kb)

Additional file 3: Table S3. Baseline characteristics according to tertiles of plasma fluorescent oxidation products (FlOPs) (N = 1,000): cross-sectional analysis in the Health Professional Follow-up Study, 1993–1995. (DOCX 13 kb)

Additional file 4: Table S4. Association between plasma fluorescent oxidation products (FlOPs) and erectile dysfunction (N = 1,000): cross-sectional analysis in the Health Professional Follow-up Study, 1993–1995.

Competing interests
The authors declare that they have no competing interests.

Authors' contribution
S.Y. carried out the study design, drafted the manuscript, and analyzed the data. T.W. supervised the study design, manuscript drafting, data collection, data analyses and interpretation. E.G. participated data collection and interpretation, and manuscript revision. B.B. and S.H. helped with data

collection, data interpretation and manuscript revision. All authors read and approved the final manuscript.

Acknowledgements
This study was supported by funded by Dr. Wu's K07-CA138714 from the National Institute of Health and by American Heart Association grant 0430202 N. The HPFS cohort and prostate cancer case–control study was supported by grant Nos. P01CA055075 and P01CA133891 from the National Institute of Health (NIH)/National Cancer Institute.

Author details
¹Division of Epidemiology and Biostatistics, Department of Environmental Health, University of Cincinnati Medical Center, Kettering Complex, 3223 Eden Ave, Cincinnati, OH, USA, 45267-0056. ²Department of Surgery, University of Cincinnati Medical Center, Cincinnati, OH, USA. ³Division of Environmental Genetics and Molecular Toxicology, Cincinnati, OH, USA. ⁴Center for Environmental Genetics, University of Cincinnati Medical Center, Cincinnati, OH, USA. ⁵Departments of Nutrition and Epidemiology, Harvard School of Public Health, Boston, MA, USA. ⁶The Channing Division of Network Medicine, Department of Medicine, Brigham and Women's Hospital, Harvard Medical School, Boston, MA, USA.

References
1. Rebholz CM, Wu T, Hamm LL, Arora R, Khan IE, Liu Y, et al. The association of plasma fluorescent oxidation products and chronic kidney disease: a case–control study. Am J Nephrol. 2012;36(4):297–304.
2. Fortner RT, Tworoger SS, Wu T, Eliassen AH. Plasma florescent oxidation products and breast cancer risk: repeated measures in the Nurses' Health Study. Breast Cancer Res Treat. 2013;141(2):307–16.
3. Jensen MK, Wang YS, Rimm EB, Townsend MK, Willett W, Wu TY. Fluorescent Oxidation Products and Risk of Coronary Heart Disease: A Prospective Study in Women. J Am Heart Assoc. 2013;2(5).
4. Frankel EN. Lipid oxidation 2nd eidtion. Dundee, Scotland: The Oily Press LTD; 2005.
5. Wu TY, Willett WC, Rifai N, Rimm EB. Plasma fluorescent oxidation products as potential markers of oxidative stress for epidemiologic studies. Am J Epidemiol. 2007;166(5):552–60.
6. Wu T, Rifai N, Willett WC, Rimm EB. Plasma fluorescent oxidation products: independent predictors of coronary heart disease in men. Am J Epidemiol. 2007;166(5):544–51.
7. Wu TY, Rifai N, Roberts LJ, Willett WC, Rimm EB. Stability of measurements of biomarkers of oxidative stress in blood over 36 h. Cancer Epidem Biomar. 2004;13(8):1399–402.
8. Singh U, Jialal I. Oxidative stress and atherosclerosis. Pathophysiology. 2006;13(3):129–42.
9. Harrison D, Griendling KK, Landmesser U, Hornig B, Drexler H. Role of oxidative stress in atherosclerosis. Am J Cardiol. 2003;91(3):7A–11A.
10. Agarwal A, Nandipati KC, Sharma RK, Zippe CD, Raina R. Role of oxidative stress in the pathophysiological mechanism of erectile dysfunction. J Androl. 2006;27(3):335–47.
11. Azadzoi KM, Schulman RN, Aviram M, Siroky MB. Oxidative stress in arteriogenic erectile dysfunction: prophylactic role of antioxidants. J Urology. 2005;174(1):386–93.
12. Aldemir M, Okulu E, Neselioglu S, Erel O, Ener K, Kayigil O. Evaluation of serum oxidative and antioxidative status in patients with erectile dysfunction. Andrologia. 2012;44 Suppl 1:266–71.
13. Barassi A, Colpi GM, Piediferro G, Dogliotti G, D'Eril GV, Corsi MM. Oxidative stress and antioxidant status in patients with erectile dysfunction. J Sex Med. 2009;6(10):2820–5.
14. Ciftci H, Yeni E, Savas M, Verit A, Celik H. Paraoxonase activity in patients with erectile dysfunction. Int J Impot Res. 2007;19(5):517–20.
15. Weber MF, Smith DP, O'Connell DL, Patel MI, de Souza PL, Sitas F, et al. Risk factors for erectile dysfunction in a cohort of 108 477 Australian men. Med J Aust. 2013;199(2):107–11.
16. Feldman HA, Goldstein I, Hatzichristou DG, Krane RJ, Mckinlay JB. Impotence and Its Medical and Psychosocial Correlates - Results of the Massachusetts Male Aging Study. J Urology. 1994;151(1):54–61.
17. Wu T, Wang Y, Ho SM, Giovannucci E. Plasma levels of nitrate and risk of prostate cancer: a prospective study. Cancer epidemiol, biomarkers prev : a publication of the American Association for Cancer Research, cosponsored by the American Society of Preventive Oncology. 2013;22(7):1210–8.
18. Farankel EN. Lipid oxidation. Dundee: The Oily Press; 1998.
19. Jeremy JY, Jones RA, Koupparis AJ, Hotston M, Persad R, Angelini GD, et al. Reactive oxygen species and erectile dysfunction: possible role of NADPH oxidase. Int J Impot Res. 2007;19(3):265–80.
20. Burnett AL, Lowenstein CJ, Bredt DS, Chang TS, Snyder SH. Nitric oxide: a physiologic mediator of penile erection. Science. 1992;257(5068):401–3.
21. Jones RW, Rees RW, Minhas S, Ralph D, Persad RA, Jeremy JY. Oxygen free radicals and the penis. Expert Opin Pharmacother. 2002;3(7):889–97.
22. Li Y, Batool-Anwar S, Kim S, Rimm EB, Ascherio A, Gao X. Prospective study of restless legs syndrome and risk of erectile dysfunction. Am J Epidemiol. 2013;177(10):1097–105.
23. Selvin E, Burnett AL, Platz EA. Prevalence and risk factors for erectile dysfunction in the US. Am J Med. 2007;120(2):151–7.

9

Correlation between penile cuff test and pressure-flow study in patients candidates for trans-urethral resection of prostate

Daniele Bianchi[1*], Angelo Di Santo[2], Gabriele Gaziev[1], Roberto Miano[3], Stefania Musco[4], Giuseppe Vespasiani[3] and Enrico Finazzi Agrò[3]

Abstract

Background: Aim of this study was to make a comparison between penile cuff test (PCT) and standard pressure-flow study (PFS) in the preoperative evaluation of patients candidates for trans-urethral resection of prostate (TURP) for benign prostatic obstruction (BPO).

Methods: We enrolled male patients with lower urinary tract symptoms candidates for TURP. Each of them underwent a PCT and a subsequent PFS. A statistical analysis was performed: sensitivity (SE), specificity (SP), positive predictive value (PPV), negative predictive value (NPV), likelihood ratio and ratio of corrected classified were calculated. Fisher exact test was used to evaluate relationships between PCT and maximal urine flow (Q_{max}): a p-value < 0.05 was considered statistically significant.

Results: We enrolled 48 consecutive patients. Overall, at PCT 31 patients were diagnosed as obstructed and 17 patients as unobstructed. At the subsequent PFS, 21 out of 31 patients diagnosed as obstructed at PCT were confirmed to be obstructed; one was diagnosed as unobstructed; the remaining 9 patients appeared as equivocal. Concerning the 17 patients unobstructed at PCT, all of them were confirmed not to be obstructed at PFS, with 10 equivocal and 7 unobstructed. The rate of correctly classified patients at PCT was 79% (95%-CI 65%-90%). About detecting obstructed patients, PCT showed a SE of 100% and a SP of 63%. The PPV was 68%, while the NPV was 100%.

Conclusions: PCT can be an efficient tool in evaluating patients candidates for TURP. In particular, it showed good reliability in ruling out BPO because of its high NPV, with a high rate of correctly classified patients overall. Further studies on a huger number of patients are needed, including post-operative follow-up as well.

Keywords: Bladder isovolumetric pressure, Non-invasive urodynamics, Penile cuff test, Prostate, Trans-urethral resection of prostate

Background

The role of urodynamics (UD) in the diagnosis of benign prostate obstruction (BPO) has been intensively investigated [1,2].

In clinical practice, when required, a proper evaluation and quantification of BPO is performed by invasive UD, in particular pressure-flow study (PFS) [1].

Over the last two decades, some alternative, less invasive tests have been proposed [3], based on equipment consisting of an external condom catheter [4], an intra-urethral device [5] or an inflatable cuff around the penis – penile cuff test (PCT) – with inflation-deflation cycles [6].

Instead of the direct intravesical sampling used in PFS, non-invasive UD aims to give information about bladder pressure by evaluating the equal urine pressure either along the urethra (in penile cuff), or at the external meatus (in external condom catheter).

In the PCT with inflation-deflation cycles [6], the pressure needed to stop the flow (p_{cuff}) represents the bladder isovolumetric pressure (BIP) e.g. the bladder pressure during an isovolumetric contraction. This pressure is detected by a cuff placed around the penis before micturition [6].

* Correspondence: danielebianchimail@yahoo.it
[1]School of Specialization in Urology, University of Rome Tor Vergata, Viale Oxford, 81-00133 Rome, Italy
Full list of author information is available at the end of the article

The cuff is automatically inflated during the voiding phase, in order to stop urine flow, and then deflated again. The inflation-deflation cycle is repeated several times during a single micturition, thus allowing to correctly assess BIP (see Figure 1).

PCT results can be plotted on the nomogram proposed by Griffiths [7] which is designed on a cartesian plane with maximal urine flow (Q_{max}) on the x-axis and p_{cuff} on y-axis, with an ascending straight line, with y-intercept equal to 80 cm H_2O, separating obstructed from non-obstructed patients.

Recently, a new prototype of PCT has been proposed [8], using an automatically controlled inflatable cuff which detects bladder voiding pressure at constant low urine flow instead of inflation-deflation cycles.

The purpose of this study was to compare the data of PCT with inflation-deflation cycles with those of a standard PFS in patients candidates for trans-urethral resection of prostate (TURP).

Methods

Male patients who previously received indication to undergo a TURP in our or in a different center were included. Indication for TURP had been made on referral urologist opinion, generally on the basis of the presence of lower urinary tract symptoms (LUTS) and a reduced flow rate, independently by other aspects as prostate volume and alpha-blockers effectiveness.

A urine sample for urine culture was collected by spontaneous micturition within 7 days before the tests in order to rule out possible infections. Exclusion criteria were diabetes mellitus, any neurological disease, use of drugs impairing bladder contractility or impacting on lower urinary tract function, an indwelling bladder catheter over the previous six months, presence of urinary tract infection, suspect of malignancies.

Approval of the study by Ethics Committee of Policlinico Tor Vergata was obtained, and all patients signed a written informed consent to be included. For each patient, we

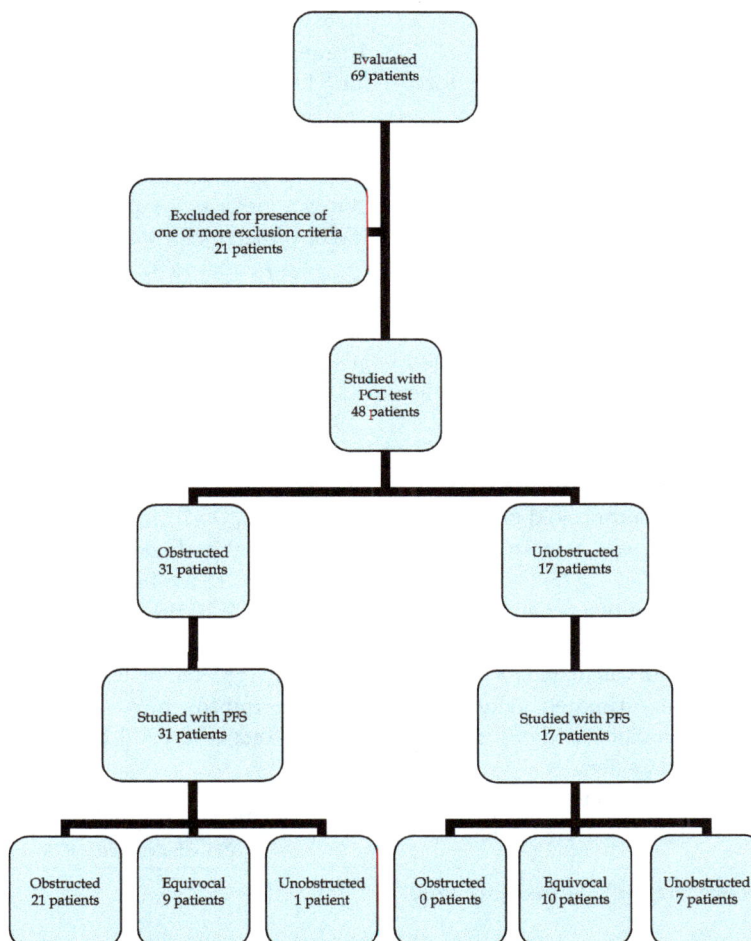

Figure 1 The principal of the test is similar to bladder pressure measurement. A small cuff is placed around the penis. When micturition has commenced, the cuff is inflated. The cuff pressure required to stop flow should equal bladder pressure. p iso: Isovolumetric pressure.

performed a PCT followed by a subsequent PFS and both procedures were conducted by the same urodynamicist.

PCT was performed by Mediplus CT3000 Cuff Machine®, which allows multiple inflation-deflation cycles during a single micturition, getting several BIP measurements.

The patients were instructed to perform a micturition without abdominal straining.

For each inflation cycle we applied the exclusion rules proposed by Drinnan et al. [9], thus a cycle was immediately excluded in case of one of the following conditions:

- No flow recovery after cuff deflation, meaning that the micturition ended during the last cycle, so the cuff pressure could have been not responsible for urine flow stop;
- There was an 'erratic' flow trace, which could be related to straining or maybe to contractions by the pelvic floor or membranous urethra;
- The urine flow was not interrupted at the device maximum pressure, which is set at 200 cm H_2O for safety reasons. This situation is associated with highly contractile bladder.

Furthermore, we repeated any test showing a total bladder volume less than 150 mL.

PFS was performed by a urodynamic equipment (Life-Tech®, Stafford, TX, USA) with water-filled bladder catheter and rectal balloon (Life-Tech®, Stafford, TX, USA), after a filling phase with non-physiological filling rate (30–50 mL/s).

The examination was conducted according to the *International Continence Society* recommendations [10,11].

PFS data were plotted on the Abrams-Griffiths modified nomogram [12,13], while PCT results were plotted on the nomogram proposed by Griffiths [7].

For each of two categories – obstructed versus non-obstructed – patients were subdivided into two subgroups according to their Q_{max}, with a threshold of 10 mL/s [14], in order to evaluate if Q_{max} was able to improve accuracy.

Sensitivity (SE), specificity (SP), positive predictive value (PPV), negative predictive value (NPV), likelihood ratio and ratio of corrected classified were calculated.

In order to assess accuracy of estimated value, 95% confidence interval (95%-CI) was calculated for SE, SP, PPV, NPV and ratio of corrected classified.

Fisher exact test was used to evaluate relationships between PCT and Q_{max}: a p-value < 0.05 was considered statistically significant.

Software Stata 13.0 (College Station®, Texas) was used for all analysis.

Results have been reported according to *Standards for Reporting of Diagnostic accuracy* (STARD) flow-chart [15].

The research was carried out in compliance with the Helsinki Declaration - Ethical Principles for Medical Research Involving Human Subjects.

Results

We enrolled 48 consecutive male patients – mean age 61.5 ± 13.1 years.

On uroflowmetry, median Q_{max} was 11.6 mL/s (range 4.0-25.0 mL/s), with a median post-void residual urine volume (PVR) of 42 mL (range 0–430 mL) detected by ultrasound scan. PSA mean value was 2.35 ng/mL (range 0.80-4.10 ng/mL).

No adverse events occurred during or after the tests.

Overall, at PCT 31 patients were diagnosed as obstructed and 17 patients as unobstructed on Griffiths nomogram [7].

On the subsequent PFS, according to Abrams-Griffiths nomogram [12,13], 21 out of 31 patients diagnosed as obstructed at PCT were confirmed to be obstructed; one was diagnosed as unobstructed; the remaining 9 patients appeared as equivocal.

Concerning the 17 patients unobstructed at PCT, all of them were confirmed not to be obstructed on PFS, with 10 equivocal and 7 unobstructed (see Table 1 and Figure 2 for STARD flow-chart).

The rate of correctly classified patients at PCT was 79% (95%-CI 65%-90%).

About pressure measurements, overall at PCT we obtained a mean p_{cuff} equal to 133.75 cm H_2O (SD 33.45 cm H_2O), while at PFS we had a mean detrusorial pressure at Q_{max} flow equal to 52.69 cm H_2O (SD 21.94 cm H_2O).

Focusing on obstructed patients, at PCT we had a mean p_{cuff} =157.00 cm H_2O (SD 26.83 cm H_2O), while at PFS the mean detrusorial pressure was 74.00 cm H_2O (SD 14.13 cm H_2O).

With regard to the further subdivision according to Q_{max}, 15 patients out of the 31 obstructed at PCT showed a $Q_{max} < 10$ mL/s, with the other 16 patients having a $Q_{max} \geq 10$ mL/s.

On the other hand, among the 17 unobstructed patients on PCT, we had 5 with a $Q_{max} < 10$ mL/s and 12 with a $Q_{max} \geq 10$ mL/s.

Patients categorization into subgroups according to their Q_{max} greater or less than 10 mL/s did not produce a further improvement of PCT ability to diagnose BPO (Fisher exact test, $p = 0.2362$).

Table 1 Results of penile cuff test (PCT) compared with pressure-flow studies (PFS)

	PFS obstructed	PFS Unobstructed/Equivocal	Total
PENILE CUFF obstructed	21	10	31
PENILE CUFF unobstructed	0	17	17
Total	21	27	48

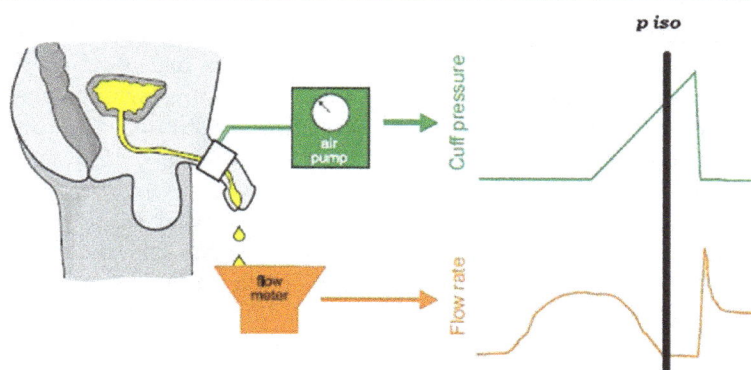

Figure 2 Results according to *Standards for Reporting of Diagnostic accuracy* (STARD) flow-chart. PCT: Penile Cuff Test. PFS: Pressure-Flow Studies.

About detecting obstructed patients, PCT showed a SE of 100% (95%-CI 84-100%) and a SP of 63% (95%-CI 42-81%), with a positive likelihood ratio of 2.7 (95%-CI 1.65-4.42). The PPV was 68% (95%-CI 49-83%), while the NPV was 100% (95%-CI 80-100%). Results are summarized in Table 2.

Discussion

Over the last century, a simple evaluation of PVR has been proposed as an appealing tool for diagnosing BPO. Nevertheless, a huge PVR may be due to an impaired detrusor contractility (IDC) [16]. In fact, it has been pointed out that up to one half of unobstructed patients with LUTS could have elevated PVR, while up to one forth of severely obstructed patients could show no PVR [1].

Thus, the association between elevated PVR and BPO is not strong enough to be used as a useful clinical tool [17].

In some papers, the role of uroflow trace has been investigated as well, but no reliable relation between its profile and BPO was found out [18].

Some Authors have shown that uroflowmetry could be able to assess the presence of BPO in the vaste majority of patients with Q_{max} less than 10 mL/s, with a progressively decreasing rate of BPO in case of Q_{max} major than 10 mL/s [1,2,14].

Accordingly, *European Association of Urology* guidelines have considered PFS as an optional test before surgery for BPO, usually indicated in the preoperative evaluation of patients showing a $Q_{max} > 15$ mL/s [19].

Conversely, 25-30% of men with decreased Q_{max} at uroflowmetry are unobstructed [1]. Indeed, decreased uroflow can result from either impaired detrusor contractility (IDC) or BPO; thus, only detrusor pressure measurement is able to distinguish between those conditions [18,20].

Furthermore, there are no tips on uroflowmetry trace shape that allows a distinction between BPO and IDC [18]; on the other hand, a normal uroflow test does not rule out BPO [20].

As a consequence, PFS still represents the gold standard for a proper evaluation of BPO in male patients, above all when an IDC is suspected [1].

In clinical practice, the nomogram proposed by Abrams and Griffiths for the diagnosis of obstruction in males at PFS has been widely used [16].

A further nomogram proposed by Abrams [13] aims to give a more accurate patients categorization by the

Table 2 Results of penile cuff test (PCT) compared with pressure-flow studies (PFS)

PCT O		PCT U						
PFS O (n)	PFS U (n)	PFS O (n)	PFS U (n)	SE %	SP %	PPV %	NPV %	LR + %
21	10	0	17	100,0	63,0	67,7	100,0	2,7

PCT: Penile Cuff Test.
PFS: Pressure-Flow Studies.
O: Obstructed.
U: Unobstructed.
n: Number of patients.
SE: Sensitivity.
SP: Specificity.
PPV: Positive Predictive Value.
NPV: Negative predictive Value.
LR+: Positive Likelihood Ratio.

introduction of bladder outlet obstruction index (BOOI) and bladder contractility index (BCI).

Thus, PFS represents the gold standard for the evaluation of BPO [1]. Nevertheless, this test is not used as a routine examination before surgery for BPO [19], because it is considered time-consuming, not cost-effective overall [1] and a potential cause of morbidity [21].

Over the last 30 years, no simple tool proved to be reliable in distinguishing between BPO and IDC.

The role of non-invasive UD in clinical practice is still unclear [19] and few data have been published about correlation between PCT and PFS findings [6,7,22,23].

Aim of our study was to make a comparison between PCT and PFS in the diagnostic work-up on patients candidates for TURP: summarizing our results, PCT showed a SE of 100% and a SP of 63% in detecting obstructed patients, with a PPV of 68% and a NPV of 100%.

Overall, the rate of correctly classified patients at PCT was 79%. In particular, non-obstructed patients at PCT were confirmed as non-obstructed at PFS.

Using the nomogram modified for non-invasive pressure measurement, Griffiths et al. [7] obtained with PCT a PPV of 68% and a NPV of 78% for PFS diagnosis of BPO. Besides, they noticed that predictive accuracy for obstruction could be improved by the additional criterion of Q_{max} less than 10 mL/s, thus obtaining a PPV of 88% and a NPV of 86%.

In our study, patients categorization into subgroups according to their Q_{max} (threshold 10 mL/s) did not add any further information as it did not get confirmation of its statistical significance at Fisher exact test.

The difference between Griffiths' and our results could be due to a different selection of patients: in our study, only patients who were candidates for a TURP [24] were enrolled, while in Griffiths' paper the Authors intended to analyze patients complaining with LUTS [7]. Nevertheless, further studies are needed to investigate this aspect.

Our data seem to confirm those ones obtained in another, more recent paper based on 30 consecutive patients complaining with LUTS. In this study, Borrini L et al. [22] found for PCT a PPV of 82% and a NPV of 88% for BPO at PFS.

According to our experience, non-invasive UD, in particular PCT, can be a useful diagnostic tool in patients candidates for TURP, suggesting a possible solution to the thorny problem about urodynamic tests before surgery for BPO. In fact, compared to PFS, PCT appeared as a quick and accurate test to rule out a BPO condition because of its high NPV. Thus it could be used to run a selection of non-obstructed patients suspected for an eventual IDC condition. Indeed, such patients are the most critical ones in BPO surgery [25], with some papers reporting about one forth of them showing no symptoms improvement after a surgical treatment [24,26].

In a paper by Harding et al. [27], a consecutive cohort of 208 men undergoing TURP were previously evaluated by PCT: 87% of patients diagnosed with BPO had a clinical improvement after surgery, while only 56% of patients deemed as not obstructed had a good outcome.

By such diagnostic pathway, non-obstructed patients (probably with IDC) could be easily recognized and adequately counseled in advance about the prospect of poor or partial symptoms improvement after surgery for BPO, avoiding a PFS.

Furthermore, the rate of correctly classified patients at PCT was high, confirming that most obstructed patients can be adequately evaluated by PCT.

We should also consider that PCT categorization does not allow for 'equivocal' patients, who finally represent the mismatch between the two urodynamic tests. Anyway, those patients can be mostly considered eligible to surgery, so PFS could be neglected in such cases.

Only patients with an unclear diagnosis could be suggested to undergo PFS, while the other ones could be probably evaluated just by PCT, getting the amount of pre-operative information useful both to the surgeon and to the patient, in terms of preoperative counseling.

Limitations of our study are the relatively small sample size and the lack of a post-operative follow-up to assess TURP efficacy in different categories of patients.

On the other hand, this is, to our knowledge, the first study comparing PCT to PFS in patients candidates for TURP.

Further papers on large series of patients including post-operative follow-up are needed, in order to assess the real role of PCT in the pre-operative evaluation for BPO.

Conclusions

PCT can be an efficient tool in evaluating patients candidates for TURP. In particular, it showed good reliability in ruling out BPO because of its high NPV, with a high rate of correctly classified patients overall. Further studies based on a bigger sample size are needed, including post-operative follow-up.

Competing interests
The authors declare that they have no competing interests.

Authors' contributions
DB participated in the design of the study, performed the statistical analysis, reviewed the literature and drafted the manuscript. ADS participated in the design and coordination of the study, performed the urodynamic tests, collected the data. GG participated in the design of the study, collected the data and reviewed the literature. RM collected the data and participated in the coordination of the study. SM participated in the design of the study and reviewed the literature. GV conceived of the study, and participated in its design and coordination. EFA conceived of the study, participated in its design and coordination and the statistical analysis, supervised the draft. All authors read and approved the final manuscript.

Author details

[1]School of Specialization in Urology, University of Rome Tor Vergata, Viale Oxford, 81-00133 Rome, Italy. [2]NeuroUrology Unit, IRCCS Fondazione Santa Lucia, Rome, Italy. [3]Department of Experimental Medicine and Surgery, University of Rome Tor Vergata, Rome, Italy. [4]Neuro-Urology Unit, Careggi Hospital, Florence, Italy.

References

1. Nitti VW: **Pressure Flow Urodynamic Studies: The Gold Standard for Diagnosing Bladder outlet Obstruction.** *Rev Urol* 2005, **7**(Suppl 6):S14–S21.
2. Mangera A, Osman NI, Chapple CR: **Assessment of BPH/BOO.** *Indian J Urol* 2014, **30**(2):177–180. doi:10.4103/0970-1591.126902.
3. Blake C, Abrams P: **Noninvasive techniques for the measurement of isovolumetric bladder pressure.** *J Urol* 2004, **171**(1):12–19.
4. Huang Foen Chung JW, Bohnen AM, Pel JJ, Bosch JL, Niesing R, van Mastrigt R: **Applicability and reproducibility of condom catheter method for measuring isovolumetric bladder pressure.** *Urology* 2004, **63**:56–60.
5. D'Ancona CAL, Bassani JWM, de Oliveira Querne FA, Carvalho J, Oliveira RR, Netto NR Jr: **New method for minimally invasive urodynamic assessment in men with lower urinary tract symptoms.** *Urology* 2008, **71**:75–78.
6. Griffiths CJ, Rix D, MacDonald AM: **Noninvasive measurement of bladder pressure by controlled inflation of a penile cuff.** *J Urol* 2002, **167**(3):1344–1347.
7. Griffiths CJ, Harding C, Blake C, McIntosh S, Drinnan MJ, Robson WA, Abrams P, Ramsden PD, Pickard RS: **A nomogram to classify men with lower urinary tract symptoms using urine flow and noninvasive measurement of bladder pressure.** *J Urol* 2005, **174**(4 Pt 1):1323–1326.
8. Clarkson B, Griffiths C, McArdle F: **Continuous non-invasive measurement of bladder voiding pressure using an experimental constant low-flow test.** *Neurourol Urodyn* 2012, **31**:557–563.
9. Drinnan MJ, McIntosh SL, Robson WA, Pickard RS, Ramsden PD, Griffiths CJ: **Inter-observer agreement in the estimation of bladder pressure using a penile cuff.** *Neurourol Urodyn* 2003, **22**:296–300.
10. Schafer W, Abrams P, Liao L, Mattiasson A, Pesce F, Spangberg A, Sterling AM, Zinner NR, van Kerrebroeck P, International Continence Society: **Good urodynamic practices: uroflowmetry, filling cystometry and pressure-flow studies.** *Neurourol Urodyn* 2002, **21**(3):261–274.
11. Abrams P, Cardozo L, Fall M, Griffiths D, Rosier P, Ulmsten U, van Kerrebroeck P, Victor A, Wein A, Subcommittee of the International Continence Society: **The standardisation of terminology of lower urinary tract function: report from the Standardistion Sub-committee of the International Continence Society.** *Neurourol Urodyn* 2002, **21**:167–178.
12. Griffiths D, Hofner K, van Mastrigt R, Rollema HJ, Spangberg A, Gleason D: **Standardisation of terminology of lower urinary tract function: pressure flow studies of voiding, urethral resistance and urethral obstruction.** *Neurourol Urodyn* 1997, **6**:1–18.
13. Abrams P: **Bladder outlet obstruction index, bladder contractility index and bladder voiding efficiency: three simple indices to define bladder voiding function.** *BJU Int* 1999, **84**:14–15.
14. Reynard JM, Yang Q, Donovan JL, Peters TJ, Schafer W, de la Rosette JJ, Dabhoiwala NF, Osawa D, Lim AT, Abrams P: **The ICS-'BPH' Study: uroflowmetry, lower urinary tract symptoms and bladder outlet obstruction.** *Br J Urol* 1998, **82**(5):619–623.
15. Bossuyt PM, Reitsma JB, Bruns DE, Gatsonis CA, Glasziou PP, Irwig LM, Moher D, Rennie D, de Vet HC, Lijmer JG: **Standards for Reporting of Diagnostic accuracy. The STARD statement for reporting studies of diagnostic accuracy: explanation and elaboration.** *Ann Intern Med* 2003, **138**(1):W1–W12.
16. Abrams PH, Griffiths D: **The assessment of prostatic obstruction from urodynamic measurements and from residual urine.** *BJU* 1979, **51**:129–134.b.
17. Griffiths DJ: **Pressure-flow studies of micturition.** *Urol Clin North Am* 1996, **23**:279–297.
18. Chancellor MB, Blaivas JG, Kaplan SA, Axelrod S: **Bladder outlet obstruction versus impaired detrusor contractility: the role of outflow.** *J Urol* 1991, **145**(4):810–812.
19. Oelke M, Bachmann A, Descazeaud A, Emberton M, Gravas S, Michel MC, N'dow J, Nordling J, de la Rosette JJ: **Guidelines on the management of**

male lower urinary tract symptoms, incl. benign prostatic obstruction. *Eur Assoc Urol* 2013, 8–9.
20. Gerstenberg TC, Andersen JT, Klarskov P, Ramirez D, Hald T: **High flow infravesical obstruction in men: symptomatology, urodynamics and the results of surgery.** *J Urol* 1982, **127**:943–945.
21. Porru D, Madeddu G, Campus G, Montisci I, Scarpa RM, Usai E: **Evaluation of morbidity of multi-channel pressure-flow studies.** *Neurourol Urodyn* 1999, **18**(6):647–52.22.
22. Borrini L, Lukacs B, Ciofu C, Gaibisso B, Haab F, Amarenco G: **Predictive value of the penile cuff-test for the assessment of bladder outlet obstruction in men.** *Prog Urol* 2012, **22**(11):657–664.
23. Arnolds M, Oelke M: **Positioning invasive versus non invasive urodynamics in the assessment of bladder outlet obstruction.** *Curr Opin Urol* 2009, **19**(1):55–62.
24. Neal DE, Ramsden PD, Sharples L, Smith A, Powell PH, Styles RA, Webb RJ: **Outcome of elective prostatectomy.** *BMJ* 1989, **299**(6702):762–767.
25. Losco G, Keedle L, King Q: **Non-invasive urodynamics predicts outcome prior to surgery for prostatic obstruction.** *BJU Int* 2013, **112**(Suppl 2):61–64.
26. Emberton M, Neal DE, Black N: **The effect of prostatectomy on symptom severity and quality of life.** *Br J Urol* 1996, **77**(2):233–247.
27. Harding C, Robson W, Drinnan M, Sajeel M, Ramsden P, Griffiths C, Pickard R: **Predicting the outcome of prostatectomy using non-invasive bladder pressure and urine flow measurements.** *Eur Urol* 2007, **52**:186–192.

10

Socio-occupational class, region of birth and maternal age: influence on time to detection of cryptorchidism (undescended testes)

Karin Sørig Hougaard[1*], Ann Dyreborg Larsen[1,2], Harald Hannerz[1], Anne-Marie Nybo Andersen[3], Kristian Tore Jørgensen[1,4], Gunnar Vase Toft[2], Jens Peter Bonde[4] and Morten Søndergaard Jensen[5]

Abstract

Background: Cryptorchidism (undescended testes) is associated with poor male fertility, but can be alleviated and fertility preserved to some degree by early detection and treatment. Here we assess the influence of socio-occupational class, geographical region, maternal age and birth cohort on time to detection and correction of cryptorchidism.

Methods: All boys born in Denmark, 1981 to 1987 or 1988 to 1994, with a diagnosis of cryptorchidism were identified in nationwide registers. The boys were followed for a diagnosis until their 16th birthday. The age at first diagnosis was noted and used as proxy for time to detection of cryptorchidism. Parental employment in the calendar year preceding birth was grouped into one of five socio-occupational classes. Geographical region was defined by place of birth in one of 15 Danish counties. Detection rate ratios of cryptorchidism were analyzed as a function of parental socio-occupational group, county, maternal age and birth cohort by use of Poisson regression.

Results: Some 6,059 boys in the early and 5,947 boys in the late cohort received a diagnosis of cryptorchidism. Time to detection was independent of parental socio-occupational group and maternal age but differed slightly between geographical regions. A similar pattern was obtained for surgical correction after a diagnosis. Age at diagnosis decreased by 2.7 years from the early to the late cohort.

Conclusions: These results indicate that childhood socio-occupational inequality in detection and correction of cryptorchidism would play a negligible role in male infertility in a life course perspective. Geographical region may have exerted some influence, especially for the oldest cohort.

Keywords: Cryptorchidism, Fertility, Diagnosis, Orchiopexy, Geography, Register, Public health

Background

Maldevelopment of the male reproductive tract is a major determinant of poor fertility later in life. Congenital cryptorchidism (undescended testes) is one such condition. Early treatment may alleviate the adverse effects of cryptorchidism on fertility, and the earlier orchiopexy is performed, the less the effect on future semen quality [1,2]. Adverse influence on gonadal cell populations in

cryptorchid boys has been observed already at 3–6 months of age [3], and based on current literature, it is recommended that cryptorchidism is treated between 6 and 12 months of age [4].

Different long-term outcomes of cryptorchidism may arise from genetic, biological and environmental determinants, interacting with social, cultural and economic factors [5]. The Danish health care system is tax-financed and accessible for all Danish citizens. Therefore economic factors related directly to contact and treatment within the health care system would not be expected to significantly influence time to detection. A tax-financed

* Correspondence: ksh@nrcwe.dk
[1]The National Research Centre for the Working Environment, Lersø Parkallé 105, DK-2100 Copenhagen, Denmark
Full list of author information is available at the end of the article

health care system does however not remove all barriers to detection of disease. Time to detection of cryptorchidism might therefore be hypothesized to vary with parental socioeconomic factors such as competing priorities and time restraints, lack of information and knowledge, communication barriers, medical mistrust, health professionals' perception of patients relative to socioeconomic status, and age [5-7]. Children of parents with low socioeconomic status are less likely to participate in the free preventive child examinations that are offered at the general practitioner until the age of five years [8]. The overall incidence of hospital referrals for cryptorchidism increases after each examination [9] and it has been estimated that testis palpation is performed in 60%-90% of these visits [10]. Non-adherence to routine prophylactic visits in low social classes may be an important reason for a delayed diagnosis and treatment. Furthermore, Danish hospitals (with few exceptions) were owned by the counties, and the treatments as well as the criteria for treatment may vary between counties as may regional differences in distance to hospital care [11-13].

Delayed diagnosis and treatment of cryptorchidism may affect male fertility in a life-course perspective. The present study investigates whether social class, maternal age and geographical region influence time to detection and surgical treatment of cryptorchidism. The study was performed in two cohorts, i.e. boys born in 1981 to 1987 or in 1988 to 1994, to investigate potential changes in the influence of social class and geographical region between these two time periods.

Methods

Study population and outcome

The study population consisted of singleton boys diagnosed with cryptorchidism before their 16th birthday. The boys were born in Denmark (excluding Greenland) from 1981 to 1987 and 1988 to 1994, i.e., the population was divided into two cohorts. At least one of the parents had to be employed in the calendar year preceding the year of birth.

The boys were identified through the Danish Civil Registration System [14], by the unique 10-digit identification number assigned at birth (CPR-number). The number is used across all public services in Denmark and enables linkage through population based registries, ensuring almost complete follow-up [15]. Cryptorchidism diagnoses were obtained from the Danish National Patient Registry, with nationwide coverage of all inpatient clinic diagnoses since 1977, and from 1995 also diagnoses from outpatient hospital clinics [16].

The boys were considered to have received a diagnosis if they had a record in the Danish National Patient Registry before their 16th birthday of a principal diagnosis of cryptorchidism according to the International

Classification of Diseases version 8 (ICD-8) codes 752.10-752.11 and 752.19 or ICD version 10 codes Q53, Q531, Q531A, Q532, Q532A, and Q539. All diagnoses were made by hospital physicians, primarily paediatricians, general surgeons, urologists and paediatric urologists [14,17]. In diagnosed boys, treatment was defined by completion of the surgical procedure of orchiopexy (fastening of the undescended testicle inside the scrotum) as indicated by the corresponding surgical codes (described in [14]). Orchiopexy indicates that the cryptorchidism is persistent, while a general diagnosis of cryptorchidism may include transient cases of undescended testes that subsequently descend spontaneously.

We followed all boys for a diagnosis or surgery until their 16th birthday, which ensured comparable follow-up between cohorts and ascertainment of almost all cases of cryptorchidism (>95% of all cases presenting until the age of 30, in the oldest cohort). The age at principal diagnosis or surgery was noted. Since the earliest possible time for detection of cryptorchidism is at birth, time of detection corresponds to the age at detection. Age at detection was therefore used as a proxy for time to detection (TTD).

Statistics Denmark administered the data linkage and regulated data access. The data aggregation and analysis were approved by Statistics Denmark, the National Board of Health and the Danish Data Protection Agency. In accordance with Guidelines for Good Epidemiological Practice [18], a protocol outlining the methods was approved by the authors before the actual analyses were initiated.

Explanatory variables

Parental socio-occupational status at birth of the child

Each boy was linked to his parents using the CPR-number in the Fertility Database [19], which enabled identification of parental employment as the basis for socioeconomic position [20,21]. In Denmark, all persons are classified annually according to occupation by Statistics Denmark from 16 years of age onwards. Specifically, socioeconomic position was defined by the NYSTGR classification, a specialised version of the Danish version the International Standard Classification of Occupations (ISCO) 1968 version, used from 1980 to 1995 by Statistics Denmark [22,23]. Socioeconomic position was defined the year before birth of the child, to avoid change in maternal occupational status due to maternity leave and change of occupational status, e.g. to become an (unemployed) house wife. The groups were defined and ranked as: white collar group 1 (senior salaried staff including managers etc. with more than 20 employees), white collar group 2 (leading salaried positions requiring higher academic education, i.e. generally more than 4 years beyond high school), white collar group 3 (other salaried staff, e.g.

office and service workers, nurses, laboratory technicians, pre-school teachers), skilled workers, and unskilled workers. Since both maternal and paternal occupational levels contribute to the socioeconomic environment of the family, one common variable was constructed, using the highest occupational level from either the father or the mother as default [21]. In cases where the father could not be identified, maternal social class was used. Self-employed and individuals outside the workforce constitute two very heterogeneous groups that cannot readily be ranked with respect to socioeconomic position; the latter contains students, unemployed with various skilled background, house wives, and recipients of social security. We therefore included only children with at least one employed parent in the study population. If one parent was self-employed or outside the workforce, socioeconomic status of the employed (not self-employed) parent was used. Accordingly, children for which both parents were self-employed, outside the workforce, or self-employed combined with assisting spouse, were excluded from the study population. In total 730 out of 12,006 boys with cryptorchidism were excluded due to the above criteria. Table 1 presents the social status of the father and mother of the excluded boys.

Geographical region at birth

TTD was assessed by region of birth, i.e. one of 15 Danish counties in existence between 1970 and 2006: Copenhagen, Frederiksborg, Roskilde, Western Zealand, Storstrøm, Bornholm, Funen, Southern Jutland, Ribe, Vejle, Ringkøbing, Aarhus, Viborg, Northern Jutland and the combined municipalities of Copenhagen and Frederiksberg. In essence, the region of birth corresponded to maternal region of living at the time of parturition. This variable was available for more than 99% of all children.

Maternal age at birth of the child

TTD was assessed by maternal age, divided into four categories (<25, 25–29, 30–34, ≥35 years).

Table 1 Exclusion of boys with cryptorchidism when none of the parents were registered as employee

Father	Mother			
	Missing	Not economically active	Self employed	Total
Missing	55	61	3	119
Not economically active	15	298	6	319
Self employed	4	116	172	292
Total	74	475	181	730

Statistical analysis

As stated, the age at principal diagnosis or surgery was used as a proxy for TTD. The detection rate of cryptorchidism (number of detected cases per person-year of in the cohorts of cryptorchid boys) as a function of socio-occupational group, county and maternal age was analysed by use of Poisson regression. Detection Rate Ratios (DRR) were estimated with unskilled manual workers as reference in analysis of socio-occupational status, and Copenhagen County as reference for geographical region. Maternal age at delivery was treated as a categorical variable with less than 25 years of age as reference. The DRR is a measure of relative difference that compares the detection rate of cryptorchidism in the group of interest with the detection rate in the reference group. The analysis was controlled for age of the child (in 1 year classes). Proportional hazards were assumed. Brothers were treated as repeated measurements. A first order autoregressive correlation structure AR(1) was assumed. The DRR estimates were stratified by birth cohort (1981–1987 and 1988–1994). Two-way interaction tests were performed to test whether effects of socio-occupational group, region, and maternal age at birth were independent of birth cohort. Follow-up ended at the time of diagnosis or surgical correction of cryptorchidism. The same statistical procedure was performed for cases with the surgical procedure of orchiopexy. Median TTD was estimated among the boys, by social group and region of birth.

The Poisson regression was performed by use of the GENMOD procedure in the statistical software package SAS version 9.2. The empiric standard error estimates was used. The significance level was set to 0.05.

Results

In the early and the later cohorts, 6,059 and 5,947 boys, respectively, received a diagnosis of cryptorchidism. The mother's personal identification number was missing for 19 of the boys and 730 boys were excluded due to parental occupational status, as described. The remaining 11,276 boys were included in the analysis. DRRs with 95% confidence interval (95% CI) are presented in Table 2.

The effect of socio-occupational group was not statistically significant in any of the birth cohorts (P = 0.15 among the boys born in 1981 – 87; P = 0.85 among the boys born in 1988 – 94).

The detection rates were highly dependent on birth cohort (P < 0.0001). The median TTD decreased from 8.37 years among the boys born 1981– 87 to 5.59 years among the boys born in 1988 – 94. The cumulative distribution of TDD for children in white collar group 1 and in unskilled manual workers by birth cohort is given in Figure 1.

Table 2 Detection rate ratios and median time to detection of cryptorchidism among cryptorchidism cases born in Denmark 1981–1994, by socio-occupational group, birth region and maternal age

	1981-1987				1988-1994			
	N	TTD (years)	DRR	95% CI	N	TTD (years)	DRR	95% CI
Socio-occupational group								
White collar 1	641	8.51	0.97	0.88 - 1.08	757	5.33	0.96	0.87 - 1.07
White collar 2	1112	8.20	1.00	0.92 - 1.08	1083	5.51	0.98	0.90 - 1.07
White collar 3	2203	8.27	1.02	0.95 - 1.09	1842	5.75	0.97	0.90 - 1.04
Skilled manual workers	658	7.92	1.11	1.01 - 1.21	617	5.59	1.00	0.91 - 1.11
Unskilled manual workers	1147	8.37	1.00		1216	5.45	1.00	
County								
Copenhagen (County)	665	7.71	1.00		725	5.43	1.00	
Copenhagen and Frederiksberg municipalities	411	8.03	0.98	0.86 - 1.11	480	5.48	0.95	0.84 - 1.07
Frederiksborg	328	8.89	0.76	0.67 - 0.86	352	5.76	0.95	0.84 - 1.07
Roskilde	220	8.04	0.91	0.78 - 1.07	189	6.45	0.83	0.72 - 0.96
Western Zealand	258	9.63	0.69	0.61 - 0.79	268	6.18	0.90	0.79 - 1.03
Storstrøm	263	8.39	0.75	0.65 - 0.87	286	5.31	1.04	0.90 - 1.21
Bornholm	48	9.58	0.65	0.49 - 0.85	27	5.63	0.90	0.65 - 1.25
Funen	557	7.57	0.92	0.82 - 1.04	546	6.07	0.90	0.81 - 1.00
Southern Jutland	307	8.86	0.76	0.66 - 0.86	266	5.24	1.17	1.02 - 1.34
Ribe	282	7.41	0.95	0.81 - 1.12	242	5.41	1.07	0.92 - 1.23
Vejle	381	8.15	0.86	0.76 - 0.98	335	5.88	0.90	0.79 - 1.03
Ringkøbing	338	8.81	0.77	0.68 - 0.88	319	5.91	0.89	0.78 - 1.02
Aarhus	853	8.06	0.90	0.81 - 1.00	764	5.14	1.07	0.96 - 1.20
Viborg	284	7.34	0.93	0.79 - 1.09	239	5.33	1.01	0.87 - 1.18
Northern Jutland	566	9.03	0.79	0.71 - 0.88	477	6.02	0.83	0.73 - 0.94
Maternal age								
<25	2033	8.24	1.00		1413	5.70	1.00	
25-29	2215	8.22	0.97	0.91 - 1.03	2248	5.46	1.04	0.97 - 1.12
30-34	1150	8.34	1.01	0.94 - 1.09	1391	5.64	0.96	0.89 - 1.04
>35	363	8.40	0.96	0.86 - 1.07	463	5.43	1.07	0.96 - 1.20

TTD: Time to detection (median value). DRR: Detection rate ratios.

Detection rates varied with county (P < 0.0001). The median TTD, by county, ranged from 7.3 to 9.63 years among the boys born 1981 – 87 and from 5.1 to 6.5 years among the boys born 1988 – 94. A statistically significant interaction between birth cohort and county (P < 0.0001) indicated that the effect of county was not constant and that some counties were slow in one period but faster in the other, and vice versa.

Maternal age at delivery was not statistically significantly associated with detection rate in any of the cohorts.

The analysis of orchiopexy was based on 4761 and 3705 boys from the early and later cohort, respectively. Results from this analysis did not challenge any of the statistical conclusions given above. These data are shown in Additional file 1: Table S1.

Discussion and conclusions

The present study investigated the influence of socio-occupational class, geographical region and maternal age on time to detection of cryptorchidism. Rate of detection was independent of socio-occupational group in both birth cohorts. In fact, the cumulative distribution of TTD of cryptorchidism in children of employed parents in white collar group 1 almost exactly matched that in children of unskilled manual workers. There was no indication of a change in the influence of socio-occupational group between boys born 1981 to 1987 and 1988 to 1994. Detection rates did, however, vary between geographical regions. A similar pattern were obtained for surgical correction after a diagnosis.

These findings indicate that inequality in childhood socio-occupational status does not influence time to

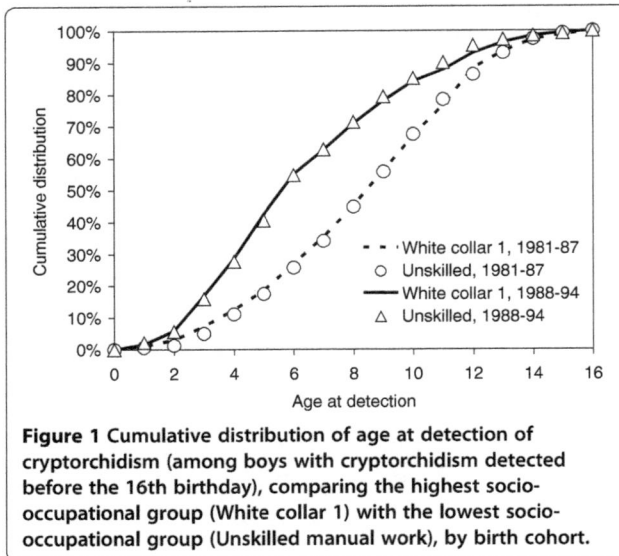

Figure 1 Cumulative distribution of age at detection of cryptorchidism (among boys with cryptorchidism detected before the 16th birthday), comparing the highest socio-occupational group (White collar 1) with the lowest socio-occupational group (Unskilled manual work), by birth cohort.

detection and correction of cryptorchidism in Denmark. The overall tendency of non-adherence to routine prophylactic visits by parents of low social classes thus seem to have only minor impact, if any, on the diagnosis and treatment of cryptorchidism [8,9]. It has, however, been shown, that although low income and education predict fewer contacts with specialist care, this may not be so for hospital referral. Actually, patients of low socioeconomic status may be referred relatively more frequently to hospital care than patients of high status [24,25]. This may somewhat compensate the less frequent use of preventive examinations in childhood at the general practitioners. Furthermore, detection of cryptorchidism does not entirely depend on visits at the general practitioner; A trained nurse specialised in child and family health care provides home visits following childbirth [11], and school-aged boys regularly attend the school nurse during the years of primary and lower secondary school in Denmark.

Some 7-20% of cryptorchidism cases cannot be detected at birth, and are said to be acquired [26,27]. Our study therefore implicitly assumes that potential differences in the incidence of acquired cryptorchidism have a negligible influence on the calculated rate ratios (including both congenital and acquired cryptorchidism). Knowledge about risk factors specific to acquired cryptorchidism is lacking but most cases of cryptorchidism, including acquired cases, are believed to occur due to prenatal causes [28]. We cannot rule out that the prevalence of acquired cryptorchidism differs by socio-occupational group, but the time-lag to detection of acquired cases may likely be similar to that of congenital cases; parents and general practitioners who act fast on congenital cryptorchidism may likely also act fast on acquired cryptorchidism. Taken together, we consider bias

due to an uneven distribution of acquired cryptorchidism (if present) unlikely.

We observed shorter TTD in the more recent 1988–1994 cohort compared with the 1981–87 cohort. Median TTD decreased by more than 2.5 years (33%) between cohorts. This is in accordance with a similar trend in complete 1995–2009 birth cohorts [9]. Here mean age at diagnosis, when followed for 6 years, decreased from 3.3 years for boys born 1995 to 1997, to 2.9 years for children born 2001 to 2003 [9]. Collectively these data suggest a steadily decreasing median age at diagnosis and surgery throughout the period from 1981 to 2009. In addition, we observed a reduced variance in mean TTD between counties over time; in the 1981–87 cohort the difference between the fastest and slowest county was 2.5 years (mean TTD) and in the 1988–1994 cohort it was 1.3 years. This may indicate a more similar approach to cryptorchidism in all counties in the more recent cohort, as this difference decreased relatively (48%) more than the reduction in time to detection between cohorts. Among small children a difference in mean TTD of, e.g., one year may likely be clinically relevant [1,2]. Geographical region may therefore have exerted some influence on cryptorchid boys' fertility later in life, especially in the oldest cohort.

The time to detection of cryptorchidism may be quite long. In the oldest cohort, 5% of the diagnosed cases remained to be found at the age of 16 years compared to the (full) follow-up of 30 years. In the most recent cohort, an even more complete follow-up would be expected to have occurred after 16 years, based on observations of the shift towards earlier diagnosis of cryptorchidism in recent years [9]. Follow-up was sufficient for almost complete case ascertainment. This allowed us to estimate the rates of diagnosis (time to detection) in different socio-occupational groups during the period of follow-up without bias from the total incidence [9,29]. Furthermore, the observed similar time to detection pattern in various socio-occupational groups allows for study of prevalence ratios of cryptorchidism across socio-occupational groups using a much shorter follow-up than in the present study.

The strengths of this study include diagnostic registry data based on standardised diagnostic reporting procedures and diagnosis by specialised hospital physicians [17]. The sample size was large and based on administrative registries of high quality with information on all Danish citizens, follow-up was almost complete, and a common coding system for socio-occupational class was used for all parents. The population based prospective birth cohort approach ensued that bias due to self-selection into the study was negligible, and e.g. language barriers were overcome. Boys, whose parents were both outside the workforce, students, self-employed or any combination hereof, were, however, not included. In total, 6% of the cryptorchid boys were excluded on these grounds. Our analyses do therefore not permit specific conclusions regarding boys from families where both parents were unemployed etc. High risk of delayed treatment in these non-participating groups seems unlikely, based on the almost exact match in age at detection of cryptorchidism between the most extreme socio-occupational groups in our study, but it cannot be ruled out completely.

The accuracy of the cryptorchidism diagnosis and surgery has been validated, based on review of a subset of medical records from 452 children born between 1995 and 2009 with a registry diagnosis of cryptorchidism, of which 249 underwent orchiopexy. The overall positive predictive value of a cryptorchidism diagnosis was 80%, and it was 99% for corrective surgery [17]. These children were born shortly after closure of our cohorts, and diagnoses were according to ICD-10. Otherwise this validation was performed on data with similar characteristics as in the present study.

In our oldest cohort, diagnosis and surgery were given on the same day for approximately half of the boys. In the younger cohort, less than 15% presented with diagnosis and orchiopexy on the same day. Until 1995, only inpatient diagnoses were available in the Danish National Patient Registry, where after also diagnoses for hospital outpatients became accessible. Inpatient admissions generally correspond to overnight hospital stays or daily hospital visits over an extended period, whereas outpatient admissions correspond to visits at hospital clinics on a less regular basis [29]. Most likely the diagnoses were given when the boys became inpatients due to surgery in the older cohort, whereas in the youngest cohort diagnoses were probably given already upon diagnostic consultation as outpatient. This may have contributed to the shift towards lower age at detection (diagnosis) in the younger cohort, but would not affect time to orchiopexy (which showed similar results).

We investigated effects of social status and geographical region in time to detection of cryptorchidism. Our findings indicate that childhood socio-occupational inequality in time to detection and correction of cryptorchidism would play a negligible role in male infertility in a life course perspective, which is reassuring from a public health perspective. Neither did we observe any association with maternal age. However, geographical region may have exerted some influence, especially for the oldest cohort.

Competing interests
The authors declare that they have no competing interests.

Authors' contributions
KSH prepared the first protocol and manuscript together with HHA who conceived the idea and furthermore designed and performed the statistical analysis. KSH, HHA, ADL and MS contrived the coupling of data. Protocols and manuscripts were modified and adapted by ADL, MS, AMNA, KJ, GT and JPB. All authors read and approved the final manuscript.

Acknowledgements
The study is part of the Danish collaborative MINERVA project (www.minervanet.dk) addressing occupational risks to human reproduction, supported by a grant from the Danish Working Environment Research Fund (grant 20080016458).

Author details
[1]The National Research Centre for the Working Environment, Lersø Parkallé 105, DK-2100 Copenhagen, Denmark. [2]Department of Occupational Medicine, Aarhus University Hospital, Aarhus, Denmark. [3]Department of Public Health, University of Copenhagen, Copenhagen, Denmark. [4]Department of Occupational and Environmental Medicine, Bispebjerg Hospital, Copenhagen University Hospital, Copenhagen, Denmark. [5]Perinatal Epidemiology Research Unit, Department of Paediatrics, Aarhus University Hospital, Aarhus, Denmark.

References
1. Canavese F, Mussa A, Manenti M, Cortese MG, Ferrero L, Tuli G, Macchieraldo R, Lala R: Sperm count of young men surgically treated for cryptorchidism in the first and second year of life: fertility is better in children treated at a younger age. Eur J Pediatr Surg 2009, 19:388–391.
2. Kollin C, Karpe B, Hesser U, Granholm T, Ritzen EM: Surgical treatment of unilaterally undescended testes: testicular growth after randomization to orchiopexy at age 9 months or 3 years. J Urol 2007, 178:1589–1593.
3. Huff DS, Fenig DM, Canning DA, Carr MG, Zderic SA, Snyder HM III: Abnormal germ cell development in cryptorchidism. Horm Res 2001, 55:11–17.
4. Ritzen EM, Bergh A, Bjerknes R, Christiansen P, Cortes D, Haugen SE, Jorgensen N, Kollin C, Lindahl S, Lackgren G, et al: Nordic consensus on treatment of undescended testes. Acta Paediatr 2007, 96:638–643.
5. Freeman HP, Chu KC: Determinants of cancer disparities: barriers to cancer screening, diagnosis, and treatment. Surg Oncol Clin N Am 2005, 14:655–669. v.
6. Kataoka-Yahiro MR, Munet-Vilaro F: Barriers to preventive health care for young children. J Am Acad Nurse Pract 2002, 14:66–72.
7. Chung JM, Lee CY, Kang DG, Kim JS, Cho WY, Cho BM, Lee SD: Parental perception of optimal surgical age for correction of cryptorchidism: a multicenter surveillance study. Urology 2011, 78:1162–1166.
8. Sondergaard G, Biering-Sorensen S, Michelsen SI, Schnor O, Andersen AM: Non-participation in preventive child health examinations at the general practitioner in Denmark: a register-based study. Scand J Prim Health Care 2008, 26:5–11.
9. Jensen MS, Olsen LH, Thulstrup AM, Bonde JP, Olsen J, Henriksen TB: Age at cryptorchidism diagnosis and orchiopexy in Denmark: a population based study of 508,964 boys born from 1995 to 2009. J Urol 2011, 186:1595–1600.
10. Michelsen SI, Kastanje M, Flachs EM, Søndergaard G, Biering-Sorensen S, Madsen M, Andersen A-MN: Evaluering af de forebyggende børneundersøgelser i almen praksis. Copenhagen: Sundhedsstyrelsen; 2007:1–163.
11. Olejaz M, Juul NA, Rudkjobing A, Okkels BH, Krasnik A, Hernandez-Quevedo C: Denmark health system review. Health Syst Transit 2012, 14:i-192.
12. Soll-Johanning H, Hannerz H, Tuchsen F: Referral bias in hospital register studies of geographical and industrial differences in health. Dan Med Bull 2004, 51:207–210.
13. Paananen R, Santalahti P, Merikukka M, Ramo A, Wahlbeck K, Gissler M: Socioeconomic and regional aspects in the use of specialized psychiatric

care–a Finnish nationwide follow-up study. *Eur J Public Health* 2013, **23**:372–377.

14. Jensen MS, Toft G, Thulstrup AM, Henriksen TB, Olsen J, Christensen K, Bonde JP: Cryptorchidism concordance in monozygotic and dizygotic twin brothers, full brothers, and half-brothers. *Fertil Steril* 2010, **93**:124–129.

15. Pedersen CB: The Danish Civil Registration System. *Scand J Public Health* 2011, **39**:22–25.

16. Lynge E, Sandegaard JL, Rebolj M: The Danish National Patient Register. *Scand J Public Health* 2011, **39**:30–33.

17. Jensen MS, Snerum TM, Olsen LH, Thulstrup AM, Bonde JP, Olsen J, Henriksen TB: Accuracy of cryptorchidism diagnoses and corrective surgical treatment registration in the Danish National Patient Registry. *J Urol* 2012, **188**:1324–1329.

18. The Chemical Manufacturers Association's Epidemiology Task Group: Guidelines for Good Epidemiology Practices for Occupational and Environmental Epidemiologic Research. *J Occup Med* 1991, **33**:1221–1229.

19. Blenstrup LT, Knudsen LB: Danish registers on aspects of reproduction. *Scand J Public Health* 2011, **39**:79–82.

20. Varela MM, Nohr EA, Llopis-Gonzalez A, Andersen AM, Olsen J: Socio-occupational status and congenital anomalies. *Eur J Public Health* 2009, **19**:161–167.

21. Morgen CS, Mortensen LH, Rasmussen M, Andersen AM, Sorensen TI, Due P: Parental socioeconomic position and development of overweight in adolescence: longitudinal study of Danish adolescents. *BMC Public Health* 2010, **10**:520.

22. Statistics Denmark: *Beskrivelse af NYSTGR og sammenhæng til SOCIO og DISCOALLE_INDK.* Copenhagen: Statistics Denmark; 2010:1–3.

23. Statistics Denmark: *Stillingsgruppering 1980–1995 - NYSTGR.* Copenhagen: Statistics Denmark. http://www.dst.dk/tilsalg/forskningsservice/ Dokumentation/hkt4forsker/hkt4_variabel_liste_forsker/hkt4_variabel.aspx? fk=107191. Downloaded May 2013.

24. Sorensen TH, Olsen KR, Vedsted P: Association between general practice referral rates and patients' socioeconomic status and access to specialised health care a population-based nationwide study. *Health Policy* 2009, **92**:180–186.

25. Halldorsson M, Kunst AE, Kohler L, Mackenbach JP: Socioeconomic differences in children's use of physician services in the Nordic countries. *J Epidemiol Community Health* 2002, **56**:200–204.

26. Wohlfahrt-Veje C, Boisen KA, Boas M, Damgaard IN, Kai CM, Schmidt IM, Chellakooty M, Suomi AM, Toppari J, Skakkebaek NE, *et al*: Acquired cryptorchidism is frequent in infancy and childhood. *Int J Androl* 2009, **32**:423–428.

27. Meij-de VA, Hack WW, Heij HA, Meijer RW: Perioperative surgical findings in congenital and acquired undescended testis. *J Pediatr Surg* 2010, **45**:1874–1881.

28. Hack WW, Goede J, van der Voort-Doedens LM, Meijer RW: Acquired undescended testis: putting the pieces together. *Int J Androl* 2012, **35**:41–45.

29. Parner ET, Schendel DE, Thorsen P: Autism prevalence trends over time in Denmark: changes in prevalence and age at diagnosis. *Arch Pediatr Adolesc Med* 2008, **162**:1150–1156.

11

Overexpression of NIMA-related kinase 2 is associated with progression and poor prognosis of prostate cancer

Yan-Ru Zeng[1†], Zhao-Dong Han[2†], Cong Wang[3†], Chao Cai[1], Ya-Qiang Huang[1], Hong-Wei Luo[1], Ze-Zhen Liu[2], Yang-Jia Zhuo[1,5], Qi-Shan Dai[1], Hai-Bo Zhao[4], Yu-Xiang Liang[2,7*] and Wei-De Zhong[1,2,5,6,7*]

Abstract

Background: The NIMA-related kinase 2 (NEK2) is a serine/threonine kinase that is involved in regulation of centrosome duplication and spindle assembly during mitosis. Dysregulation of these processes causes chromosome instability and aneuploidy, which are hallmark changes of many solid tumors. However, whether aberrant expression of NEK2 is associated with outcome of prostate cancer (PCa) patients remains to be determined.

Methods: Expression of NEK2 in human PCa cells and primary PCa tissues was assessed by quantitative RT-PCR. Expression of NEK2 in human PCa cells was depleted with siRNA. Effects of the depletion on cell proliferation, survival, and tumorigenicity were assessed both *in vitro* with cell cultures and *in vivo* with subcutaneous implantation of xenografts. *In silico* analyses of the online Taylor dataset were carried out to determine whether the expression level of NEK2 correlated with the clinicopathological characteristics of prostate cancer.

Results: Compared with benign human prostatic epithelial cells and tissues, the expression of NEK2 was elevated in human PCa cells and primary PCa tissues. Depleting NEK2 expression inhibited human PCa cell proliferation *in vitro* and xenograft growth *in vivo*. Expression level of NEK2 in PCa positively correlated with the Gleason score and pathologic stage of the patient.

Conclusion: The results suggest that overexpression of NEK2 has the potential to serve as a biomarker for PCa prognosis. Further validation with large sample pool is warrant.

Background

The centrosome is the primary site of microtubule nucleation in cells, which plays a critical role in mitotic spindle formation and chromosome segregation [1, 2]. Normally, cells enter mitosis with two properly duplicated centrosomes. The process ensures bipolarity and correct axial positioning of the spindle. However, cancer cells often exhibit multipolar spindles associating with abnormal centrosome numbers or architectures [3–5]. A number of cell cycle-regulated protein kinases located at the centrosomes have been identified, which are required

for mitotic progression and correct bipolar spindle formation [6]. Among them is NIMA-related kinase 2 (NEK2) that has three alternative splice isoforms (NEK2A, NEK2B and NEK2C). The expression of these three isoforms is tightly regulated in a cell cycle-dependent manner, suggesting that they may have isoform-specific roles in mitosis [7, 8].

NEK2 is a constitutive active serine and threonine kinase that phosphorylates multiple proteins involved in centrosome duplication and cell cycle regulation. It binds to microtubules and is enriched in the centrosome, where it contributes to centrosome splitting during the G2/M phase of the cell cycle [9]. Aberrant NEK2 activities cause failure in regulating centrosome duplication, resulting aneuploidy, and, therefore, are oncogenic [10]. Increased NEK2 expression causes premature splitting of centrosomes in human cells. Expression of a kinase-dead mutant of NEK2 induces centrosome abnormalities and

---

* Correspondence: doctorbaby@126.com; zhongwd2009@live.cn
†Equal contributors
2Department of Urology, Guangdong Key Laboratory of Clinical Molecular Medicine and Diagnostics, Guangzhou First People's Hospital, Guangzhou Medical University, Guangzhou 510180, China
1Guangdong Provincial Institute of Nephrology, Southern Medical University, Guangzhou 510515, China
Full list of author information is available at the end of the article

aneuploidy [11, 12]. Similar to other kinases that are involved in spindle assembly or duplication, overexpression of NEK2 has been reported in several neoplastic diseases, such as preinvasive and invasive breast carcinomas [10], lung adenocarcinomas [13], testicular seminomas [14], and diffuse large B cell lymphomas [15]. Overexpression of NEK2 in non-transformed breast epithelial cells induces over duplication of the centrosome [10]. Increased expression of NEK2 causes centrosome amplification in breast cancer cells that express oncogenic K-RAS [16]. Furthermore, NEK2-dependent phosphorylation is required for kinetochore localizations of HEC1, a protein essential for faithful chromosome segregation [17]. In addition, NEK2 is also involved in regulation of viability and apoptosis. Depletion of NEK2 sensitizes HeLa cells to apoptosis and induces alternative splice of SRSF1 target genes [18].

Although a large number of data demonstrate elevated expression as well as reduced stability of NEK2 in cancer cells, whether NEK2 upregulation plays a role in PCa is not clearly. In this study, we investigated expression patterns of NEK2 in tissue microarrays (TMAs) of human PCa and the effect of NEK2 depletion on cell proliferation in PCa cells. The data showed strong correlation of NEK2 expression with the prognostic outcome of PCa patients. Together, our results indicate that NEK2 has a promising value for predicting outcome of PCa recurrence. Future studies with large sample pools are warranted to determine whether the expression level of NEK2 can serve as a biomarkers for PCa prognosis, which still needs prospective validation.

Methods

Patients and tissue samples

The study was approved by the Research Ethics Committee of Guangzhou First People's Hospital, Guangzhou Medical University, China. An informed consent was obtained from all of the patients. All specimens were handled and remained anonymous according to the ethical and legal standards.

For immunohistochemistry analyses, TMAs with detail clinical information were purchased from Shanghai Outdo Biotech Co, LTD (Cat#: HPro-Ade180PG-01), which includes 99 primary PCa tissues and 81 adjacent non-cancerous prostate tissues from patients without chemotherapy or radiotherapy before surgery. The Taylor dataset (http://www.ncbi.nlm.nih.gov/geo/query/acc.cgi?acc=GSE21032) contains microarray data for mRNAs from 149 primary PCa tissues and 29 adjacent noncancerous prostate tissues [19]. The dataset contains patient survival time and follow-up examination between from 1 to 175 months with a median of 51 months postsurgery. The date of prostatectomy was considered as day 1 for the survival analyses. The PSA recurrence was defined as three successive PSA rises (final value >0.2 ng/ml), single PSA >0.4 ng/ml, or use of secondary therapy administered for detectable PSA >0.1 ng/ml, which was considered as the biochemical recurrence-free endpoint. The overall survival that was determined from the date of surgery to the time of the last follow-up or death.

Cell culture, transfection, and treatment

For cell viability assays, human PCa LNCaP cells were seeded in 96-well plates (2×10^3/well) and cultured for 24, 48, and 72 h. Cells were then incubated with 20 µl CCK-8 solution (Cat No: C0038, Beyotime, China) for 4 h at 37 °C. The absorbance was measured at the wavelength of 495 nm with a spectrophotometer. Data were expressed as mean ± SD of three independent samples. For RNA interference experiments, cells were transfected with siRNAs using Lipofectamine RNAi-MAX (Invitrogen) according to manufacturer's instructions and harvested at 24, 48, and 72 h after the transfection for protein and RNA analyses. Sequences of NEK2 siRNAs and scrambled siRNA are listed in Table 1.

Quantitative real-time RT-PCR

Total RNAs were isolated from cells and prostate tissues using the TRIzol reagent (Invitrogen, Carlsbad, CA, USA) according to the manufacturer's instructions. Reverse transcription was carried out using the ReverTra Ace reagents kit (TOYOBO, Osaka, Japan). Real-time RT-PCR was carried out with the MiniOpticon real-time PCR detection system (Bio-Rad, Hercules, CA, USA) using the SYBR Green master mix (TaKaRa, Otsu, Japan). The thermal cycling conditions comprised of one cycle at 94 °C for 4 min, 40 cycles at 94 °C for 15 s, 60 °C for 15 s, and 72 °C for 15 s. All data were analyzed using the Opticon Monitor software (ver3.1, Bio-Rad). The expression of NEK2 was calculated as relative expression level to the GAPDH internal control using the comparative cycle threshold (CT) method. The primer sequences for NEK2 are GCTTAGGTAGCCCTTTTCATTTACA and GCCTCAGGTCTATGAACCCAG. The primer sequences for GAPDH are CATGGGTGTGAACCATGAGAAGT and ACAGTAGAGGCAGGGATGATGTTCT.

Table 1 Sequences of the tested NEK2 siRNA targets

siRNA	mRNA target
Scr	ATAGTTCGTCCACTTCAGC
NEK2 .1	CGGAGGAAGAGTGATGGCAAGATAT
NEK2 .2	GAAGTGATGGTGGTCATACCGTATT
NEK2 .3	GCTGTATGAGTTATGTGCATTAATG

Western blotting analysis

Proteins were extracted 48-hours post-transfection for Western blot analyses. Proteins (40 µg) were fractioned on SDS-PAGE and transferred onto Hybond nitrocellulose membranes (GE Healthcare). The membranes were blocked with 5 % skim milk in PBS-Tween 20 and probed with anti-NEK2 (bs-5732R, Bioss Co Ltd., China) or anti-β-actin antibody (sc-47778, Santa Cruz, USA). The specifically bound antibodies were detected with horse radish peroxidase-conjugated secondary antibody and visualized with the SuperSignal West PICO Chemiluminescent Detection Kit (Pierce Biotechnology). β-actin was used as an internal loading control.

Tumor growth

All nude mice with an average age of 6–8 weeks were purchased from the Guangdong Medical Laboratory Animal Center. The NEK2 silenced cells were injected on the left side flank and the control cells on the right side flank. Briefly, 2×10^6 cells were suspended in 0.1 ml culture medium, and then mixed with Matrigel (BD Biosciences,NO.356234) at the ratio of 1:1. The injections were carried out in a sterilized hood. Five mice per group were used and the experiments were repeated three times. The tumor size was measured with caliper at three time points and the means were

calculated. The tumor tissues were harvested at day 43 after the implantation for histology and biochemistry analyses.

Immunohistochemistry analysis

The specimens were fixed in 10 % neutral buffered formalin and subsequently embedded in paraffin. The paraffin-embedded tissues were sectioned at 4 µm thickness and then deparaffinized with xylene and rehydrated for subsequence analyses. For immunohistochemistry staining, the sections were subjected to a brief proteolytic digestion and a peroxidase blocking, the sections were incubated overnight with the primary antibody against NEK2 at a dilution of 1:400, at 4 °C. After washing, the sections were then incubated with peroxidase labeled polymer and substrate–chromogen from DAKO EnVision System (Dako Diagnostics, Switzerland) to detect the specifically bound antibodies as suggested by the manufacturer. No primary antibodies were used as the negative controls. The sections were then lightly counterstained with hematoxylin. The staining was scored by two independent experienced pathologists, who were blinded to the clinicopathological data and clinical outcomes of the patients. The scores of the two pathologists were compared. Any discrepant scores were trained through re-examining the staining by both pathologists to achieve a consensus

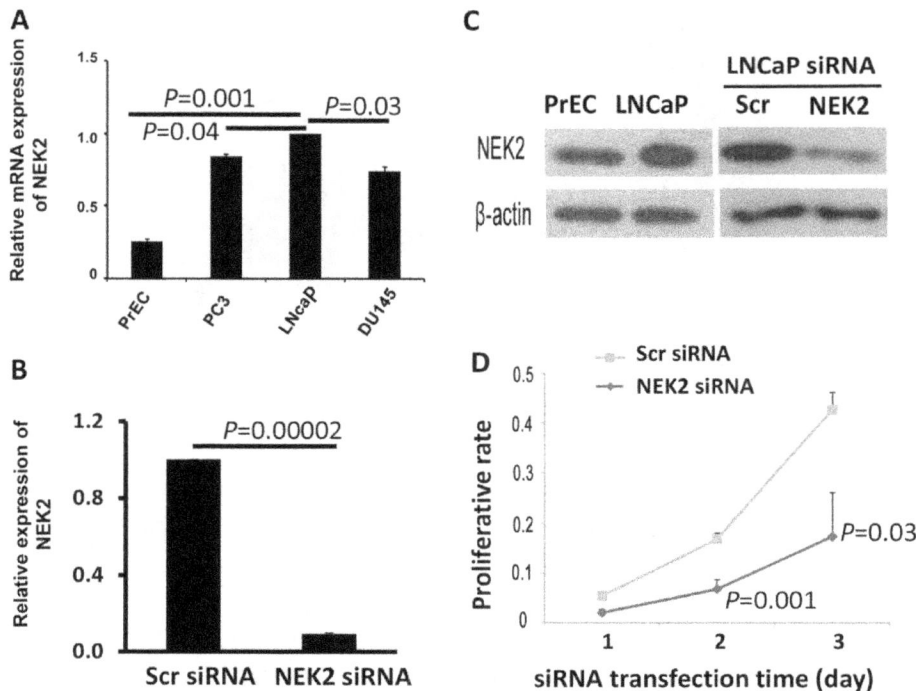

Fig. 1 NEK2 expression and function in prostate epithelial cell lines. **a** & **b** Real-time RT-PCR analyses of NEK2 expression in benign human prostatic epithelial cells and PCa cells (**a**) or NEK2-depleted LNCaP cells. **c** Western blot analysis for NEK2 protein expression in PrEC and siRNA treated LNCaP cells. **d** Proliferation analyses of LNCaP cells with or without depletion of NEK2

score. The number of positive-staining cells in ten representative microscopic fields was counted, and the percentage of positive cells was calculated. The staining was subjected to arbitrative categorized to 5 groups based on the percentage of positive cells for semi-quantitative analyses as following: 0 (0 %), 1 (1–10 %), 2 (11–50 %), 3 (51–80 %) and 4 (>80 %). The staining intensity was visually scored and stratified as follows: 0 (negative), 1 (weak), 2 (moderate) and 3 (strong). A

final immunoreactivity scores (IRS) were obtained for each case by adding the percentage and the intensity score [20, 21].

Statistical analysis

The statistical analyses was carried out with the SPSS software (Version 13.0 for Windows, SPSS Inc., IL, USA) and SAS 9.1 (SAS Institute, Cary, NC, USA). Continuous variables were expressed as mean ± SD. The

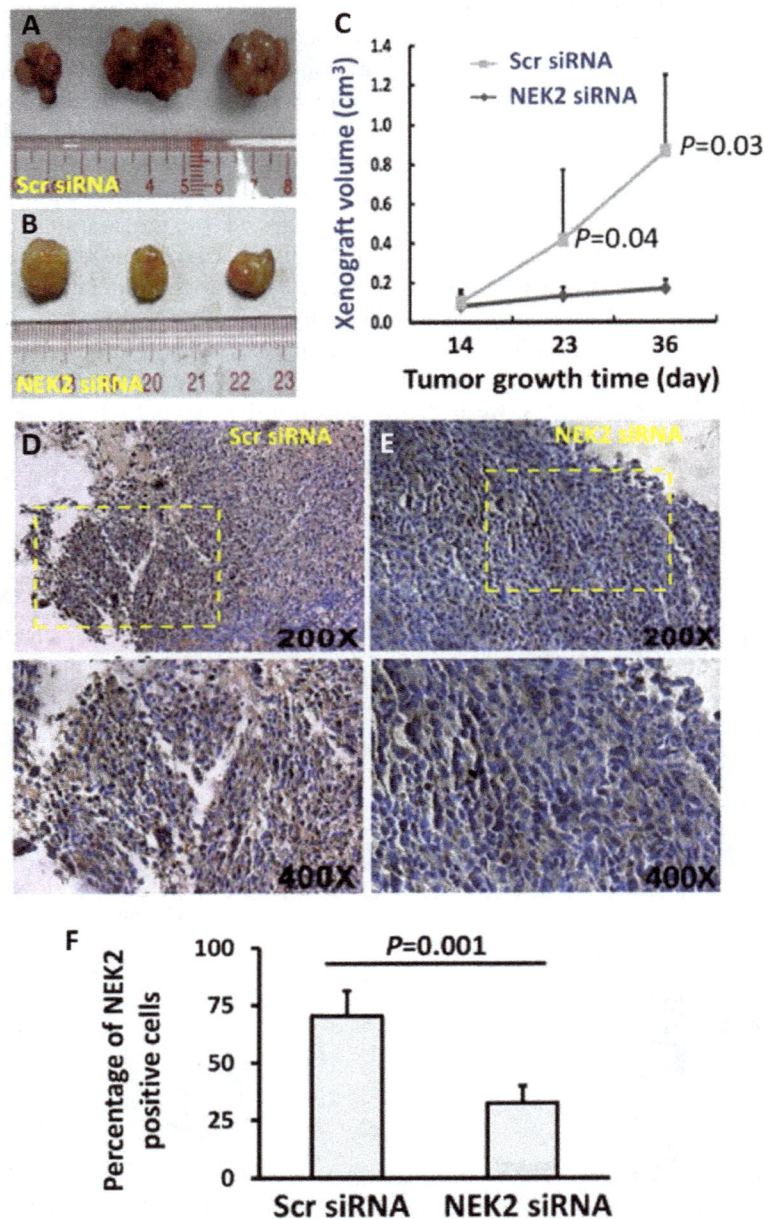

Fig. 2 Depletion of NEK2 by siRNA inhibits the growth of LNCaP subcutaneous xenograft growth in nude mice. **a** & **b** Representative images of LNCaP xenografts. **c** Tumor growth curves of LNCaP xenografts. **d** & **e** Immunostaining of NEK2 in LNCaP xenografts. The figure magnification is × 200 and × 400, respectively. **f** Statistical analysis of the NEK2 positive cells in the immunostaining

Kaplan–Meier method was used for the survival analyses and a log-rank test was used to analyze the difference of survival. The chiquest trend test was used for ordinal data analysis. Differences were considered statistically significant when *P* was smaller than 0.05.

Results

Depleting NEK2 expression reduces cell proliferation in PCa cells

To determine whether human PCa cells had aberrant NEK2 expression at the mRNA level, quantitative real-time RT-PCR was performed to assess the expression of NEK2 in three human PCa and one benign human prostatic epithelial cell lines. As shown in Fig. 1a, expression of NEK2 was higher in all three PCa cells than in benign human prostatic epithelial cells at the mRNA level, especially in LNCaP cell line. Then we chose LNCaP cells for the further study to determine whether high expression of NEK2 contributed to cell proliferation, siRNA was used to deplete the expression of NEK2 in LNCaP cells. Both real time RT-PCR and Western blot analyses showed that the expression of NEK2 was reduced at both mRNA and protein levels (Fig. 1b&c). Cell proliferation assays demonstrated that LNCaP cells with NEK2

depletion had a lower proliferation rate than the cells transfected with scramble siRNAs (Fig. 1d). The results suggest that high expression of NEK2 promotes cell proliferation.

Depletion of NEK2 expression suppresses tumorigenicity of LNCaP cells

To determine whether depletion of NEK2 affected the tumorigenicity of LNCaP cells, the silenced and control cells were implanted to the flanks of the same mice. The tumor sizes were measured at day 14, 23, and 36 post the implantation. It was apparent that tumors derived from NEK2 silenced cells were smaller than those from control cells (Fig. 2a, b&c). The tumors were harvested at day 43 after the implantation for further analyses. In addition to smaller size, the tumors with NEK2 silenced cells were relatively pale than the tumors from control cells (Fig. 2b). Immunostaining revealed that expression of NEK2 protein was reduced compared with the tumors derived from scramble siRNA transfected control cells. High magnification images showed that nuclear and cytosol staining of NEK2 staining was visible in control cells, but was absent in NEK2 depleted cells (Fig. 2d&e). The percentage of NEK2 positive

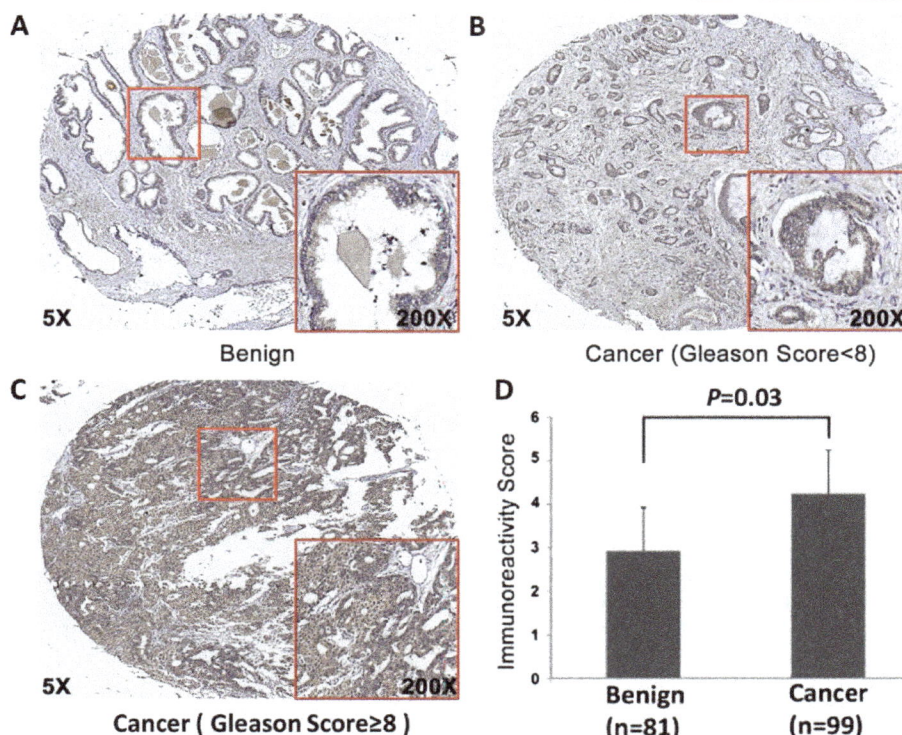

Fig. 3 Immunohistochemical staining for NEK2 expression in PCa and adjacent non-cancerous tissues (original magnification × 50). **a** Benign prostate tissue. **b** PCa with a Gleason score <8. **c** PCa with a Gleason score ≥8. **d** statistical analyses showing higher immunoreactivity scores in cancerous tissues than in adjacent non-cancerous tissues. (IRS: Ca = 4.25 ± 1.36 vs Benign = 2.93 ± 1.51, *P* =0.03). **a**, **b**, and **c** were from TMA sample NO. A5, J8, and H8, respectively

cells was dramatically decreased in NEK2 siRNA group (Fig. 2f).

The expression level of NEK2 is associated with the clinicopathological characteristics of PCa and tumor recurrence time of PCa patients

We then analyzed the expression pattern and localization of NEK2 in a PCa TMA comprised of 99 PCa and 81 adjacent non-cancerous prostate tissues by immunohistochemistry staining. Representative pictures of immunohistochemistry staining of NEK2 are shown in Fig. 3a-c. NEK2 immunostaining was weak or undetectable in adjacent noncancerous prostate tissues (Fig. 3a). In contrast, strong staining of NEK2 was readily seen in the cytoplasm and nucleus of PCa tissues (Fig. 3b-c). A summary of NEK2 immunostaining in PCa tissues was shown in Table 2. Apparently, the PCa with a Gleason Score ≥8 had higher NEK2 expression than those with a Gleason Score <8. In addition, the PCa at high pathological stages showed increased NEK2 expression compared with PCa at low pathological stages. Moreover, statistical analyses of the Taylor dataset also showed that PCa with a Gleason Score ≥ 8 had higher expression of NEK2 than those with a Gleason Score <8 ($P = 0.011$) at the mRNA level. In addition, overexpression

of NEK2 was also associated with metastasis, PSA failure, and overall survival time of patient, although no correlation between NEK2 expression at the mRNA level and pathological stages was seen in the Taylor dataset (Table 2).

We then use the Kaplan–Meier method to analyze the association of NEK2 expression levels with the biochemical recurrence-free time and the overall survival time of PCa patients. The median of NEK2 expression in all PCa tissues of the Taylor dataset was used as the cutoff to divide all PCa tissues into high ($n = 80$) and low ($n = 80$) NEK2 expression groups. As shown in Fig. 4, the biochemical recurrence-free time of PCa patients with high NEK2 expression levels was shorter than those with low NEK2 expression levels. However, no correlation of the overall survival time of PCa patients with NEK2 expression levels was seen.

Discussion

PCa affects one in nine men over the age of 65 and is the most frequently diagnosed cancer in American males [22, 23]. Early diagnosis through detection of serum prostate specific antigen (PSA) and improved procedures for surgical intervention and radiation therapy have significantly reduced the number of fatalities [24–27].

Table 2 Association of NEK2 expression with the clinicopathological characteristics of prostate cancer

Clinical feature	IRS of NEK2 in our cohort			NEK2 expression in Taylor dataset		
	Case	$\bar{X} \pm s$	p	Case	$\bar{X} \pm s$	p
Age(years)						
<71 years	85	3.67 ± 1.43	0.904	146	7.54 ± 0.29	0.717
≥71 years	95	3.64 ± 1.70		4	7.48 ± 0.26	
Serum PSA						
<4 (ng/ml)	-	-	-	24	7.58 ± 0.32	0.440
≥4 (ng/ml)	-	-		123	7.53 ± 0.29	
Gleason score						
<8	70	3.81 ± 1.08	<0.001	117	7.48 ± 0.25	0.011
≥8	28	5.36 ± 1.39		22	7.71 ± 0.37	
Pathological Stage						
T2	70	3.81 ± 1.08	<0.001	86	7.48 ± 0.23	0.063
T3	29	5.31 ± 1.39		55	7.58 ± 0.35	
Metastasis						
No	99	4.25 ± 1.35	-	122	7.47 ± 0.25	<0.001
Yes	0	-		28	7.81 ± 0.33	
Overall survival						
Alive	-	-	-	131	7.51 ± 0.27	0.086
Die	-	-		19	7.68 ± 0.38	
PSA failure						
Negative	-	-	-	104	7.46 ± 0.25	<0.001
Positive	-	-		36	7.66 ± 0.31	

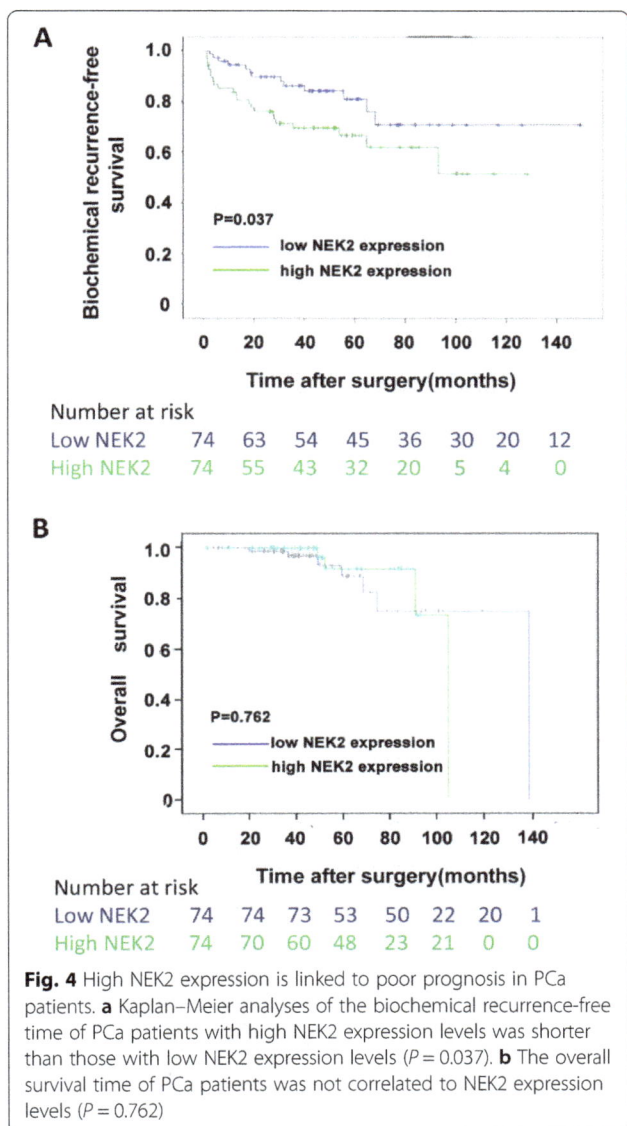

Fig. 4 High NEK2 expression is linked to poor prognosis in PCa patients. **a** Kaplan–Meier analyses of the biochemical recurrence-free time of PCa patients with high NEK2 expression levels was shorter than those with low NEK2 expression levels (*P* = 0.037). **b** The overall survival time of PCa patients was not correlated to NEK2 expression levels (*P* = 0.762)

need further investigation to elucidate. The expression level of NEK2 was associated with the clinicopathological characteristics of PCa and tumor recurrence time of PCa patients. However, analyses of Taylor dataset revealed no statistical difference of NEK2 expression at the mRNA level in different pathological PCa group. Therefore, post translational modification of NEK is likely account for the differential expression of NEK proteins in normal prostate and PCa cells and tissues.

Aberrant NEK2 activity has been documented in multiple malignancies, including pediatric Ewing's sarcoma, follicular lymphoma (FL), diffuse large B cell lymphoma (DLBCL), mammary gland tumor, leukemia, cervical, ovarian, breast cancers [10, 15, 16, 29–33].tumori Previous studies have shown that NEK2 contributes to assembly and maintenance of centrosomes and to bipolar spindle formation [12, 34, 35]. Therefore, inappropriately high expression of NEK2 might interfere with either centrosome integrity or chromosome segregation. However, the underlying cause for the increase in NEK2 expression is still unclear. This has led to a hypothesis that deregulation of centrosome function could be a major contributory factor to the genetic instability and loss of tissue differentiation that drive most cancer progression. Similar findings from other study indicate that aberrant expression and activity of NEK2 drive the progression and transformation of lymphomas that ultimately causes a more aggressive disease [31]. Specifically, overexpression of NEK2 in the ARP-1 multiple myeloma cells causes reduced treatment efficacy of bortezomib, doxorubicin, and etoposide [28]. Downregulation of NEK2 by shRNA inhibited myeloma cell growth and decreased drug resistance *in vitro* and in NOD-Rag/null gamma mice [19]. Paclitaxel and doxorubicin in combination with Nek2 siRNA or ASO treatment promote breast cancer cell apoptosis [36].

In summary, we reported that NEK2 was highly expressed in PCa cells and tissues. Depletion of NEK2 inhibited proliferation and tumorigenicity of the cells. In addition, expression of NEK2 was associated with poor outcome of PCa patients. Thus, the expression level of NEK2 has the potential for predicting PCa progression. A large study with more patient pool is warranted to determine whether expression of NEK2 can serve as a biomarker for PCa diagnosis and prognosis.

Conclusions

The findings demonstrate that the overexpression of NEK2 is associated with progression in PCa and suggest that NEK2 has the potential to serve as a biomarker for PCa prognosis. Further validation with large sample pool is warrant.

Abbreviations
NEK2: NIMA-related kinase 2; PCa: Prostate cancer; PSA: Prostate specific antigen; TMA: Tissue microarray.

However, there is still no effective cure for men with advanced PCa that is often castration-resistant. Many studies have been dedicated to identifying prognostic markers that can be used to distinguish indolent versus aggressive forms of PCa. NEK2 is a centrosomal locating serine/threonine kinase required for centrosome duplication in mitosis. Expression of NEK2 is frequently upregulated in human cancers [9]. Recent evidence suggests that nuclear localization of NEK2 represents a strong predictor for drug resistance and poor prognosis in cancer [28]. Yet, the function of NEK2 in PCa progression is still obscure. Here, we reported the expression of NEK2 was elevated in PCa both at the mRNA and protein levels. As we just use one representative cell line for the study, the results could not completely reflect the relationship of NEK2 with androgen, which

Competing interests

The authors declare that they have no competing interests.

Authors' contributions

CW, ZDH, YXL and WDZ participated in study design and coordination, analysis and interpretation of data, material support for obtained funding, and supervised study. YRZ, YQH and ZZL: performed most of the experiments and statistical analysis and drafted the manuscript. Other authors: carried out the experiment and sample collection. All authors read and approved the final manuscript.

Acknowledgements

This work was supported by grants from National Natural Science Foundation of China (81170699, 81272813, 81270761, and 81101712), Projects of Guangdong Key Laboratory of Clinical Molecular Medicine and Diagnostics, Guangzhou Medical Key Subject Construction Project.

Author details

[1]Guangdong Provincial Institute of Nephrology, Southern Medical University, Guangzhou 510515, China. [2]Department of Urology, Guangdong Key Laboratory of Clinical Molecular Medicine and Diagnostics, Guangzhou First People's Hospital, Guangzhou Medical University, Guangzhou 510180, China. [3]School of Pharmacy, Wenzhou Medical University, Wenzhou 325035, China. [4]Department of Urology, The Fifth Affiliated Hospital of Guangzhou Medical University, Guangzhou 510799, China. [5]Department of Urology, Huadu District People's Hospital, Southern Medical University, Guangzhou 510800, China. [6]Urology Key Laboratory of Guangdong Province, The First Affiliated Hospital of Guangzhou Medical University, Guangzhou Medical University, Guangzhou 510230, China. [7]Department of Urology, Guangzhou First People's Hospital, Guangzhou Medical University, Guangzhou 510180, China.

References

1. Doxsey S. Re-evaluating centrosome function. Nat Rev Mol Cell Biol. 2001;2(9):688–98.
2. Bornens M. Centrosome composition and microtubule anchoring mechanisms. Curr Opin Cell Biol. 2002;14(1):25–34.
3. Pihan GA, Purohit A, Wallace J, Knecht H, Woda B, Quesenberry P, et al. Centrosome defects and genetic instability in malignant tumors. Cancer Res. 1998;58(17):3974–85.
4. Lingle WL, Lutz WH, Ingle JN, Maihle NJ, Salisbury JL. Centrosome hypertrophy in human breast tumors: implications for genomic stability and cell polarity. Proc Natl Acad Sci U S A. 1998;95(6):2950–5.
5. Pihan GA, Purohit A, Wallace J, Malhotra R, Liotta L, Doxsey SJ. Centrosome defects can account for cellular and genetic changes that characterize prostate cancer progression. Cancer Res. 2001;61(5):2212–9.
6. Nigg EA. Mitotic kinases as regulators of cell division and its checkpoints. Nat Rev Mol Cell Biol. 2001;2(1):21–32.
7. Fry AM. The Nek2 protein kinase: a novel regulator of centrosome structure. Oncogene. 2002;21(40):6184–94.
8. Hames RS, Fry AM. Alternative splice variants of the human centrosome kinase Nek2 exhibit distinct patterns of expression in mitosis. Biochem J. 2002;361(Pt 1):77–85.
9. Hayward DG, Fry AM. Nek2 kinase in chromosome instability and cancer. Cancer Lett. 2006;237(2):155–66.
10. Hayward DG, Clarke RB, Faragher AJ, Pillai MR, Hagan IM, Fry AM. The centrosomal kinase Nek2 displays elevated levels of protein expression in human breast cancer. Cancer Res. 2004;64(20):7370–6.
11. Fry AM, Meraldi P, Nigg EA. A centrosomal function for the human Nek2 protein kinase, a member of the NIMA family of cell cycle regulators. EMBO J. 1998;17(2):470–81.
12. Faragher AJ, Fry AM. Nek2A kinase stimulates centrosome disjunction and is required for formation of bipolar mitotic spindles. Mol Biol Cell. 2003;14(7):2876–89.
13. Landi MT, Dracheva T, Rotunno M, Figueroa JD, Liu H, Dasgupta A, et al. Gene expression signature of cigarette smoking and its role in lung adenocarcinoma development and survival. PLoS ONE. 2008;3(2):e1651.
14. Barbagallo F, Paronetto MP, Franco R, Chieffi P, Dolci S, Fry AM, et al. Increased expression and nuclear localization of the centrosomal kinase Nek2 in human testicular seminomas. J Pathol. 2009;217(3):431–41.
15. Andreasson U, Dictor M, Jerkeman M, Berglund M, Sundstrom C, Linderoth J, et al. Identification of molecular targets associated with transformed diffuse large B cell lymphoma using highly purified tumor cells. Am J Hematol. 2009;84(12):803–8.
16. Zeng X, Shaikh FY, Harrison MK, Adon AM, Trimboli AJ, Carroll KA, et al. The Ras oncogene signals centrosome amplification in mammary epithelial cells through cyclin D1/Cdk4 and Nek2. Oncogene. 2010;29(36):5103–12.
17. Chen Y, Riley DJ, Zheng L, Chen PL, Lee WH. Phosphorylation of the mitotic regulator protein Hec1 by Nek2 kinase is essential for faithful chromosome segregation. J Biol Chem. 2002;277(51):49408–16.
18. Naro C, Barbagallo F, Chieffi P, Bourgeois CF, Paronetto MP, Sette C. The centrosomal kinase NEK2 is a novel splicing factor kinase involved in cell survival. Nucleic Acids Res. 2014;42(5):3218–27.
19. Taylor BS, Schultz N, Hieronymus H, Gopalan A, Xiao Y, Carver BS, et al. Integrative genomic profiling of human prostate cancer. Cancer Cell. 2010;18(1):11–22.
20. Remmele W, Stegner HE. Recommendation for uniform definition of an immunoreactive score (IRS) for immunohistochemical estrogen receptor detection (ER-ICA) in breast cancer tissue. Pathologe. 1987;8(3):138–40.
21. Kaemmerer D, Peter L, Lupp A, Schulz S, Sanger J, Baum RP, et al. Comparing of IRS and Her2 as immunohistochemical scoring schemes in gastroenteropancreatic neuroendocrine tumors. Int J Clin Exp Pathol. 2012;5(3):187–94.
22. Abate-Shen C, Shen MM. Molecular genetics of prostate cancer. Genes Dev. 2000;14(19):2410–34.
23. Ruijter E, van de Kaa C, Miller G, Ruiter D, Debruyne F, Schalken J. Molecular genetics and epidemiology of prostate carcinoma. Endocr Rev. 1999;20(1):22–45.
24. Peskoe SB, Joshu CE, Rohrmann S, McGlynn KA, Nyante SJ, Bradwin G et al. Circulating total testosterone and PSA concentrations in a nationally representative sample of men without a diagnosis of prostate cancer. Prostate. 2015;75(11):1167–76.
25. Jackson WC, Schipper MJ, Johnson SB, Foster C, Li D, Sandler HM et al. Duration of Androgen Deprivation Therapy Influences Outcomes for Patients Receiving Radiation Therapy Following Radical Prostatectomy. Eur Urol. 2015. doi:10.1016/j.eururo.2015.05.009.
26. Demirkol MO, Acar O, Ucar B, Ramazanoglu SR, Saglican Y, Esen T. Prostate-specific membrane antigen-based imaging in prostate cancer: Impact on clinical decision making process. Prostate. 2015;75(7):748–57.
27. Hoyer M, Muren LP, Glimelius B. The evolution of radiotherapy techniques in the management of prostate cancer. Acta Oncol. 2015;54(6):821–4.
28. Zhou W, Yang Y, Xia J, Wang H, Salama ME, Xiong W, et al. NEK2 induces drug resistance mainly through activation of efflux drug pumps and is associated with poor prognosis in myeloma and other cancers. Cancer Cell. 2013;23(1):48–62.
29. Matsuhashi A, Ohno T, Kimura M, Hara A, Saio M, Nagano A, et al. Growth suppression and mitotic defect induced by JNJ-7706621, an inhibitor of cyclin-dependent kinases and aurora kinases. Curr Cancer Drug Targets. 2012;12(6):625–39.
30. Liu X, Gao Y, Lu Y, Zhang J, Li L, Yin F. Upregulation of NEK2 is associated with drug resistance in ovarian cancer. Oncol Rep. 2014;31(2):745–54.
31. de Vos S, Hofmann WK, Grogan TM, Krug U, Schrage M, Miller TP, et al. Gene expression profile of serial samples of transformed B-cell lymphomas. Lab Invest. 2003;83(2):271–85.
32. Cappello P, Blaser H, Gorrini C, Lin DC, Elia AJ, Wakeham A, et al. Role of Nek2 on centrosome duplication and aneuploidy in breast cancer cells. Oncogene. 2014;33(18):2375–84.
33. Koch M, Wiese M. Gene expression signatures of angiocidin and darapladib treatment connect to therapy options in cervical cancer. J Cancer Res Clin Oncol. 2013;139(2):259–67.
34. Twomey C, Wattam SL, Pillai MR, Rapley J, Baxter JE, Fry AM. Nek2B stimulates zygotic centrosome assembly in Xenopus laevis in a kinase-independent manner. Dev Biol. 2004;265(2):384–98.
35. Uto K, Sagata N. Nek2B, a novel maternal form of Nek2 kinase, is essential for the assembly or maintenance of centrosomes in early Xenopus embryos. EMBO J. 2000;19(8):1816–26.
36. Lee J, Gollahon L. Nek2-targeted ASO or siRNA pretreatment enhances anticancer drug sensitivity in triplenegative breast cancer cells. Int J Oncol. 2013;42(3):839–47.

miRNAs associated with prostate cancer risk and progression

Hung N. Luu[1,2], Hui-Yi Lin[3], Karina Dalsgaard Sørensen[4], Olorunseun O. Ogunwobi[5], Nagi Kumar[6], Ganna Chornokur[6], Catherine Phelan[6], Dominique Jones[7], LaCreis Kidd[7], Jyotsna Batra[8], Kosj Yamoah[6,9], Anders Berglund[10], Robert J. Rounbehler[11], Mihi Yang[12], Sang Haak Lee[13], Nahyeon Kang[13], Seung Joon Kim[13], Jong Y. Park[6*] and Giuliano Di Pietro[6,14]

Abstract

Prostate cancer is the most common malignancy among men in the US. Though considerable improvement in the diagnosis of prostate cancer has been achieved in the past decade, predicting disease outcome remains a major clinical challenge. Recent expression profiling studies in prostate cancer suggest microRNAs (miRNAs) may serve as potential biomarkers for prostate cancer risk and disease progression. miRNAs comprise a large family of about 22-nucleotide-long non-protein coding RNAs, regulate gene expression post-transcriptionally and participate in the regulation of numerous cellular processes. In this review, we discuss the current status of miRNA in studies evaluating the disease progression of prostate cancer. The discussion highlights key findings from previous studies, which reported the role of miRNAs in risk and progression of prostate cancer, providing an understanding of the influence of miRNA on prostate cancer. Our review indicates that somewhat consistent results exist between these studies and reports on several prostate cancer related miRNAs. Present promising candidates are miR-1, −21, 106b, 141, −145, −205, −221, and −375, which are the most frequently studied and seem to be the most promising for diagnosis and prognosis for prostate cancer. Nevertheless, the findings from previous studies suggest miRNAs may play an important role in the risk and progression of prostate cancer as promising biomarkers.

Background

Prostate cancer (PCa) is the most common malignancy among men in the US. In 2016, there were approximately 180,890 new cases and 26,120 PCa related deaths [1]. Over the past two decades, PCa detection with serum prostate specific antigen (PSA/KLK3) has led to a significant increase in the detection of low-grade PCa (Gleason < 6), a disease that has been shown to pose little risk of either metastatic spread or death. Active surveillance has thus evolved as a recommended management strategy for men with low grade disease. On the other hand, in 10 to 15% of cases, the cancer is aggressive and advances beyond the prostate, sometimes turning lethal, characterized by recurrence and early metastasis through the bloodstream and lymphatic system. Moreover, distant disease is associated with a low 5-year survival rate of 28% (2014–2015 ACS Cancer Treatment and Survivorship Facts and Figures). It should also be noted that racial differences may influence the diagnosis and also the progression and PCa treatment [2].

The most important clinical challenge is to distinguish men who have a potentially lethal form of PCa from those with an indolent disease [3]. Given the significant morbidity associated with treatment interventions, active surveillance could help identify men with aggressive disease who would benefit from intensive treatment compared to those in which conservative measures would suffice. Currently, the stratification of PCa patients is guided by the PSA kinetics, clinical stage, and the grade of tumor (Gleason score). Although these parameters are still clinically useful, they have limitations in detecting cases, predicting disease outcomes and guiding clinical management decisions. For example, the sensitivity of PSA with standard cut-off of 4 ng/mL is only 20.5% while the specificity is 93.6% [4]. Thus new biomarkers are

* Correspondence: Jong.Park@moffitt.org
[6]Department of Cancer Epidemiology, H. Lee Moffitt Cancer Center and Research Institute, Tampa, FL 33612, USA
Full list of author information is available at the end of the article

urgently needed to improve existing diagnostic, prognostic and treatment management plans. Results from numerous reports suggest a critical role of microRNAs (miRNAs) in PCa progression (reviewed in [5]). These studies reveal expression of miRNAs are dysregulated in prostate tumor and indicated miRNAs may serve as promising PCa risk stratification biomarkers [5].

miRNAs comprise a large family of ~22-nucleotide-long non-protein coding RNAs that regulate gene expression post-transcriptionally by both destabilizing mRNA transcripts and repressing their translation. Since the discovery of the first miRNA (lin-4) in 1993 [6], many other miRNAs have been identified [5, 7]. Reportedly, miRNAs normally regulate cellular processes such as development and differentiation in multicellular organisms [8, 9]. Subsequent studies found that expression of miRNAs are significantly associated with various human cancers, including prostate cancer. For example, miR-143, miR-145, and miR-375 were identified as biomarkers with a high-level sensitivity and specificity in PCa detection [10], albeit unequivocally [5].

Most miRNAs bind at the 3′ untranslated regions (3′ UTR), 5′ UTR and coding mRNA regions, which leads to mRNA degradation or translational inhibition [11–13]. miRNAs regulate the activity of more than 60% of all human gene products [9, 14, 15]. Biological functional studies suggest miRNAs are involved in the regulation a plethora of cellular processes, including those essential to tumorigenesis [14]. Each miRNA may regulate hundreds of genes with varying specificities through base pairing to mRNAs [16]. Moreover, a certain gene may serve as a targeted by multiple miRNAs via different binding sites [17, 18]. Therefore, a miRNA can play a role in multiple biological cell signaling pathways by regulating the expressions and functions of their target genes [19]. Currently, there are over 1,800 human miRNAs identified. Many of them are expressed in a tissue-specific manner and changes in the expression of certain miRNAs are associated with various cancers including PCa (miRBase Release 21, www.mirbase.org) [14].

In this review, we will provide overview information on the current status of miRNA studies in PCa. The discussion will highlight key findings from human studies, examine the expression of miRNA in prostate tumor tissues with a view to understand the influence of miRNAs on prostate carcinogenesis or possibly the modulation of the clinical course of the disease. We will also review studies comparing the expression of miRNAs in different biological states of PCa via tumor tissue and biological fluid relative to controls. The review will conclude with a discussion of the therapeutic potential of miRNAs in PCa and on future directions of miRNA research in PCa.

miRNA and prostate cancer

miRNAs affect gene expression significantly and their dysregulation may cause tumorigenesis and its progression. The first report of miRNA's role in human cancer came from a study that characterized chromosome 13q14 in chronic lymphocytic leukemia (CLL) [20]. Since the first report of aberrant miRNA expression in CLL, the dysregulation of a number of miRNAs is closely associated with the development and progression of various cancers. Furthermore, about 50% of miRNA sequences are located in cancer-related regions (including fragile sites, breakpoint regions, viral integration sites and regions frequently linked with loss of heterozygosity or amplification) in the human genome, suggesting a role of miRNAs in cancer [21]. Moreover, recent studies indicated the dysregulation of miRNA profiles in PCa based on high-throughput methodologies (i.e., microarrays, RNA-Seq, proteomic arrays).

Further, miRNA expression profiles may help to distinguish between normal and tumor tissues [22–28]. miRNA profiles appear to have a better accuracy to differentiate between tumor and normal tissues when compared to mRNA profiling [29]. Expression profiles of miRNAs often correspond with clinic-pathological parameters and predict patient outcome or response to treatment [22, 30, 31]. These observations underscore the potential of miRNAs as new diagnostic or prognostic biomarkers. Additionally, the oncogenic or tumor-suppressive functions of miRNAs [24, 32] suggested that miRNAs may be new candidates for cancer drug treatment. Beyond that, miRNAs has also been shown to be more stable than the mRNA and are therefore more suitable to be measured in formalin-fixed paraffin-embedded (FFPE) samples [33, 34]. The stability of miRNAs also makes miRNAs better candidates for blood-based markers [35, 36].

Dysregulation of miRNA in cancer could be caused by several genomic aberrations. These genomic anomalies may include, chromosomal modification, such as translocation, change of transcriptional factors and aberrant expression, epigenetic alterations, and changes in miRNA processing [22]. Several studies reveal miR-155 is induced at the transcriptional level by transforming growth factor β (TGFB1)/Smad, nuclear factor-κB (NFKB1) and activator protein-1 (AP1) family transcription factors (JUN/JUNB/JUND/FOS/FOSB) through direct interaction with the miR-155 promoter [37–39].

miRNAs as oncogenes and tumor suppressors

miRNAs are divided into two types, oncogenes or tumor suppressors based upon whether their targets. Several miRNAs have been characterized as oncogenes and tumor suppressors in PCa. miRNAs inhibit the expression of tumor suppressor genes via their up-regulation in tumor cells, and are commonly termed oncogenic miRNAs or onco-miRs. The oncogenic miRNAs in PCa may enhance proliferative function by down-regulation of cell-cycle dependent kinase inhibitors p21 and p27 [40–42], as well as members of the E2F family of transcription factors [40, 43]. For example, miR-17-92 cluster contains six miRNAs (miR-17, –18a, –19a, –19b-1, –20a, and -92a-1) that are over-expressed in PCa [44], particularly miR-20a is over-expressed in prostate tumor tissues [45]. miR-20a decreases apoptosis in PCa PC-3 cells through repression of E2F2 and E2F3 and inhibition of miR-20a by antisense oligonucleotide, inducing the cell death [43]. Others PCa-associated onco-miRs, miR-1, –21, –106b, –125b, –221 and –222 are known.

The expression of miR-1, also considered an onco-miRNA, is inversely related to the WDR6, XPO6 and SMARCA4 expression. However, miR-1 expression correlates positively with TWF1 transcription (PTK9) in PCa cells, suggesting that microRNAs binding may lead to mRNA cellular accumulation and sequestration of the inhibited mRNA. miR-1 also inhibit expression of exporter-6 and protein tyrosine kinase 9 (also referred to as A6/twinfilin) in PCa cells [40]. Chang et al. [46] showed that decreased miR-1 levels was modulate by the activation of EGFR, leading to invasiveness and the involvement of TWIST1 in facilitating metastasis bone in PCa cell lines. These results indicated that EGFR functions as a transcription factor, repressing miR-1, which has an onco-suppressive role [46]. Kojima et al. [47] showed a down-regulation of miR-1, miR-15a, miR-16-1, and miR-133a in PCa tissues, and these negative regulations contributed to the proliferation, migration and invasion in PC3 and DU145 cells. miR-1 and miR-133a may functioned as tumor suppressors that regulate PNP, an oncogenic gene in Pca [47]. Ambs et al. [40] and Martens-Uzunova et al. [48] observed down-regulation in PCa tissues and linked to PCa progression, castration-resistant disease, and metastasis. Therefore, miR-1 was also suggested at candidate prognostic biomarker for Pca [46, 47, 49–53].

The miR-21 is overexpressed and plays an important role in PCa tumorigenesis, stimulating invasion and metastasis [45, 54–58], and induced invasion and motility of prostate tumor cells [59]. Ribas et al. [57] demonstrated androgen-induced Androgen Receptor binding to the miR-21 promoter that showed a direct transcriptional regulation, even after castration. Their results demonstrated that miR-21 contribute to PCa androgen receptor-driven proliferation and was overexpressed in LNCaP and LAPC-4 cells and in human tumors, but not correlate with stage, grade, or PSA [57]. The coordinated action of miR-21 and androgen receptor signaling, suppresses TGFBR2 levels through binding to its 3'UTR, enhancing androgen receptor signaling, thereby exerting

its oncogenic effects on prostate tumors, through inhibition the suppressor activity of the tumor by TGFβ pathway [59]. The miR-21 may be implicated in the resistance to apoptosis, in motility and invasion in PCa cells [60]. miR-21 is able to downregulate Cyclin dependent kinase inhibitors expression by targeting the coding region of the gene, being able to attenuate the p57Kip2 action, which is inhibit the cell cycle [59]. An overexpressed miR-21 can lead to a decrease in the levels of RECK (Reversion-inducing cysteine-rich protein with Kazal motifs, a key inhibitor of several metaloproteinases) as well, and consequently cause an increase in the PCa promotion and progression [58].

miR-106b which targets the p21 (CDKN1A) and E2F1, displays an anti-apoptotic role in PCa cells by inhibiting caspase activation. Thus miR-106 suppressed E2F1 and p21/WAF1 protein expression [40]. Ambs et al. [40] and Szczyrba et al. [61] observed over-expression of miR-106b in gene expression profiling of prostate tumors. miR-106b appears to be a PCa oncogene, and was suggested as a candidate prognostic marker for PCa [62–64].

miR-125b is usually was over-expressed in androgen-independent PCa cells, but was downregulated in androgen-dependent LNCaP cells. Ectopic expression of miR-125b in LNCaP cells stimulates growth as a consequence of downregulation of its major target BAK1, a pro-apoptotic gene belonging to the Bcl-2 family [65, 66]. The miR-145 binds to the 3'UTR of MYO6 gene and regulated negatively, resulting in a decrease in myosin VI (involved in cancer-related cell migration), and β-actin in LNCaP cell line [61].

Poliseno et al. [62] has shown that miR-25, miR-93, and miR-106b are up-regulated in PCa and are inversely correlated with PTEN (phosphatase and tensin homolog deleted on chromosome 10, is a tumor suppressor that antagonizes signaling via the phosphatidylinositol-3-kinase-Akt pathway) abundance in prostate cancer. The authors also observed that miR-22 transformed MEFs (mouse embryonic fibroblasts) when combined with c-MYC (a regulatory gene encoding a transcription factor), as well as the miR-106b-25 cluster when combined with c-MYC or when combined with MCM7 (mini-chromosome maintenance protein 7). The expression of MCM7 correlated with tumor progression [62].

Hudson et al. [49] have observed that miR-32, miR-106b-25, and miR-375 are up-regulated in primary tumor tissues and miR-106b-25 showed an additional increased in metastatic lesions especially in bones. On the other hand, miR-101 was down-regulated in tumors and metastases. The caspase-7, a novel candidate target of miR-106b-25, and its inhibition may be important in anti-apoptotic and oncogenic functions, promote cell cycle progression and hyper-proliferation, and miR-

106b-25 can also alter the cell adhesion properties in PCa. miR-106b-25 negatively regulates Fas-activated kinase involved in apoptosis. The authors hypothesized that the combined inhibition of pro-apoptotic E2F1, Bim (apoptosis regulator), Fas-activated kinase (serine/threonine transferase kinase/transferase), caspase-7 and PTEN provides miR-106b-25 expressing in cancer cells. In addition, the down-regulation of cell death-inducing integrin-beta 8, which is a target of miR-106b-25, and miR-93, can still support independent growth anchorage [49]. Liang et al. [64] have observed that REST (RE-1 Silencing Transcription Factor) expression decreases with overexpression of miR-93 and miR-106b-25 induced in LNCaP and PC3 cells hypoxia, and elevated expression of pro-neural Phox2a, as well the ASH-1 transcription factors and TH and ChgA NE markers. On the other hand, under conditions of hypoxia, excessive expression of miR-93 led to the destruction of REST [64].

The miR-200c also is upregulation, and it's targets with ZEB1 and ZEB2, that are transcription factors, that also are able to negatively regulate the miR-200c expression, thus increasing E-cadherin expression [61]. miR-205 has an onco-suppressive function by inhibiting the transition from epithelial to mesenchymal tissue, cell migration, and invasion in the human prostate [48]. Knockdown of miR-221 and miR-222, which are upregulated in the androgen-independent PCa cancer cell line, reduced the clonogenecity and tumorigenicity of androgen-independent PC-3 cells [41, 42]. Ectopic expression of miR-221 and miR-222 enhanced the colony forming potential and in vivo growth of androgen-dependent LNCaP cells by inducing a G1-S shift in the cell cycle [41].

In contrast to onco-miRs, tumor suppressor miRNAs were down-regulated in tumor cells to permit tumor progression. For example, the miR-15a/16-1 cluster located on chromosome 13q14 was frequently deleted in about 50% of PCa tumors [67]. Decreased activity of these two miRNAs resulted in hyperplasia of the prostate in mice and increased expression through intra-tumoral delivery resulted in the regression of PCa xenografts [67, 68]. miR-15a−miR-16-1 cluster controlled cell survival, proliferation and invasion by suppressing cyclin D1 (CCND1) and WNT3A [67]. Similarly, miR-101 expression in PCa was decreased during progression of the disease mainly due to the loss of one or both of its genomic loci. Moreover, miR-101 inhibited the expression and function of EZH2, a member of the polycomb protein group [69].

The tumor-suppressive role of miRNAs in PCa has generally been ascribed to their ability to interfere with cell migration, invasion and pro-apoptotic functions. Ectopic expression of miR-126* significantly reduced the translation of prostein (SLC45A3), which is a prostate-specific protein involved in PCa motility and invasiveness. Presumably, miR-126 binds to the 3′ UTR of prostein mRNA, resulted in reduced invasiveness of LNCaP cells [70]. Similarly, ectopic miR-34a expression induced cell cycle arrest and senescence, inhibited cell growth, and attenuated resistance to the chemotherapeutic agent camptothecin. miR-126 increased chemotherapy sensitivity by inducing apoptosis through suppression of the deacetylase sirtuin (SIRT1) and cyclin dependent kinase 6 (CDK6) and aggressive cellular behavior [71, 72].

Moreover, miR-146a reduced cell proliferation, invasion and metastasis of PC-3 cells to human bone marrow endothelial cell monolayers through the suppression of the Rho-associated protein kinase ROCK1 [73]. Other tumor suppressor-associated miRNAs evaluated in PCa cell models included miR-23b, miR-145, and miR-205. Ectopic expression of miR-23b, and miR-145 in LNCaP cells significantly reduced proliferation [74–77]. Similarly, ectopic expression of miR-205 in PCa cells resulted in reduction of cell locomotion and invasion and down-regulation of several oncogenes involved in PCa progression [78].

Although functional studies might define certain miRNAs as onco-miRNAs or tumor suppressor miRNAs, their expression in prostate tumors might not correlate with these classifications. For instance, miR-125b, miR-221, miR-222, miR-373 and miR-520c as onco-miRs in experimental models [41, 42, 65, 66]; however, these miRs were down-regulated in prostate tumor tissue relative to normal prostate tissue [76, 79–81]. miR-373 and miR-520c play a critical role in PCa by inhibiting expression of CD44 RNA [82]. Other miRNAs also defied their given classification as either a tumor suppressor or oncogenic miRNAs. Previous functional studies demonstrated a dual role for miRs-133b and −375 in different PCa cell lines [83–85].

Normally, miR-133b is downregulated as a tumor suppressor miR and miR-375 is upregulated as an oncomiR in PCa tumor tissue relative to normal tissue. However, forced expression of miR-133b increased proliferation in androgen-dependent cells (LNCaP, 22Rv1) [84] while miR-375 decreased proliferation and invasion of androgen-independent PC-3 cells [85]. Thus functional studies performed in experimental models might not perfectly recapitulate clinical disease [86]. In the same way, miR-373 was 1.5 times more prevalent in benign glandular and benign stromal cells, than in the same tissues from PCa patients, as well as miR-520c showed reduced in primary tumors and metastases. Never the less, miR-373 and miR-520c act as pro-invasive agents, mediated by binding with CD44 3'UTR [82].

In summary, miRNAs have an important role in human cancer. More than 50% of miRNA genes are located in cancer-associated regions in the human genome and the expressions of miRNAs are dysregulated in various human cancers, including PCa. Certain miRNAs are upregulated in cancer (onco-miRs), while others are downregulated (tumor suppressors). However, expression profiles and functional studies of miRNAs in PCa cell lines do not always correlate with expression in prostate tumor tissue.

miRNAs in prostate cancer

Numerous biomarkers have been proposed as promising predictors for risk and/or progression of PCa. However, most biomarkers could not clearly demonstrate their independent clinical potential and, therefore, these biomarkers fail to enhance accuracy of current nomograms. Since the first discovery of miRNAs [6] in 1993, many studies have investigated whether dysregulation of miRNA expression in PCa may correlate with the risk and progression of this disease. These studies reported a number of differentially expressed miRNAs in biological samples from patients with PCa. Tables 1 and 2 summarize results from studies of miRNA expression in PCa.

Diagnosis/progression of prostate cancer based on tissue

MicroRNA profiling in PCa tissues shows different expression patterns as compared with normal tissues. These unique miRNA expression profiling may provide tools for better prediction of diagnosis and progression of PCa. These data also assist to determine treatment strategies of PCa.

Porkka et al. [87] reported that differential expression of 51 miRNAs between BPH and prostate tumor tissues based on data from oligonucleotide array hybridization. Eight of these miRNAs were upregulated, while 22 were down-regulated in tumor tissues as compared with ones in BPH tissues. The authors observed an expression of several miRNAs, Let-7f, miR-19b, −184, and −198, were associated with advanced disease. Ambs et al. [40] evaluated mRNAs profiles detected in 60 LCM prostate tumors and 16 non-tumor prostate tissues using genome-wide expression assays. Expression of some miRNAs was significantly different comparing prostate tumors and non-tumor samples (miR-32, −133a-1, −490, −494, −520 h) as well as patients with organ-confined PCa vs. extra prostatic disease extension (miR-101-1/2, −200a, and -200b). These data suggested that miRNA dysregulation was related to development and progression of PCa. Further, the mRNA and miRNA analyses revealed influence the expression of cancer related genes by miRNAs in PCa cells. For example, the miR-106b-25 cluster maps to intron 13 of MCM7, which was significantly up-regulated in prostate tumors [40].

Ozen et al. [79] analyzed the expression of 480 human miRNAs between 10 benign peripheral zone tissues and 16 prostate tumors using microarrays and observed and validated down-regulation of several miRNAs including let-7c, miR-125b, and miR-145 in localized prostate tumor samples compared to benign peripheral zone tissue, and demonstrated miR-145 expression has a heterogeneous pattern in PCa tissue [79]. Mercateli et al. [42] showed overexpression of miR-221 is sufficient to strongly induce growth of LNCaP xenografts in mice. The tumor growth advantage in miR-221 expressing was significantly higher than mice in the referent group ($p = 0.01$). The average volume fold increase of miR-221 expressing tumors was higher than control tumors ($p = 0.025$) [42].

With high-throughput liquid phase hybridization (mirMASA) reactions and 114 miRNA probes, Tong et al. [76] observed downregulation of miR-221 and other miRNAs (miR-23b, −100, −145, and −222) in malignant prostate tissue ($n = 40$). They developed the 48 miRNA signature (including miR-135b and miR-194) that predicted biochemical recurrence after prostatectomy. Further evidence was provided for the growth modulatory roles of miRNAs by showing reduced ectopic expression of miR-23b, −145, −221 and −222 in LNCaP cell [76]. Khan et al. [88] analyzed over 1,000 proteins with multidimensional liquid phase peptide fractionation followed by tandem mass spectrometry, using 15 tissues samples, 5 of the prostate tumor, 5 of adjacent benign tissue and 5 of distant metastatic tissues. The study revealed the involvement of miR-128-a/b in regulating progression of PCa, where the miR-128 levels were elevated in lines of BPH prostatic epithelial cells, when compared to invasive PCa cells. The findings were validated in an independent set of 15 clinical specimens. Furthermore, transient overexpression of miR-128 in PCa cell lines attenuated cellular invasion, which suggest miR-128 as an important negative regulator of cellular invasiveness in vitro [88].

Prueitt et al. [80] showed a role of miRNAs in PCa progression by demonstrating a higher expression of 19 miRNAs (particularly miR-224) and downregulation of 34 miRNAs (particularly metallothioneins and proteins with mitochondrial localization and involvement in cell metabolism) in patients with progression than those with a locally confined disease [80]. However, Kristensen et al. [89] reported epigenetic downregulation of miR-224 and miR-452 (which are located in an intron of the GABRE) was a significant independent adverse predictor for time to BCR after radical prostatectomy in two large PCa patient cohorts ($n = 293$ and 198, respectively) [89]. Wang et al. [90] analyzed about 273 miRNAs using cell lines from 62 PCa patients with aggressive phenotype (Gleason score ≥ 8) and 63 PCa patients with nonaggressive

Table 1 Summary of miRNA expression studies on samples from prostate cancer patients

Author year (reference)	Tissue/serum	Outcome	miRNA identified
Risk/Diagnostic			
Ozen, 2008 [79]	Tissue	Risk/Diagnostic	Let-7b-g, 26a-b, 29a-c, 30a-e, 99a-b, 125a-b
Gandellini, 2009 [78]	Tissue	Risk/Diagnostic	miR-205
Mahn 2011 [118]	Tissue/Serum	Diagnostic	let7i, 16, 26a, 195
Wach, 2012 [10]	Tissue	Diagnostic	miR-143, 145, 375
Avgeris, 2013 [101]	Tissue	Diagnostic	miR-145
Srivastava, 2013 [105]	Tissue/Urine	Diagnostic	miR-205, 221, 99b
Tsuchiyama, 2013 [106]	Tissue	Diagnostic	miR-182-5p
Guzel 2015 [107]	Tissue	Diagnostic	miR-361-3p, 133b, 221, 203
Roberts, 2015 [128]	Tissue/Serum	Diagnostic	miR-200b, 200c, 375
Kristensen 2016 [112]	Tissue	Diagnostic	Up: miR-375, 663b, 615-3p, 425-5p, 663a, 182-5p, 183-5p. Down: miR-205-5p, 221-3p, 222-3p, 376c-3p, 136-5p, 455-3p, 455-5p, −154-5p
Mitchell, 2008 [35]	Serum	Diagnostic	miR-141
Lodes, 2009 [137]	Serum	Diagnostic	miR-16, 92a, 103, 107
Moltzahn, 2011 [99]	Serum	Diagnostic	miR-26b, 223, 874, 1274a
Yaman Agaoglu, 2011 [54]	Plasma	Diagnostic	miR-21, 141, 221
Selth, 2012 [114]	Serum	Diagnostic	miR-141, 298, 346, 375
Chen 2012 [119]	Plasma	Diagnostic	let7c, let7e, 30c, 622, 1285
Cheng, 2013 [120]	Serum	Diagnostic	miR-210
Haldrup, 2014 [113]	Serum	Diagnostic	miR-141, 375
Westermann, 2014 [121]	Serum	Diagnostic	miR-141
Kachakova, 2015 [122]	Plasma	Diagnostic	let-7c, 375
Haj-Ahmad, 2014 [126]	Urine	Diagnostic	miR-182-5, 484
Korzeniewski, 2014 [127]	Urine	Diagnostic	miR-483-5p, 1275, 1290
Risk/Progression			
Porkka, 2007 [87]	Tissue	Risk/Progression	Let-7a-d, Let-7f, 19b, 145, 184, 198, 202, 210,
Ambs, 2008 [40]	Tissue	Risk/Progression	miR-1, 32, 101, 106b, 182, 200a, 200b, 494, 520 h
Mercatelli, 2008 [42]	Tissue	Progression	miR-221, 222
Prueitt, 2008 [80]	Tissue	Progression	miR-2, 10, 125b, 224
Tong, 2009 [76]	Tissue	Risk/Progression	miR-23b, 100, 135b, 145, 194, 221, 222
Wang, 2009 [90]	Tissue	Progression	miR-9*, 16, 221, 222, 331-3p, 145, 551a
Szczyrba, 2010 [61]	Tissue	Progression	miR-143
Shaefer, 2010 [81]	Tissue	Risk/Progression	miR-96, 205
Pesta, 2010 [93]	Tissue	Progression	miR-20a
Khan, 2010 [88]	Tissue	Progression	miR-128
Spahn, 2010 [91]	Tissue	Progression	miR-221
Hagman, 2010 [92]	Tissue	Risk/Progression	miR-34c
Brase, 2011 [115]	Tissue/Serum	Progression	miR-141, 375
Barnabas, 2011 [103]	Tissue	Progression	miR-151
Leite, 2011 [138]	Tissue	Progression	let7c, miR-100, miR-145, miR-191
Martens-Uzunova, 2012 [48]	Tissue	Progression	miR-1, 133a, 133b, 143, 143*, 145, 145*, 204, 221, 222
Li, 2012 [55]	Tissue	Progression	miR-21
Tsuchiyama, 2013 [106]	Tissue	Progression	miR-182-5p
Amankwah, 2013 [102]	Tissue	Progression	miR-21

Table 1 Summary of miRNA expression studies on samples from prostate cancer patients (Continued)

He, 2013 [134]	Tissue	Progression	miR-19a, miR-374b
Kristensen, 2014 [89]	Tissue	Progression	miR-224, 452
Wang, 2014 [124]	Tissue/Serum	Progression	miR-19, miR-345, miR-519c-5p
Dip, 2015 [139]	Tissue	Progression	Let-7c
Zhang, 2011 [100]	Serum	Progression	miR-21
Yaman Agaoglu, 2011 [54]	Plasma	Progression	miR-21, miR-221
Shen, 2012 [56]	Plasma	Progression	miR-20a, miR-21, miR-145, miR-221
Watahiki, 2013 [123]	Plasma	Progression	miR-21, −126, −141, −151-3p, −152, −200c,-375, −423-3p
Nguyen, 2013 [116]	Serum	Progression	miR-141, miR-375, miR-378, miR-409-3p
Diagnostic/Progression			
Hao, 2011 [95]	Tissue	Diagnostic/Progression	miR-21
Mihelich, 2011 [98]	Tissue	Diagnostic/Progression	miR-96, miR-182, miR-183
Bryant 2012 [117]	Serum/Urine	Diagnostic/Progression	miR-181a-2, miR-625, miR-107, miR-574-3p, miR-20a, miR-23a, miR-624
Mavridis, 2013 [109]	Tissue	Diagnostic/Progression	miR-224
Larne, 2013 [108]	Tissue	Diagnostic/Progression	miR-96-5p, miR-183-5p, miR-145-5p, miR-221-5p
Walter, 2013 [110]	Tissue	Diagnostic/Progression	Up: miR-122, miR-335, miR-184, miR-193, miR-34, miR-138, Down: miR-373, −9, −198, −144 -215, −96, −222, −148, −92, −27, −125, −126, −27
Casanova-Salas, 2014 [111]	Tissue/Serum	Diagnostic/Progression	miR-187 and miR-182
Mihelich, 2015 [125]	Serum	Diagnostic/Progression	let-7a, −24, −26b, −30c, −93, −100, −103, −106a, −107, −130b, −146a, −223, −451, −874,
Kristensen, 2016 [112]	Tissue	Diagnostic/Progression	miR185-5p, miR-221-3p, miR-326
Treatment response			
He, 2013 [134]	Tissue	Treatment Response	miR-23b, miR-220, miR-221, miR-222, and miR-205
Lichner, 2013 [135]	Tissue	Treatment Response	miR-152
Gonzales, 2011 [133]	Plasma	Treatment Response	miR-141
Cheng, 2013 [120]	Serum	Treatment Response	miR-210
Someya, 2015 [136]	Blood	Treatment Response	miR-99a

phenotype (Gleason grade ≤ 5) and identified a significant association with PCa grade in 7 miRNAs included miR–16, −9*, −145, 222, −221, −331-3p, and -551a, especially the miR-145 and miR-331-3p, showed significantly down-regulated in aggressive PCa [90].

Schaefer et al. [81] analyzed tumor tissue and normal adjacent tissue from two groups of 76 and 79 men with untreated PCa. This study demonstrated miR-130b with a significantly different expression between normal and tumor tissues. miRs-125b, −205 and −222 were significantly related to tumor stage while miRs-31, −96 and −205 showed a significant correlations with Gleason score. When the combination of six miRNAs (miR-96, −149, −181b, −182, −205 and −375) was used, the AUC was significant (0.88) in discriminating normal and tumor tissue [81]. Spahn et al. [91] analyzed samples from BPH, primary PCa of a high risk group and corresponding metastatic tissues by microarray analysis. A PCa specific miRNA expression signature was generated based on the differential expression of 66 (48 downregulated and 18 upregulated) miRNAs between tumor and BPH tissues ($p < 0.01$). They observed a progressive downregulation of miR-221 in aggressive and metastatic PCa. Downregulation of miR-221 was also associated with Gleason score and clinical recurrence [91].

Hagman et al. [92] found the relative expression of miR-34c was significantly lower in the PCa samples compared to the BPH samples ($p = 0.0005$) and decreased with higher grade. The miR-34c level in patients with metastasis was found to be significantly lower than patients without metastasis ($p = 0.02$). The expression of miR-34c distinguishes aggressive from non-aggressive PCa ($p = 0.012$) and was inversely correlated with PSA level. Although there was no significant correlation between miR-34c expression levels and treatment/response to treatment, the expression of miR-34c was significantly correlated with survival [92].

Table 2 Summary of miRNA expression studies on prostate tumor/serum samples

miRNA investigated	Expression	Tissue	Reference
let-7a-2,let-7i,16-1,17-5p,20a,21,24-1,25,27a,29a,29b-2,30c,32, 34a,92-2,93-1, 95,101-1, 106a, 124a-1,126a-1,135-2,146,149, 181b-1,184,187,191,196-1 197, 199a-1, 214,128a, 195,198, 199a-1,199a-2,203,206,214,218-2,223,	up	tumor	Volina, 2006 [45]
202,210,296,320,370,373*,498,503	up	tumor	Porkka, 2007 [87]
let-7i,25,26a-1/2,31,32,34b,92-1/2,93,99b,106b,125a,181a-1/2,182, 188,194-1/2,196a/2,200c, 370, 375,425,449	up	tumor	Ambs, 2008 [40]
221,222	up	tumor	Mercatelli, 2008 [42]
16,19b,24,100,125b,141,143,296	up	serum	Mitchell, 2008 [35]
141,200b, 200c	up	prostate cells	Mitchell, 2008 [35]
221	up	PCa cells	Mercatelli, 2008 [42]
221	up	tumor	Spahn, 2009 [91]
9*,15a,16,145,221,222,331,551a	up	PCa cells	Wang, 2009 [90]
128	up	PCa cells	Khan, 2010 [88]
let-7a,let-7c,let-7f,15b,20a,21,25,26b,30b,106a, 106b, 126*,148a,200c,218,375,	up	tumor	Szczyrba, 2010 [61]
25,93,106b	up	tumor	Poliseno, 2010 [61]
96,182,182*,183	up	tumor	Schaefer, 2010 [81]
141	up	plasma	Gonzales, 2011 [133]
182	up	Prostate cells	Mihelich, 2011 [98]
100,145,191,let7c	up	tumor	Leite, 2011 [138]
9*,141,200b,375,516a-3p	up	serum	Brase, 2011 [115]
21	up	plasma	Yaman Agaoglu, 2011 [54]
34c	up	PCa cells	Hao, 2011 [95]
20a,21,221	up	plasma	Shen, 2012 [56]
107,141,301a,326,432,484,574-3p,625*,2110	up	plasma	Bryant, 2012 [117]
21	up	tumor	Li, 2012 [55]
let-7b,7,9*,17,19b,20a,21,25,30d,32,92a-1*,93,95,96,106a*,106b, 106b*,130b, 142-3p,141*, 148a, 153,182,182*,183,183*,200b*, 200c*, 210,301b,363,375, 425,512-3p,583,615-3p,663,801,	up	tumor	Martens-Uzunova, 2012 [48]
let-7a,20a,21,106a,106b,375,	up	tumor	Wach, 2012 [10]
96,124,141,302b,375,378*,489,520d-5p,548a-3p,548c-3p, 875-5p,892b,	up	serum	Nguyen, 2013 [116]
96-5p,183-3p,183-5p	up	tumor	Larne, 2013 [108]
10b,15a,15b,16,18a,18b,20b,25,30c,32,34a,34c-5p, 92a, 122, 124,125a-5p, 125b,128a,133b, 134, 135b,146b-5p,148b,181a,181b,181c,184,193a-5p, 193b,206,214, 215,301a,372	up	tumor	Walter, 2013 [110]
19a,188-5p,574-5p,663,939,1224-5p,1225-5p,1249,1915,K12-3,UL70-3p,	up	tumor	He, 2013 [134]
21	up	tumor	Amankwah, 2013 [102]
32,106b-25,375	up	tumor	Hudson, 2013 [53]
96-5p,182-5p,183-5p,	up	tumor	Tsuchiyama, 2013 [106]
141,200a,200c,210,375	up	serum	Cheng, 2013 [120]
19a,19b,20a,20b,26a,26b,29c,106a,125a,125b,135a, 141, 148a,151–5p,174b, 193a, 196b, 331-3p,365, 374a, 374b, 1274b,	up	tumor	Lichner, 2013 [135]
19b	up	tumor	Wang, 2014 [124]
182,SNORD78,U17b,U78_s,U78_x	up	tumor	Casanova-Salas 2014 [111]
17*,200b*,210,297,375,501-3p,551b,562	up	serum	Haldrup, 2014 [113]
345,519c-5p	up	serum	Wang, 2014 [124]
93,106b-25	up	PCa cells	Liang, 2014 [61]
Let-7a,103,107,130b,106a,26b,451,223,93,24,30c,874,100, 146a	up	serum	Mihelich, 2015 [125]

Table 2 Summary of miRNA expression studies on prostate tumor/serum samples *(Continued)*

miRNA	Direction	Sample	Reference
let-7a-5p,let-7d-3p,let-7d-5p,7-5p,7b-5p,20a-5p,21-3p,25-3p, 29b-2-5p,30d-3p, 92a-3p, 92b-3p, 93-3p,96-5p,103a-3p,107, 130b-3p, 182-5p,183-5p,191-5p, 196b-5p,200b-3p, 200b-5p, 200c-3p 329, 331-3p,339-3p,342-5p,375,421, 423-3p,423-5p, 425-5p, 484, 615-3p,663a,663b,664a-3p, 1248,1260a	up	tumor	Kristensen, 2016 [112]
Let-7a,let-7b,let-7c,let-7d,let-7 g,16,23a,23b,26a,92,99a,103,125a,125b,143, 145,195,199a, 199a*,221,222,497	down	tumor	Porkka, 2007 [87]
let-7b,1-2,34a,145,7-1/2,126,128a,133a-1,145,205,218-2,220,221,329,340,345, 410, 487,490,494,499,520 h	down	tumor	Ambs, 2008 [40]
let-7b-g, 26a-b,29a-c,30a-e,99a-b,125a-b,145, 200a-b	down	tumor	Ozen, 2008 [79]
22,24,27a,27b,29a,30e,101,125a-5p,125b,143, 145, 152, 199a-5p,221,223, 320,424,	down	tumor	Szczyrba, 2010 [61]
16,31,125b,145,149,181b,184,205,221,222	down	tumor	Schaefer, 2010 [81]
34c	down	tumor	Hagman, 2010 [92]
34c	down	PCa cells	Hao, 2011 [95]
30c,100,223,346	down	Prostate cells	Mihelich, 2011 [98]
141	down	plasma	Yaman Agaoglu, 2011 [54]
143,145,221	down	tumor	Wach, 2012 [10]
1,15a,16-1,133a	down	tumor	Kojima, 2012 [52]
1,10b,27b,29a,29b,34b,126,126*,130a,133a,133b,139-5p,142-3p,142-5p,143, 143*,145,145*, 146a,149,150,155,181b,193b,193b*,204,205,221,221*,222,223, 224,328,338-3p, 342-5p, 361-3p 378,378*,455-3p,455-5p,483-3p,485-3p,551b	down	tumor	Martens-Uzunova, 2012 [48]
181a-2*	down	plasma	Bryant, 2012 [117]
31-5p,34c-5p,205-5p,221-3p,222-3p	down	tumor	Tsuchiyama, 2013 [106]
101	down	tumor	Hudson, 2013 [49]
221,222	down	tumor	Amankwah, 2013 [102]
23b,26b,30c,155,181d,193a-5p,200b-5p,205,221,221-5p,222,224,335,374a, 374b, 455-3p,505	down	tumor	He, 2013 [134]
145-5p,205-5p,221-5p,409-5p	down	tumor	Larne, 2013 [108]
224	down	tumor	Mavridis, 2013 [109]
222	down	serum	Cheng, 2013 [120]
409-3p,623,	down	serum	Nguyen, 2013 [116]
19a,19b	down	serum	Wang, 2014 [124]
34a*,34c-3p,187,221*,221,224,	down	tumor	Casanova-Salas 2014 [111]
1,133b	down	tumor	Karatas, 2014 [55]
1	down	Prostate cells	Chang, 2015 [46]
15a-5p,16-5p,19b-3p,22-3p,23a-3p,23b-3p,24-3p,26a-5p, 27a-3p, 27b-3p, 29a-3p, 29b-3p,30a-3p,30a-5p,30c-5p,30e-3p, 30e-5p, 33a-5p,34a-5p,99a-3p, 99a-5p,101-3p, 125b-2-3p, 125b-5p, 127-3p,130a-3p,132-3p,136-5p,143-3p, 149-5p, 152, 154-5p,155-5p, 181a-5p,181b-5p,195-5p, 199a-3p,199a-5p, 199b-5p, 205-5p, 214-5p,218-5p,221-3p,222-3p, 223-3p,335-5p,338-3p,362-3p, 363-3p376a-3p,376c-3p,424-5p, 451a,455-3p, 455-5p,497-5p,502-3p,660-5p	down	tumor	Kristensen, 2016 [112]

Pesta et al. [93] evaluated the expression of four miR-NAs, miR- let-7a, −15a, −16, and 20a in 53 prostate tumor and 85 benign prostatic hyperplasia (BPH) tissues to investigate whether miRNA expression is related to clinic-pathological features of PCa. They observed a difference in expression for miR-20a in patients with a Gleason score of 7–10 compared with patients with a low Gleason score of less than 6, suggesting an onco-genic role for miR-20a in PCa development [93].

Although the previous study demonstrated the potential of miR-20a to distinguish between more and less aggressive PCa disease, the use of BPH tissue is not the most appropriate control relative to normal tissue and potentially impede the identification of unique miRNAs in PCa. On the other hand, Taylor et al. [94] reported that, the copy-number alterations in prostate tumors modestly revealed distinct subgroups with substantial differences in time to biochemical recurrence while unsupervised hierarchical clustering of mRNA and miRNA data failed to identify robust clusters of patients with significant differences in prognosis [94].

Szczyrba et al. [61] found 16 miRNAs upregulated by at least 1.5-fold and 17 miRNAs downregulated by at least 1.5-fold in snap frozen prostate tumor tissue. Strong upregulation was found for miR-148a, −200c, −375, and the miR-143, −145 and −223 were downregulated [61]. In another study by Hao et al. [95], miR-21, and miR-141 were upregulated at least 2-fold, while miR-10, −16, −34c, and -125b, were downregulated in formalin fixed paraffin embedded (FFPE) tumor tissues as compared with BPH specimens [95]. The positive predictive value was enhanced from 40 to 87.5% when the PSA variable was added with expression variable of miR-21 and miR-141. After analysis of tumor samples from Caucasians and African-Americans, miR-182 level tended to be higher in PCa tissues and miR-30c, −100, −223, and −346 were expressed at lower levels in PCa tissue in Caucasians.

Therefore, miR-21 may indicate a potential role of carcinogenesis in prostate tissue [57]. In addition, multiple studies reported that miR-21 is an oncogene in prostate cancer and over-expression may be related to the development of castration-resistance PCa [57–60, 96]. In addition, Bonci et al. [97] recently reported over-expression in PCa metastasis.

A RNA microarray profiling analysis of a patient cohort with organ-confined prostate tumors indicated the overexpression of miR-96, −182, and −183 with at least 2-fold in laser captured micro-dissected (LCM) PCa tissue compared with normal adjacent prostate tissue [98]. Moltzahn et al. [99] identified miRNA signatures which can distinguish healthy controls from patients and correlate with a prognosis. Cluster and ROC analyses indicated the diagnostic potential and the ability to further separate PCa patients according to their risk of recurrence by their miRNA signatures [99]. Zhang et al. [100] assessed a potential role of serum miR-21 in the progression of PCa with 56 patients, including 20 localized PCa, 20 with androgen-dependent PCa (ADPC), 10 with hormone-refractory PCa (HRPC), and 6 with BPH. Significantly higher levels of miR-21 were detected in patients with ADPC and HRPC, especially in those resistant to docetaxel-based chemotherapy. These findings suggest miR-21 may be a biomarker at the transition to hormone refractory disease and a potential indicator for response to treatment in PCa patients [100].

Martens-Uzunova et al. [48] analyzed the expression of miRNAs in 102 prostate tumor tissues, adjacent normal tissues, lymph and trans-urethral resection from normal and PCa patients. Regarding the miRNAs, the authors analyzed 80 miRNA species, where 22 were

identified with significant differences between the two groups with or without PCa that can serve as a diagnosis markers. The authors also identified a miR profile consist of 25 miRNAs, which 12 overexpressed and 13 under-expressed in prostate tumor tissues with poor outcome. This 25 miRNA profile is very accurate to predict a recurrence (AUC = 0.991, $p < 0.0001$ Kaplan-Meier analysis). They also observed that the overall expression of miRNA was lower in PCa malignant lymphoma compared to the PCa prostate tissues. 19 miRNAs have been upregulated in metastatic lymph node while 69 miRNAs, including miR-1, −133a, −133b, −143, −143*, −145, −145*, −204, −221 and −222, have been downregulated in comparison to PCa tissue [48].

Li et al. [55] confirmed the miR-21 expression in 169 PCa tissue samples was significantly associated with clinical variables, such as stage, lymph node involvement, capsular invasion, organ confined disease, Gleason score, BCR and patient follow-up. The relationship between miR-21 as BCR persisted even after adjusting for standard clinico-pathological parameters (i.e., PSA, patient age, Gleason score, surgical margin, lymph node metastasis, capsular invasion, and pathological stage) [55].

Avgeris et al. [101] evaluated the clinical utility of miR-145 using 137 prostate tumor tissues and 64 benign samples. They found that the reduction of miR-145 expression in PCa was correlated with Gleason score, clinical stage, tumor size and PSA level and follow-up PSA levels. Further, the reduction of miR-145 expression was significantly associated with increased risk for biochemical recurrence and shorter disease-free survival (DFS) among PCa patients. This relationship remained significant after adjusting for Gleason score, clinical stage, PSA and age at diagnosis [101]. We [102], reported a significantly increased risk for recurrence ($p < 0.0001$) in patients with decreased expression of miR-21, but not for miR-221 ($p = 0.57$) or miR-222 ($p = 0.24$). An increased risk of recurrence was more prominent in obese ($p = 0.031$) than non-obese patients. After adjustment for stage and Gleason score, the results showed miR-21 expression was independently linked to disease recurrence among obese patients [102].

Barnabas et al. [103] observed a copy number gain of miR-151 gene at 8q24 in PCa tissues from African-American men who developed BCR after radical prostatectomy. These data suggested a copy number gain of miR-151 gene in primary tumor that may indicate the presence of metastatic disease [103]. Leite et al. [104] observed a 2.7-3.4 fold higher likelihood of BCR when miR-100, −145, −191, and let-7c were over-expressed. However, only miR-100 showed a significant association independently with BCR in multi-variable analysis [104].

Srivastava et al. [105] evaluated expression of 8 miR-NAs in 40 paired prostate tissues. miR-205, miR-214, miR-221 and miR-99b were significantly downregulated in PCa tumor tissue. These miRNA profiles can discriminate PCa patients from healthy individuals successfully [105]. Tsuchiyama et al. [106] tested whether levels of miRNAs were correlated with aggressiveness. Expression of miR-315p, −34c-5p, and −205-5p was significantly decreased compared to those in normal tissues regardless of Gleason pattern ($p < 0.05$). Meanwhile, in the same patients with high grade PCa, expression of miR-31-5p −182-5p, and −205-5p in tumor tissues was higher than ones obtained from intermediate Gleason tumor ($p < 0.05$) [106]. Using prostate tissues from 23 PCa and 25 BPH patients from Turkey, 4 candidate miRNAs were evaluated (i.e., miR-133b, −203, −221, and −361-3p). miR-361-3p was significantly lower in tumor tissues from PCa than BPH patients ($p = 0.004$). Both miR-133b and miR-221 were downregulated in PCa compared to BPH ($p < 0.01$ and 0.03, respectively). The levels of miR-203 were found to be significantly upregulated in PCa samples ($p = 0.0002$). The AUC values of all miRNAs, miR-133b, miR-203, miR-221, and miR-361-3p were 0.73, 0.81, 0.71, and 0.74, respectively [107].

Larne et al. [108] developed a formula which can predict early stage of PCa with aggressive progression characteristics. Using differentially expressed miRNAs in PCa tissue samples, the authors developed a miRNA signature, consisting of four miRNAs [(miR-96-5p x miR-183-5p)/(miR-145-5p x miR221-5p)], denoted as the miRNA index quote (miQ). The miQ provided an excellent diagnostic discrimination. The median of miQ is 17 times higher in the PCa group compared to the non-PCa group ($p < 0.0001$). Further, miQ level is also associated with grades ($p = 0.0067$), PSA levels ($p < 0.0001$), metastasis ($p < 0.0001$) and survival ($p = 0.0014$). More importantly, miQ distinguishes aggressive tumors from non-aggressive PCa ($p < 0.0001$) with an AUC of 0.90 (95% CI: 0.77–0.97) [108].

Mavridis et al. [109] reported that miR-224 could distinguish PCa patients from BPH patients with an AUC of 0.67 ($p = 0.001$) in tissue samples. miR-224 expression inversely correlated with aggressiveness ($p = 0.017$), thus Gleason score, advanced disease stage, PSA, risk of relapse and positively with progression-free survival [109]. Walter et al. [110] found upregulation of miR-143 and miR-146b and loss of 18 miRNAs (e.g. miR-34c, −29b, −212 and -10b) in the PCa tumors relative to normal epithelium and/or stroma ($p < 0.001$). In addition, upregulation of 11 miRNAs and downregulation of 7 miRNAs were found in the tumors with high Gleason score (≥8) when compared with ones with Gleason score 6 [110]. Casanova-Salas et al. [111] found the expression miR-182 was increased in PCa tissue samples and decreased 6 miRNAs, miR-34a*, −34c-3p, −187, −221*, −221 and. 224. Further miR-182 and miR-187 were also differentially expressed according to clinical variables, such as Gleason score, stage, status of TMPRSS2-ERG and progression [111].

In one of the largest miRNA profiling studies published for PCa, Kristensen et al. [112] analyzed the expression of 752 miRNAs in a training set of 13 non-malignant and 134 PCa tissue samples. Subsequently, a total of 93 miRNAs with diagnostic/prognostic potential were selected for further validation in two similar-sized independent patient cohorts. The authors identified several novel deregulated miRNAs in PCa as compared to nonmalignant prostate tissue samples as well as between more/less aggressive PCa subgroups, as defined by clinic-pathological parameters. Most notably, the authors also identified a novel 3-miRNA prognostic signature (miR-185-5p + miR-221-3p + miR-326) predicted time to biochemical recurrence after radical prostatectomy independently of routine clinical variables in a training cohort as well as in two independent validation cohorts. This is the first report to demonstrate independent prognostic value for a miRNA signature in three independent PCa patient cohorts, supporting the potential clinical relevance of this signature [112].

Diagnosis/progression of prostate cancer based on serum
Some studies have examined the differential expression of miRNAs in serum or plasma in an attempt to develop a blood based diagnosis, detection of progression and recurrence of PCa. Mitchell et al. [35] showed that serum levels of miR-141 can distinguish PCa patients from healthy controls, supporting the potential role of this miRNA as a diagnostic marker for PCa. The upregulation of miR-141 in PCa patients was confirmed in later studies [54, 95, 113–117]. Mahn et al. [118] found circulating oncogenic miRNAs (i.e., miR-26a, −32, −195 and let-7i), particularly miR-26a have a sensitivity of 89% and specificity of 56% (area under the curve: AUC = 0.70) for diagnosis. The diagnostic accuracy increased when these four miRNAs were analyzed in combination (sensitivity: 78.4%, specificity: 66.7%, AUC = 076). Increased levels of miR-16, −26a, and −195 were inversely associated with surgical margin positivity. miR-195 and -let7i were also inversely associated with Gleason score. They found a significant reduction of miR-16, −26a, and −195 levels after radical prostatectomy. miR-32 was found to be down-regulated in PCa tissue ($p = 0.02$) [118].

Chen et al. [119] found that a panel of five serum miRNAs (let-7c, let-7e, miR-30c, −622 and −1285) were significantly different in PCa patients as compared to healthy controls in both identification and validation cohorts. All 5 miRNAs could distinguish PCa from healthy controls individually. The respective sensitivity and specificity values were: let-7c, 68.5 and 70%; let-7e,

77.8 and 75%; miR-30c, 79.6 and 68.8%; miR- 622, 90 and 63.0%; miR-1285, 61.3 and 57.4% [119]. Wach et al. [10] reported on the detection of miR-145 in endothelial cells of blood vessels but not stromal cells. Based upon the ratio of miRNA expression, they concluded that miR-145 may be the best negative predictive biomarker suitable for diagnostic or prognostic purposes in PCa [10].

Selth et al. [114] used a mouse model of PCa as a tool to discover serum miRNAs that could be used in a clinical setting. Among 45 miRNAs identified, four miRNAs (miR-141, −298, −346, and −375) were significantly elevated in metastatic PCa samples as compared to those in healthy controls (all $p < 0.05$). miR-141 and miR-375 were associated with biochemical recurrence (BCR) [114]. Cheng et al. [120] identified five serum miRNAs (miR-141, −200a, −200c, −210, and −375) associated with metastatic castration resistant PCa in both screening and validation cohorts. In the screening cohort, serum levels of five miRNAs were significantly increased in PCa cases as compared with controls (miR-141: $p < 0.0001$, AUC = 0.90; miR-200a: $p = 0.007$, AUC = 0.70; miR-200c: $p = 0.017$, AUC = 0.72; miR-210: $p = 0.02$, AUC = 0.68; and miR-375: $p = 0.009$, AUC = 0.77), while the respective p-values of these five miRNAs were 0.001, 0.073, 0.055, 0.022, and 0.021 in a validation cohort [120].

Haldrup et al. [113] performed genome-wide miRNA profiling of serum samples from 13 BPH control and 31 PCa patients. The dysregulation of miR-141 and −375, two of the most well-documented candidate miRNA markers for PCa, was confirmed. Further, they developed three novel and highly specific miRNA panels (miR-562/-210/-501-3p/-375/-551b) able to identify 84% of all PCa patients, 80% of patients with disseminated PCa (let-7a*/miR-210/-562/-616), and 75% of disseminated PCa patients when compared to localized PC patients (miR-375/-708/-1203/-200a) [113]. miR-141 levels were significantly increased in patients with a higher Gleason score ($p = 0.05$) although the levels of miR-26a-1 and −141 in 170 pre-biopsy serum samples were similar in patients with positive and negative biopsies ($p = 0.72$, AUC = 0.52 and $p = 0.84$, AUC = 0.49, respectively) [121].

The expression levels of 4 miRNAs in plasma from 59 PCa patients with different clinic-pathological characteristics and two groups of controls, 16 BPH samples and 11 young asymptomatic men (YAM) were analyzed to evaluate their diagnostic and prognostic value in comparison to PSA. miR-375 was significantly downregulated in 83.5% of patients compared to BPH controls and showed stronger diagnostic accuracy (AUC = 0.81, 95% CI: 0.70–0.92, $p = 0.00016$) compared with PSA (AUC = 0.71, 95% CI: 0.56–0.86, $p = 0.013$). Sensitivity of 86.8% and specificity of 81.8% were reached when all

biomarkers were combined (AUC = 0.88) and YAM were used as calibrators [122].

In a study of 51 PCa patients and 20 healthy controls in Turkey, Yaman Agaoglu et al. [54] investigated the levels of miRs-21, −141, and −221 in plasma of patients and healthy controls. They found miR-21 and miR-221 levels were significantly higher in prostate patients than controls ($p < 0.001$, ROC-AUC = 88% and $p < 0.001$, AUC = 83%; respectively), but not for miR-141 ($p = 0.20$). miR-141, however, was found to be significantly higher in local advanced patients in comparison with those diagnosed with local outcome ($p < 0.001$, AUC = 76%) [54]. Brase et al. [115] observed enhanced expression of miR-375 and miR-141 in prostate tumor tissue compared to normal tissue and both miRNAs were upregulated in the sera of patients with metastatic disease compared to those with localized disease and correlated with high Gleason score or lymph-node positive status. These findings show miR-375 and miR-141 detection in serum may be associated with advanced disease [115].

Nguyen et al. [116] demonstrated over-expression miR-375, −378, and −141 were significantly in serum collected from castration resistant PCa patients compared to those with localized disease, while miR-409-3p was significantly under-expressed. In prostate tumor tissues, the expression of miR-375 and miR-141 were significantly higher than those in normal prostate tissue [116]. Relative to normal tissue, miR-205 (downregulated in mCRPC) was indicated by Watahiki et al. [123] to be associated with a lower Gleason score and a lower probability of both BCR and clinically evident metastatic events after prostatectomy. To the contrary, miR-141, 151-3p, 152 and 423-3p are inversely associated with prognosis and/or Gleason score. miR-141 and −152 may identify individuals with a high probability of recurrence after surgical treatment. miR-423-3p and miR-205 were suggested as novel prognostic factors due to their correlation with several clinical parameters [123].

Wang et al. [124] investigated whether pre-surgical serum levels of miRNAs can identify PCa patients. miR-19a and miR-19b displayed higher expression in the case group compared to controls, consistent with higher serum levels in cases. Conversely, miR-345 and -519c-5p had significantly lower expression among PCa patient. These results were consistent with lower levels in the patients' serum samples. Logistic regression models for predicting case/control status showed all four miRNAs as highly significant predictors of outcome status even when controlling for age, PSA, clinical stage, and degree of biopsy involvement. In the validation cohort, expression data of 4 miRNAs were consistent with data from the discovery cohort. Models consisting of a combination either miR-19a or -19b together with miR-345 and

- 519c-5p showed an AUC of 0.94, reaching high significance (p = 0.02 and p = 0.017 respectively) [124].

Shen et al. [56] also found miR-20a, −21 and −145 levels were significantly associated with PCa but not disease aggressiveness. The combination of these three miRNAs was a significant predictor and distinguished high risk PCa patients [56]. Martens-Uzunova et al. [48] evaluated some miRNAs significantly different in lymphocytes that could be used in the evaluation of progression of PCa, although some demonstrated an upregulation 2 fold-change or more between normal and PCa tissue (miR- 95, 96, 32, 153,182, 182*, 183) were and others (miR-133a, 133b, 221, 221*, 222, 224, 338-3p, 378*, 455-5p) were downregulation, especially miR-205 showed 6.3 fold downregulation [48]. Karatas et al., studying tissue samples from patients with recurrent and non-recurrent PCa, confirmed a negative uptake of miR-1 and miR-133b, miR-145* in recurrent Pca [51].

Mihelich et al. [125] developed the equation, miR Risk Score based on 7 miRNAs, miR, let-7a, −26b, −106a, −107, −130b, −223, and −451 in plasma samples. This scoring system showed to be highly predictive of low-grade PCa. The AUC for low-grade PCa was 0.69 across the range of miR risk scores [125]. Bryant et al. [117] reported 12 miRNAs were differentially expressed in PCa patients plasma compared with controls. Among the 12 miRNAs, 11 were significantly correlated with metastases. The association of two miRNAs, miR-141 and miR-375 with metastatic PCa was confirmed in a separate cohort. An analysis of urine samples indicated miR-107 and miR-574-3p were significantly associated with PCa risk [117].

Diagnosis/progression of prostate cancer based on urine and ejaculation

Srivastava et al. evaluated expression of 8 miRNAs in urine and tissue samples. miR-205, and miR-214 were significantly downregulated in PCa patients in both tissue and urine specimens. This miRNA profile can discriminate PCa patients from healthy individuals with 89% sensitivity and 80% specificity [105]. Haj-Ahmad et al. [126] performed miRNA expression profiling with urine samples obtained from 8 PCa patients, 12 BPH patients and 10 healthy males using whole genome expression analysis. Differential expression of two individual miRNAs between healthy males and BPH patients was detected and found to possibly target genes related to PCa development and progression among 894 miRNAs assayed. The authors found the sensitivity and specificity of miR-1825 for detecting PCa among BPH individuals were 60 and 69%, respectively. Further, the sensitivity and specificity for miR-1825 and −484 using tandem deregulation at the same time were 45 and 75%, respectively [126]. Another urine study suggested miR-483-5p was significantly associated with PCa based on samples from 71 PCa patients and 18 controls (p = 0.01; AUC = 0.69) [127].

Roberts et al. [128] evaluated the diagnostic performance of ejaculated-derived PCA3, Hepsin, and miRNAs (miR-125b, −200b, −200c, and −375) in 61 PCa patients. In stratified analysis, miR-200c (AUC = 0.79) and miR-375 (AUC = 0.76) demonstrated as the best single marker performance, while a combination of serum PSA, miR-200c and miR-125b further improved a prediction capacity for PCa status as compared to PSA alone determined by biopsy (AUC = 0.87 vs. 0.67; p < 0.05), and prostatectomy pathology (AUC = 0.81 vs. 0.70). For PCa status by biopsy, the specificity enhanced from 11% for PSA only to 67% for a combination of PSA, miR-200c, and miR-125b, with 90% specificity [128].

miRNA as predictors of therapeutic response for prostate cancer

miRNAs affect the expression of multiple genes in disease pathways and therefore represent interesting drug targets. Different experimental approaches used to validate the function of miRNAs can be potentially developed for miRNA-based therapies. For example, over-expressed oncogenic miRNAs can efficiently be inhibited using modified antisense oligonucleotides and this strategy was positively evaluated in animal models [129–131]. Expression of down-regulated tumor suppressor miRNA can be restored using synthetic precursor double stranded miRNA molecules or miRNA expression vectors delivered through lentiviral systems [67, 86]. miRNAs can also be exploited to increase the sensitivity of tumor cells to conventional anticancer agents [86]. For example, identification of miRNAs involved in the transition from androgen-independent to androgen-dependent state will aid in the modulation of the androgen-independent phenotype with the aim of increasing the responsiveness of advanced PCa to anticancer therapies. Some studies have currently demonstrated miRNAs are differentially expressed in androgen-independent compared to androgen-dependent PCa cell lines [65, 66, 73, 132].

With Low-Density Arrays (TLDA) to screen differentially expressed serum miRNAs, Cheng et al. [120] found that serum level of miR-210 were correlated with PSA level change per day during treatment (p = 0.029). Furthermore, expression of miR-210 was significantly lower in non-aggressive disease patients, as compared to those with recurrence (p = 0.001). The authors suggest that a subset of mCRPC patients may have a higher hypoxia response signaling, leading to increased miR-210 and therapy resistance. These data suggested miR-210 levels could be used to identify a distinct, subset of mCRPC patients with tumor-associated hypoxia. Gonzales et al. [133] studied in 21 PCa patients in a longitudinal manner with multiple blood draws. They determined the levels of miR-141 in PCa patients and compared it to the levels of three other conventional PCa biomarkers: PSA, lactate dehydrogenase (LDH) and circulating tumor cells (CTC). Then they found that miR-141 level changes were similar with changes observed by PSA, LDH and CTC and to the clinical assessments of the patients, suggests miR-141 can be used as a marker for therapeutic response in PCa patients. He et al. [134] reported that 28 miRNAs were differentially expressed between PCa tumor and adjacent benign tissues. The authors compared the miRNA expression profiles to non-Chinese populations and found that miR-23b, −220, −221, −222, and −205 may be common targets for treatments in all populations. This study also identified 15 specific miRNAs in Chinese patients. miR-374b and miR-19a showed significant correlations with clinical-pathological features in Chinese patients [134].

Lichnew et al. [135] confirmed results for 2 miRNAs were downregulation of miR-331-3p ($p = 0.009$) in the low-risk BCR group and miR-152 in the high-risk group ($p = 0.012$). To further confirm their results, using a second independent set of PCa cases, they observed similar results, as expected. The prediction model correctly classified high-risk individuals (33/35, 94.3%) and low-risk individuals (6/29, 20.7%) [135]. Someya et al. [136] investigated an association between miRNA expression and radio-sensitivity of PCa patients. They observed different miRNA expression among PCa patients with different radiation treatments. Three miRNAs (miR-99a, −147 and −508) in non-irradiated peripheral blood lymphocytes (PBLs) and one miRNA in irradiated PBLs (miR-199b), and significant induction of 11 miRNAs by irradiation (miR- 28, −185, −221, −340, −376c, −422a, −486, −491, −542, −652 and −660) were found. The authors concluded a combination of low ATP-dependent DNA helicase II (Ku80/XRCC5) expression and highly-induced miR-99a expression could be a promising marker for predicting radio-sensitivity after radiotherapy [136].

Conclusions

miRNAs regulate gene expression post-transcriptionally by both destabilizing mRNA and inhibiting their translation. Post-transcriptional regulation guarantees rapid and reversible changes in protein synthesis without altering transcription. Further, miRNAs can simultaneously modulate several cancer-relevant gene networks, because of their ability to bind to several targets. These attributes make miRNAs attractive candidates relevant as one-hit multi-target (polypharmacological) therapeutic agents against PCa and cancer in general. Further, miRNAs

represent a potential source of PCa diagnostic biomarkers. The stability of miRNA in serum and plasma and previous work showing differential expression of serum miRNA in normal and tumor tissue suggest the potential of miRNA as blood-based biomarkers for PCa diagnosis.

However, detailed knowledge of their expression, regulation, target genes and mechanism of action is required to achieve this goal. Moreover, it is critical to establish standard protocols for miRNA normalization and collection of tissue biospecimens. Some studies analyze miRNA expression in laser micro-dissected tumor tissue to procure tumor tissue with high purity [40, 98, 105, 106]. Unfortunately, other studies continue to analyze miRNA expression in snap frozen or FFPE tissue as observed in this review [61, 95, 101]. RNA endogenous controls (e.g., RNU44, RNU6B) can vary from study to study. The analysis of miRNA expression in non-micro-dissected tumor tissue and use of various miRNA endogenous controls, may skew miRNA expression profiles in PCa. For biological fluids (i.e., serum, plasma, urine), there is no designated endogenous control to normalization miRNA expression in cancer. However, some studies utilize stable synthetic Caenorhabditis elegans (i.e., Cel-39, −54, −238) as spike-in internal controls to normalized miRNA expression in serum [35, 115]. It is well known that African American men are 2.5 times more likely to die from PCa relative to Caucasian men [1]. In this review, majority of the miRNA profiling studies utilized pre-dominantly Caucasian populations. Given this apparent racial disparity in PCa, more miRNA profiling studies in diverse populations are needed to identify ethnic-specific miRNAs that may possibly play a role in aggressive disease among African American men. Ultimately, miRNA profiling in tumor tissue and biological fluids collected from more diverse populations using more standardized miRNA normalization protocols may lead to the identification of more key miRNAs and elucidate the role of miRNAs in PCa disease prevalence in certain populations.

Further studies in in vivo knockout or knock-in models should be helpful in understanding the pathways affected by miRNAs. Further, gene expression and proteomic analysis associated with loss- and gain-of-function studies in different model systems might contribute to a better understanding of the cellular networks affected by miRNA in the development and progression of cancer [5]. Additional investigation is also warranted to ascertain whether dysregulation of miRNA expression is causative rather than a consequence of cancer.

In summary, expression profiling studies provide evidence for the role of miRNAs in PCa diagnosis and prognosis. However, limited overlap exists between these studies and an extremely limited number of PCa-related miRNAs are currently known. Present promising candidates are miR-1, −21, 106b, 141, miR-145, miR-205, miR-221, and miR-375, which are the most frequently studied and seem to be the most promising for diagnosis and prognosis for prostate cancer.

Acknowledgment
This research was supported in part, by the National Cancer Institute grant R01CA128813 (PI: Park, JY).

Competing interests
The authors declare that they have no competing interests.

Authors' contributions
HL, GD, JP carried our the literature search and drafted the manuscript. HL, KS, OO, NK, GC, CP, DJ, LK, JB, KY, AB, RR, MY, SL, NK, SK participated in the design of the study and revision. All authors read and approved the final manuscript.

Author details
[1]Division of Epidemiology, Department of Medicine, Vanderbilt Epidemiology Center, Vanderbilt-Ingram Cancer Center, Vanderbilt University School of Medicine, Nashville, TN, USA. [2]Department of Epidemiology and Biostatistics, College of Public Health, University of South Florida, Tampa, FL, USA. [3]Biostatistics Program, School of Public Health, Louisiana State University Health Sciences Center, New Orleans, LA 70112, USA. [4]Department of Molecular Medicine, Aarhus University Hospital, Aarhus, Denmark. [5]Department of Biological Sciences, Hunter College of The City University of New York, New York, NY 10065, USA. [6]Department of Cancer Epidemiology, H. Lee Moffitt Cancer Center and Research Institute, Tampa, FL 33612, USA. [7]Department of Pharmacology and Toxicology, James Brown Cancer Center, University of Louisville School of Medicine, Louisville, KY 40202, USA. [8]Australian Prostate Cancer Research Centre-QLD, Institute of Health and Biomedical Innovation and School of Biomedical Sciences, Translational Research Institute, Queensland University of Technology, Brisbane, Australia. [9]Department of Radiation Oncology, H. Lee Moffitt Cancer Center and Research Institute, Tampa, FL 33612, USA. [10]Department of Biostatistics and Bioinformatics, H. Lee Moffitt Cancer Center and Research Institute, Tampa, FL 33612, USA. [11]Department of Tumor Biology, H. Lee Moffitt Cancer Center and Research Institute, Tampa, FL 33612, USA. [12]Research Center for Cell Fate Control, College of Pharmacy, Sookmyoung Women's University, Seoul, Republic of Korea. [13]Department of Internal Medicine, The Cancer Research Institute, College of Medicine, The Catholic University of Korea, Seoul, Republic of Korea. [14]Department of Pharmacy, Federal University of Sergipe, Rodovia Marechal Rodon, Jardim Rosa Elze, Sao Cristóvão, Brazil.

References
1. Siegel RL, Miller KD, Jemal A. Cancer statistics, 2016. CA Cancer J Clin. 2016; 66(1):7–30.
2. Pietro GD, Chornokur G, Kumar NB, Davis C, Park JY. Racial differences in the diagnosis and treatment of prostate cancer. Int Neurourol J. 2016;20 Suppl 2:S112–9.
3. Shen MM, Abate-Shen C. Molecular genetics of prostate cancer: new prospects for old challenges. Genes Dev. 2010;24(18):1967–2000.
4. Ankerst DP, Thompson IM. Sensitivity and specificity of prostate-specific antigen for prostate cancer detection with high rates of biopsy verification. Arch Ital Urol Androl. 2006;78(4):125–9.
5. Amankwah EaP, JY. miRNAs in human prostate cancer. In: Toxicology and epigenetics. edn. Edited by Sahu S. Chichester: The Wiley; 2012. p. 205–17.
6. Lee RC, Feinbaum RL, Ambros V. The C. elegans heterochronic gene lin-4 encodes small RNAs with antisense complementarity to lin-14. Cell. 1993; 75(5):843–54.
7. Bentwich I. Prediction and validation of microRNAs and their targets. FEBS Lett. 2005;579(26):5904–10.
8. Wahid F, Shehzad A, Khan T, Kim YY. MicroRNAs: synthesis, mechanism, function, and recent clinical trials. Biochim Biophys Acta. 2010;1803(11):1231–43.
9. Wienholds E, Plasterk RH. MicroRNA function in animal development. FEBS Lett. 2005;579(26):5911–22.
10. Wach S, Nolte E, Szczyrba J, Stohr R, Hartmann A, Orntoft T, Dyrskjot L, Eltze E, Wieland W, Keck B, et al. MicroRNA profiles of prostate carcinoma detected by multiplatform microRNA screening. Int J Cancer. 2012;130(3):611–21.
11. Bartel DP, Chen CZ. Micromanagers of gene expression: the potentially widespread influence of metazoan microRNAs. Nat Rev Genet. 2004;5(5):396–400.
12. Pang Y, Young CY, Yuan H. MicroRNAs and prostate cancer. Acta Biochim Biophys Sin Shanghai. 2010;42(6):363–9.
13. Rigoutsos I. New tricks for animal microRNAs: targeting of amino acid coding regions at conserved and nonconserved sites. Cancer Res. 2009;69(8):3245–8.
14. Krol J, Loedige I, Filipowicz W. The widespread regulation of microRNA biogenesis, function and decay. Nat Rev Genet. 2010;11(9): 597–610.
15. Friedman RC, Farh KK, Burge CB, Bartel DP. Most mammalian mRNAs are conserved targets of microRNAs. Genome Res. 2009;19(1):92–105.
16. Schaefer A, Jung M, Kristiansen G, Lein M, Schrader M, Miller K, Stephan C, Jung K. MicroRNAs and cancer: current state and future perspectives in urologic oncology. Urol Oncol. 2010;28(1):4–13.
17. Brennecke J, Stark A, Russell RB, Cohen SM. Principles of microRNA-target recognition. PLoS Biol. 2005;3(3):e85.
18. Filipowicz W, Bhattacharyya SN, Sonenberg N. Mechanisms of post-transcriptional regulation by microRNAs: are the answers in sight? Nat Rev Genet. 2008;9(2):102–14.
19. Santarpia L, Nicoloso M, Calin GA. MicroRNAs: a complex regulatory network drives the acquisition of malignant cell phenotype. Endocr Relat Cancer. 2010;17(1):F51–75.
20. Calin GA, Dumitru CD, Shimizu M, Bichi R, Zupo S, Noch E, Aldler H, Rattan S, Keating M, Rai K, et al. Frequent deletions and down-regulation of micro-RNA genes miR15 and miR16 at 13q14 in chronic lymphocytic leukemia. Proc Natl Acad Sci U S A. 2002;99(24):15524–9.
21. Zhang B, Pan X, Cobb GP, Anderson TA. microRNAs as oncogenes and tumor suppressors. Dev Biol. 2007;302(1):1–12.
22. Calin GA, Croce CM. MicroRNA signatures in human cancers. Nat Rev Cancer. 2006;6(11):857–66.
23. Calin GA, Croce CM. MicroRNAs and chromosomal abnormalities in cancer cells. Oncogene. 2006;25(46):6202–10.
24. Calin GA, Croce CM. MicroRNA-cancer connection: the beginning of a new tale. Cancer Res. 2006;66(15):7390–4.
25. Cummins JM, Velculescu VE. Implications of micro-RNA profiling for cancer diagnosis. Oncogene. 2006;25(46):6220–7.
26. Dalmay T. MicroRNAs and cancer. J Intern Med. 2008;263(4):366–75.
27. Dalmay T, Edwards DR. MicroRNAs and the hallmarks of cancer. Oncogene. 2006;25(46):6170–5.
28. Tricoli JV, Jacobson JW. MicroRNA: potential for cancer detection, diagnosis, and prognosis. Cancer Res. 2007;67(10):4553–5.
29. Lu J, Getz G, Miska EA, Alvarez-Saavedra E, Lamb J, Peck D, Sweet-Cordero A, Ebert BL, Mak RH, Ferrando AA, et al. MicroRNA expression profiles classify human cancers. Nature. 2005;435(7043):834–8.
30. Calin GA, Ferracin M, Cimmino A, Di Leva G, Shimizu M, Wojcik SE, Iorio MV, Visone R, Sever NI, Fabbri M, et al. A MicroRNA signature associated with prognosis and progression in chronic lymphocytic leukemia. N Engl J Med. 2005;353(17):1793–801.
31. Schetter AJ, Leung SY, Sohn JJ, Zanetti KA, Bowman ED, Yanaihara N, Yuen ST, Chan TL, Kwong DL, Au GK, et al. MicroRNA expression profiles associated with prognosis and therapeutic outcome in colon adenocarcinoma. JAMA. 2008;299(4):425–36.
32. Medina PP, Slack FJ. microRNAs and cancer: an overview. Cell Cycle. 2008; 7(16):2485–92.
33. Jung M, Schaefer A, Steiner I, Kempkensteffen C, Stephan C, Erbersdobler A, Jung K. Robust microRNA stability in degraded RNA preparations from human tissue and cell samples. Clin Chem. 2010;56(6):998–1006.
34. Dijkstra JR, Mekenkamp LJ, Teerenstra S, De Krijger I, Nagtegaal ID. MicroRNA expression in formalin-fixed paraffin embedded tissue using real time quantitative PCR: the strengths and pitfalls. J Cell Mol Med. 2012;16(4):683–90.

35. Mitchell PS, Parkin RK, Kroh EM, Fritz BR, Wyman SK, Pogosova-Agadjanyan EL, Peterson A, Noteboom J, O'Briant KC, Allen A, et al. Circulating microRNAs as stable blood-based markers for cancer detection. Proc Natl Acad Sci U S A. 2008;105(30):10513–8.

36. Chen X, Ba Y, Ma L, Cai X, Yin Y, Wang K, Guo J, Zhang Y, Chen J, Guo X, et al. Characterization of microRNAs in serum: a novel class of biomarkers for diagnosis of cancer and other diseases. Cell Res. 2008;18(10):997–1006.

37. Kong W, Yang H, He L, Zhao JJ, Coppola D, Dalton WS, Cheng JQ. MicroRNA-155 is regulated by the transforming growth factor beta/Smad pathway and contributes to epithelial cell plasticity by targeting RhoA. Mol Cell Biol. 2008;28(22):6773–84.

38. O'Connell RM, Taganov KD, Boldin MP, Cheng G, Baltimore D. MicroRNA-155 is induced during the macrophage inflammatory response. Proc Natl Acad Sci U S A. 2007;104(5):1604–9.

39. Yin Q, McBride J, Fewell C, Lacey M, Wang X, Lin Z, Cameron J, Flemington EK. MicroRNA-155 is an Epstein-Barr virus-induced gene that modulates Epstein-Barr virus-regulated gene expression pathways. J Virol. 2008;82(11):5295–306.

40. Ambs S, Prueitt RL, Yi M, Hudson RS, Howe TM, Petrocca F, Wallace TA, Liu CG, Volinia S, Calin GA, et al. Genomic profiling of microRNA and messenger RNA reveals deregulated microRNA expression in prostate cancer. Cancer Res. 2008;68(15):6162–70.

41. Galardi S, Mercatelli N, Giorda E, Massalini S, Frajese GV, Ciafre SA, Farace MG. miR-221 and miR-222 expression affects the proliferation potential of human prostate carcinoma cell lines by targeting p27Kip1. J Biol Chem. 2007;282(32):23716–24.

42. Mercatelli N, Coppola V, Bonci D, Miele F, Costantini A, Guadagnoli M, Bonanno E, Muto G, Frajese GV, De Maria R, et al. The inhibition of the highly expressed miR-221 and miR-222 impairs the growth of prostate carcinoma xenografts in mice. PLoS ONE. 2008;3(12):e4029.

43. Sylvestre Y, De Guire V, Querido E, Mukhopadhyay UK, Bourdeau V, Major F, Ferbeyre G, Chartrand P. An E2F/miR-20a autoregulatory feedback loop. J Biol Chem. 2007;282(4):2135–43.

44. He L, Thomson JM, Hemann MT, Hernando-Monge E, Mu D, Goodson S, Powers S, Cordon-Cardo C, Lowe SW, Hannon GJ, et al. A microRNA polycistron as a potential human oncogene. Nature. 2005;435(7043):828–33.

45. Volinia S, Calin GA, Liu CG, Ambs S, Cimmino A, Petrocca F, Visone R, Iorio M, Roldo C, Ferracin M, et al. A microRNA expression signature of human solid tumors defines cancer gene targets. Proc Natl Acad Sci U S A. 2006;103(7):2257–61.

46. Chang YS, Chen WY, Yin JJ, Sheppard-Tillman H, Huang J, Liu YN. EGF receptor promotes prostate cancer bone metastasis by downregulating miR-1 and activating TWIST1. Cancer Res. 2015;75(15):3077–86.

47. Kojima S, Chiyomaru T, Kawakami K, Yoshino H, Enokida H, Nohata N, Fuse M, Ichikawa T, Naya Y, Nakagawa M, et al. Tumour suppressors miR-1 and miR-133a target the oncogenic function of purine nucleoside phosphorylase (PNP) in prostate cancer. Br J Cancer. 2012;106(2):405–13.

48. Martens-Uzunova ES, Jalava SE, Dits NF, van Leenders GJ, Moller S, Trapman J, Bangma CH, Litman T, Visakorpi T, Jenster G. Diagnostic and prognostic signatures from the small non-coding RNA transcriptome in prostate cancer. Oncogene. 2012;31(8):978–91.

49. Hudson RS, Yi M, Esposito D, Watkins SK, Hurwitz AA, Yfantis HG, Lee DH, Borin JF, Naslund MJ, Alexander RB, et al. MicroRNA-1 is a candidate tumor suppressor and prognostic marker in human prostate cancer. Nucleic Acids Res. 2012;40(8):3689–703.

50. Liu YN, Yin JJ, Abou-Kheir W, Hynes PG, Casey OM, Fang L, Yi M, Stephens RM, Seng V, Sheppard-Tillman H, et al. MiR-1 and miR-200 inhibit EMT via Slug-dependent and tumorigenesis via Slug-independent mechanisms. Oncogene. 2013;32(3):296–306.

51. Karatas OF, Guzel E, Suer I, Ekici ID, Caskurlu T, Creighton CJ, Ittmann M, Ozen M. miR-1 and miR-133b are differentially expressed in patients with recurrent prostate cancer. PLoS One. 2014;9(6):e98675.

52. Stope MB, Stender C, Schubert T, Peters S, Weiss M, Ziegler P, Zimmermann U, Walther R, Burchardt M. Heat-shock protein HSPB1 attenuates microRNA miR-1 expression thereby restoring oncogenic pathways in prostate cancer cells. Anticancer Res. 2014;34(7):3475–80.

53. Liu YN, Yin J, Barrett B, Sheppard-Tillman H, Li D, Casey OM, Fang L, Hynes PG, Ameri AH, Kelly K. Loss of androgen-regulated MicroRNA 1 activates SRC and promotes prostate cancer bone metastasis. Mol Cell Biol. 2015;35(11):1940–51.

54. Yaman Agaoglu F, Kovancilar M, Dizdar Y, Darendeliler E, Holdenrieder S, Dalay N, Gezer U. Investigation of miR-21, miR-141, and miR-221 in blood circulation of patients with prostate cancer. Tumour Biol. 2011;32(3):583–8.

55. Li T, Li RS, Li YH, Zhong S, Chen YY, Zhang CM, Hu MM, Shen ZJ. miR-21 as an independent biochemical recurrence predictor and potential therapeutic target for prostate cancer. J Urol. 2012;187(4):1466–72.

56. Shen J, Hruby GW, McKiernan JM, Gurvich I, Lipsky MJ, Benson MC, Santella RM. Dysregulation of circulating microRNAs and prediction of aggressive prostate cancer. Prostate. 2012;72(13):1469–77.

57. Ribas J, Ni X, Haffner M, Wentzel EA, Salmasi AH, Chowdhury WH, Kudrolli TA, Yegnasubramanian S, Luo J, Rodriguez R, et al. miR-21: an androgen receptor-regulated microRNA that promotes hormone-dependent and hormone-independent prostate cancer growth. Cancer Res. 2009;69(18):7165–9.

58. Reis ST, Pontes-Junior J, Antunes AA, Dall'Oglio MF, Dip N, Passerotti CC, Rossini GA, Morais DR, Nesrallah AJ, Piantino C, et al. miR-21 may acts as an oncomir by targeting RECK, a matrix metalloproteinase regulator, in prostate cancer. BMC Urol. 2012;12:14.

59. Mishra S, Deng JJ, Gowda PS, Rao MK, Lin CL, Chen CL, Huang T, Sun LZ. Androgen receptor and microRNA-21 axis downregulates transforming growth factor beta receptor II (TGFBR2) expression in prostate cancer. Oncogene. 2014;33(31):4097–106.

60. Li T, Li D, Sha J, Sun P, Huang Y. MicroRNA-21 directly targets MARCKS and promotes apoptosis resistance and invasion in prostate cancer cells. Biochem Biophys Res Commun. 2009;383(3):280–5.

61. Szczyrba J, Loprich E, Wach S, Jung V, Unteregger G, Barth S, Grobholz R, Wieland W, Stohr R, Hartmann A, et al. The microRNA profile of prostate carcinoma obtained by deep sequencing. Mol Cancer Res. 2010;8(4):529–38.

62. Poliseno L, Salmena L, Riccardi L, Fornari A, Song MS, Hobbs RM, Sportoletti P, Varmeh S, Egia A, Fedele G, et al. Identification of the miR-106b ~ 25 microRNA cluster as a proto-oncogenic PTEN-targeting intron that cooperates with its host gene MCM7 in transformation. Sci Signal. 2010;3(117):ra29.

63. Hudson RS, Yi M, Esposito D, Glynn SA, Starks AM, Yang Y, Schetter AJ, Watkins SK, Hurwitz AA, Dorsey TH, et al. MicroRNA-106b-25 cluster expression is associated with early disease recurrence and targets caspase-7 and focal adhesion in human prostate cancer. Oncogene. 2013;32(35):4139–47.

64. Liang H, Studach L, Hullinger RL, Xie J, Andrisani OM. Down-regulation of RE-1 silencing transcription factor (REST) in advanced prostate cancer by hypoxia-induced miR-106b ~ 25. Exp Cell Res. 2014;320(2):188–99.

65. DeVere White RW, Vinall RL, Tepper CG, Shi XB. MicroRNAs and their potential for translation in prostate cancer. Urol Oncol. 2009;27(3):307–11.

66. Shi XB, Xue L, Yang J, Ma AH, Zhao J, Xu M, Tepper CG, Evans CP, Kung HJ, deVere White RW. An androgen-regulated miRNA suppresses Bak1 expression and induces androgen-independent growth of prostate cancer cells. Proc Natl Acad Sci U S A. 2007;104(50):19983–8.

67. Bonci D, Coppola V, Musumeci M, Addario A, Giuffrida R, Memeo L, D'Urso L, Pagliuca A, Biffoni M, Labbaye C, et al. The miR-15a-miR-16-1 cluster controls prostate cancer by targeting multiple oncogenic activities. Nat Med. 2008;14(11):1271–7.

68. Aqeilan RI, Calin GA, Croce CM. miR-15a and miR-16-1 in cancer: discovery, function and future perspectives. Cell Death Differ. 2010;17(2):215–20.

69. Varambally S, Cao Q, Mani RS, Shankar S, Wang X, Ateeq B, Laxman B, Cao X, Jing X, Ramnarayanan K, et al. Genomic loss of microRNA-101 leads to overexpression of histone methyltransferase EZH2 in cancer. Science. 2008;322(5908):1695–9.

70. Musiyenko A, Bitko V, Barik S. Ectopic expression of miR-126*, an intronic product of the vascular endothelial EGF-like 7 gene, regulates prostein translation and invasiveness of prostate cancer LNCaP cells. J Mol Med (Berl). 2008;86(3):313–22.

71. Fujita Y, Kojima K, Hamada N, Ohhashi R, Akao Y, Nozawa Y, Deguchi T, Ito M. Effects of miR-34a on cell growth and chemoresistance in prostate cancer PC3 cells. Biochem Biophys Res Commun. 2008;377(1):114–9.

72. Lodygin D, Tarasov V, Epanchintsev A, Berking C, Knyazeva T, Korner H, Knyazev P, Diebold J, Hermeking H. Inactivation of miR-34a by aberrant CpG methylation in multiple types of cancer. Cell Cycle. 2008;7(16):2591–600.

73. Lin SL, Chiang A, Chang D, Ying SY. Loss of mir-146a function in hormone-refractory prostate cancer. RNA. 2008;14(3):417–24.

74. Fuse M, Nohata N, Kojima S, Sakamoto S, Chiyomaru T, Kawakami K, Enokida H, Nakagawa M, Naya Y, Ichikawa T, et al. Restoration of miR-145 expression suppresses cell proliferation, migration and invasion in prostate cancer by targeting FSCN1. Int J Oncol. 2011;38(4):1093–101.

75. Suh SO, Chen Y, Zaman MS, Hirata H, Yamamura S, Shahryari V, Liu J, Tabatabai ZL, Kakar S, Deng G, et al. MicroRNA-145 is regulated by DNA methylation and p53 gene mutation in prostate cancer. Carcinogenesis. 2011;32(5):772–8.

76. Tong AW, Fulgham P, Jay C, Chen P, Khalil I, Liu S, Senzer N, Eklund AC, Han J, Nemunaitis J. MicroRNA profile analysis of human prostate cancers. Cancer Gene Ther. 2009;16(3):206–16.

77. Wach S, Nolte E, Szczyrba J, Stohr R, Hartmann A, Orntoft T, Dyrskjot L, Eltze E, Wieland W, Keck B et al. MicroRNA profiles of prostate carcinoma detected by multiplatform microRNA screening. Int J Cancer 2012;130(3):611-21.

78. Gandellini P, Folini M, Longoni N, Pennati M, Binda M, Colecchia M, Salvioni R, Supino R, Moretti R, Limonta P, et al. miR-205 exerts tumor-suppressive functions in human prostate through down-regulation of protein kinase cepsilon. Cancer Res. 2009;69(6):2287–95.

79. Ozen M, Creighton CJ, Ozdemir M, Ittmann M. Widespread deregulation of microRNA expression in human prostate cancer. Oncogene. 2008;27(12): 1788–93.

80. Prueitt RL, Yi M, Hudson RS, Wallace TA, Howe TM, Yfantis HG, Lee DH, Stephens RM, Liu CG, Calin GA, et al. Expression of microRNAs and protein-coding genes associated with perineural invasion in prostate cancer. Prostate. 2008;68(11):1152–64.

81. Schaefer A, Jung M, Mollenkopf HJ, Wagner I, Stephan C, Jentzmik F, Miller K, Lein M, Kristiansen G, Jung K. Diagnostic and prognostic implications of microRNA profiling in prostate carcinoma. Int J Cancer. 2010;126(5):1166–76.

82. Yang K, Handorean AM, Iczkowski KA. MicroRNAs 373 and 520c are downregulated in prostate cancer, suppress CD44 translation and enhance invasion of prostate cancer cells in vitro. Int J Clin Exp Pathol. 2009;2(4):361–9.

83. Patron JP, Fendler A, Bild M, Jung U, Muller H, Arntzen MO, Piso C, Stephan C, Thiede B, Mollenkopf HJ, et al. MiR-133b targets antiapoptotic genes and enhances death receptor-induced apoptosis. PLoS ONE. 2012;7(4):e35345.

84. Li X, Wan X, Chen H, Yang S, Liu Y, Mo W, Meng D, Du W, Huang Y, Wu H, et al. Identification of miR-133b and RB1CC1 as independent predictors for biochemical recurrence and potential therapeutic targets for prostate cancer. Clin Cancer Res. 2014;20(9):2312–25.

85. Costa-Pinheiro P, Ramalho-Carvalho J, Vieira FQ, Torres-Ferreira J, Oliveira J, Goncalves CS, Costa BM, Henrique R, Jeronimo C. MicroRNA-375 plays a dual role in prostate carcinogenesis. Clin Epigenetics. 2015; 7(1):42.

86. Gandellini P, Folini M, Zaffaroni N. Towards the definition of prostate cancer-related microRNAs: where are we now? Trends Mol Med. 2009;15(9): 381–90.

87. Porkka KP, Pfeiffer MJ, Waltering KK, Vessella RL, Tammela TL, Visakorpi T. MicroRNA expression profiling in prostate cancer. Cancer Res. 2007;67(13): 6130–5.

88. Khan AP, Poisson LM, Bhat VB, Fermin D, Zhao R, Kalyana-Sundaram S, Michailidis G, Nesvizhskii AI, Omenn GS, Chinnaiyan AM, et al. Quantitative proteomic profiling of prostate cancer reveals a role for miR-128 in prostate cancer. Mol Cell Proteomics. 2010;9(2):298–312.

89. Kristensen H, Haldrup C, Strand S, Mundbjerg K, Mortensen MM, Thorsen K, Ostenfeld MS, Wild PJ, Arsov C, Goering W, et al. Hypermethylation of the GABRE ~ miR-452 ~ miR-224 promoter in prostate cancer predicts biochemical recurrence after radical prostatectomy. Clin Cancer Res. 2014; 20(8):2169–81.

90. Wang L, Tang H, Thayanithy V, Subramanian S, Oberg AL, Cunningham JM, Cerhan JR, Steer CJ, Thibodeau SN. Gene networks and microRNAs implicated in aggressive prostate cancer. Cancer Res. 2009;69(24):9490–7.

91. Spahn M, Kneitz S, Scholz CJ, Stenger N, Rudiger T, Strobel P, Riedmiller H, Kneitz B. Expression of microRNA-221 is progressively reduced in aggressive prostate cancer and metastasis and predicts clinical recurrence. Int J Cancer. 2010;127(2):394–403.

92. Hagman Z, Larne O, Edsjo A, Bjartell A, Ehrnstrom RA, Ulmert D, Lilja H, Ceder Y. miR-34c is downregulated in prostate cancer and exerts tumor suppressive functions. Int J Cancer. 2010;127(12):2768–76.

93. Pesta M, Klecka J, Kulda V, Topolcan O, Hora M, Eret V, Ludvikova M, Babjuk M, Novak K, Stolz J, et al. Importance of miR-20a expression in prostate cancer tissue. Anticancer Res. 2010;30(9):3579–83.

94. Taylor BS, Schultz N, Hieronymus H, Gopalan A, Xiao Y, Carver BS, Arora VK, Kaushik P, Cerami E, Reva B, et al. Integrative genomic profiling of human prostate cancer. Cancer Cell. 2010;18(1):11–22.

95. Hao Y, Zhao Y, Zhao X, He C, Pang X, Wu TC, Califano JA, Gu X. Improvement of prostate cancer detection by integrating the PSA test with miRNA expression profiling. Cancer Invest. 2011;29(4):318–24.

96. Mishra S, Lin CL, Huang TH, Bouamar H, Sun LZ. MicroRNA-21 inhibits p57Kip2 expression in prostate cancer. Mol Cancer. 2014;13:212.

97. Bonci D, Coppola V, Patrizii M, Addario A, Cannistraci A, Francescangeli F, Pecci R, Muto G, Collura D, Bedini R, et al. A microRNA code for prostate cancer metastasis. Oncogene. 2016;35(9):1180–92.

98. Mihelich BL, Khramtsova EA, Arva N, Vaishnav A, Johnson DN, Giangreco AA, Martens-Uzunova E, Bagasra O, Kajdacsy-Balla A, Nonn L. miR-183-96-182 cluster is overexpressed in prostate tissue and regulates zinc homeostasis in prostate cells. J Biol Chem. 2011;286(52):44503–11.

99. Moltzahn F, Olshen AB, Baehner L, Peek A, Fong L, Stoppler H, Simko J, Hilton JF, Carroll P, Blelloch R. Microfluidic-based multiplex qRT-PCR identifies diagnostic and prognostic microRNA signatures in the sera of prostate cancer patients. Cancer Res. 2011;71(2): 550–60.

100. Zhang HL, Yang LF, Zhu Y, Yao XD, Zhang SL, Dai B, Zhu YP, Shen YJ, Shi GH, Ye DW. Serum miRNA-21: elevated levels in patients with metastatic hormone-refractory prostate cancer and potential predictive factor for the efficacy of docetaxel-based chemotherapy. Prostate. 2011; 71(3):326–31.

101. Avgeris M, Stravodimos K, Fragoulis EG, Scorilas A. The loss of the tumour-suppressor miR-145 results in the shorter disease-free survival of prostate cancer patients. Br J Cancer. 2013;108(12):2573–81.

102. Amankwah EK, Anegbe E, Park H, Pow-Sang J, Hakam A, Park JY. miR-21, miR-221 and miR-222 expression and prostate cancer recurrence among obese and non-obese cases. Asian J Androl. 2013;15(2):226–30.

103. Barnabas N, Xu L, Savera A, Hou Z, Barrack ER. Chromosome 8 markers of metastatic prostate cancer in African American men: gain of the MIR151 gene and loss of the NKX3-1 gene. Prostate. 2011;71(8):857–71.

104. Leite KR, Tomiyama A, Reis ST, Sousa-Canavez JM, Sanudo A, Camara-Lopes LH, Srougi M. MicroRNA expression profiles in the progression of prostate cancer–from high-grade prostate intraepithelial neoplasia to metastasis. Urol Oncol. 2013;31(6):796–801.

105. Srivastava A, Goldberger H, Dimtchev A, Ramalinga M, Chijioke J, Marian C, Oermann EK, Uhm S, Kim JS, Chen LN, et al. MicroRNA profiling in prostate cancer–the diagnostic potential of urinary miR-205 and miR-214. PLoS ONE. 2013;8(10):e76994.

106. Tsuchiyama K, Ito H, Taga M, Naganuma S, Oshinoya Y, Nagano K, Yokoyama O, Itoh H. Expression of microRNAs associated with Gleason grading system in prostate cancer: miR-182-5p is a useful marker for high grade prostate cancer. Prostate. 2013;73(8):827–34.

107. Guzel E, Karatas OF, Semercioz A, Ekici S, Aykan S, Yentur S, Creighton CJ, Ittmann M, Ozen M. Identification of microRNAs differentially expressed in prostatic secretions of patients with prostate cancer. Int J Cancer. 2015; 136(4):875–9.

108. Larne O, Martens-Uzunova E, Hagman Z, Edsjo A, Lippolis G, den Berg MS, Bjartell A, Jenster G, Ceder Y. miQ–a novel microRNA based diagnostic and prognostic tool for prostate cancer. Int J Cancer. 2013; 132(12):2867–75.

109. Mavridis K, Stravodimos K, Scorilas A. Downregulation and prognostic performance of microRNA 224 expression in prostate cancer. Clin Chem. 2013;59(1):261–9.

110. Walter BA, Valera VA, Pinto PA, Merino MJ. Comprehensive microRNA profiling of prostate cancer. J Cancer. 2013;4(5):350–7.

111. Casanova-Salas I, Rubio-Briones J, Calatrava A, Mancarella C, Masia E, Casanova J, Fernandez-Serra A, Rubio L, Ramirez-Backhaus M, Arminan A, et al. Identification of miR-187 and miR-182 as biomarkers of early diagnosis and prognosis in patients with prostate cancer treated with radical prostatectomy. J Urol. 2014;192:252–9.

112. Kristensen H, Thomsen AR, Haldrup C, Dyrskjot L, Hoyer S, Borre M, Mouritzen P, Orntoft TF, Sorensen KD. Novel diagnostic and prognostic classifiers for prostate cancer identified by genome-wide microRNA profiling. Oncotarget. 2016;7:30760–71.

113. Haldrup C, Kosaka N, Ochiya T, Borre M, Hoyer S, Orntoft TF, Sorensen KD. Profiling of circulating microRNAs for prostate cancer biomarker discovery. Drug Deliv Transl Res. 2014;4(1):19–30.

114. Selth LA, Townley S, Gillis JL, Ochnik AM, Murti K, Macfarlane RJ, Chi KN, Marshall VR, Tilley WD, Butler LM. Discovery of circulating microRNAs associated with human prostate cancer using a mouse model of disease. Int J Cancer. 2012;131(3):652–61.

115. Brase JC, Johannes M, Schlomm T, Falth M, Haese A, Steuber T, Beissbarth T, Kuner R, Sultmann H. Circulating miRNAs are correlated with tumor progression in prostate cancer. Int J Cancer. 2011;128(3):608–16.

116. Nguyen HC, Xie W, Yang M, Hsieh CL, Drouin S, Lee GS, Kantoff PW. Expression differences of circulating microRNAs in metastatic castration resistant prostate cancer and low-risk, localized prostate cancer. Prostate. 2013;73(4):346–54.

117. Bryant RJ, Pawlowski T, Catto JW, Marsden G, Vessella RL, Rhees B, Kuslich C, Visakorpi T, Hamdy FC. Changes in circulating microRNA levels associated with prostate cancer. Br J Cancer. 2012;106(4):768–74.

118. Mahn R, Heukamp LC, Rogenhofer S, von Ruecker A, Muller SC, Ellinger J. Circulating microRNAs (miRNA) in serum of patients with prostate cancer. Urology. 2011;77(5):1265. e1269-1216.

119. Chen ZH, Zhang GL, Li HR, Luo JD, Li ZX, Chen GM, Yang J. A panel of five circulating microRNAs as potential biomarkers for prostate cancer. Prostate. 2012;72(13):1443–52.

120. Cheng HH, Mitchell PS, Kroh EM, Dowell AE, Chery L, Siddiqui J, Nelson PS, Vessella RL, Knudsen BS, Chinnaiyan AM, et al. Circulating microRNA profiling identifies a subset of metastatic prostate cancer patients with evidence of cancer-associated hypoxia. PLoS ONE. 2013;8(7):e69239.

121. Westermann AM, Schmidt D, Holdenrieder S, Moritz R, Semjonow A, Schmidt M, Kristiansen G, Muller SC, Ellinger J. Serum microRNAs as biomarkers in patients undergoing prostate biopsy: results from a prospective multi-center study. Anticancer Res. 2014;34(2):665–9.

122. Kachakova D, Mitkova A, Popov E, Popov I, Vlahova A, Dikov T, Christova S, Mitev V, Slavov C, Kaneva R. Combinations of serum prostate-specific antigen and plasma expression levels of let-7c, miR-30c, miR-141, and miR-375 as potential better diagnostic biomarkers for prostate cancer. DNA Cell Biol. 2015;34(3):189–200.

123. Watahiki A, Macfarlane RJ, Gleave ME, Crea F, Wang Y, Helgason CD, Chi KN. Plasma miRNAs as biomarkers to identify patients with castration-resistant metastatic prostate cancer. Int J Mol Sci. 2013;14(4):7757–70.

124. Wang SY, Shiboski S, Belair CD, Cooperberg MR, Simko JP, Stoppler H, Cowan J, Carroll PR, Blelloch R. miR-19, miR-345, miR-519c-5p serum levels predict adverse pathology in prostate cancer patients eligible for active surveillance. PLoS ONE. 2014;9(6):e98597.

125. Mihelich BL, Maranville JC, Nolley R, Peehl DM, Nonn L. Elevated serum microRNA levels associate with absence of high-grade prostate cancer in a retrospective cohort. PLoS ONE. 2015;10(4):e0124245.

126. Haj-Ahmad TA, Abdalla MA, Haj-Ahmad Y. Potential urinary miRNA biomarker candidates for the accurate detection of prostate cancer among benign prostatic hyperplasia patients. J Cancer. 2014;5(3):182–91.

127. Korzeniewski N, Tosev G, Pahernik S, Hadaschik B, Hohenfellner M, Duensing S. Identification of cell-free microRNAs in the urine of patients with prostate cancer. Urol Oncol. 2015;33(1):16. e17-22.

128. Roberts MJ, Chow CW, Schirra HJ, Richards R, Buck M, Selth LA, Doi SA, Samaratunga H, Perry-Keene J, Payton D, et al. Diagnostic performance of expression of PCA3, Hepsin and miR biomarkers inejaculate in combination with serum PSA for the detection of prostate cancer. Prostate. 2015;75(5): 539–49.

129. Elmen J, Lindow M, Silahtaroglu A, Bak M, Christensen M, Lind-Thomsen A, Hedtjarn M, Hansen JB, Hansen HF, Straarup EM, et al. Antagonism of microRNA-122 in mice by systemically administered LNA-antimiR leads to up-regulation of a large set of predicted target mRNAs in the liver. Nucleic Acids Res. 2008;36(4):1153–62.

130. Krutzfeldt J, Rajewsky N, Braich R, Rajeev KG, Tuschl T, Manoharan M, Stoffel M. Silencing of microRNAs in vivo with 'antagomirs'. Nature. 2005;438(7068): 685–9.

131. Stenvang J, Kauppinen S. MicroRNAs as targets for antisense-based therapeutics. Expert Opin Biol Ther. 2008;8(1):59–81.

132. Sun T, Wang Q, Balk S, Brown M, Lee GS, Kantoff P. The role of microRNA-221 and microRNA-222 in androgen-independent prostate cancer cell lines. Cancer Res. 2009;69(8):3356–63.

133. Gonzales JC, Fink LM, Goodman Jr OB, Symanowski JT, Vogelzang NJ, Ward DC. Comparison of circulating MicroRNA 141 to circulating tumor cells, lactate dehydrogenase, and prostate-specific antigen for determining treatment response in patients with metastatic prostate cancer. Clin Genitourin Cancer. 2011;9(1):39–45.

134. He HC, Han ZD, Dai QS, Ling XH, Fu X, Lin ZY, Deng YH, Qin GQ, Cai C, Chen JH, et al. Global analysis of the differentially expressed miRNAs of prostate cancer in Chinese patients. BMC Genomics. 2013;14:757.

135. Lichner Z, Fendler A, Saleh C, Nasser AN, Boles D, Al-Haddad S, Kupchak P, Dharsee M, Nuin PS, Evans KR, et al. MicroRNA signature helps distinguish early from late biochemical failure in prostate cancer. Clin Chem. 2013; 59(11):1595–603.

136. Someya M, Yamamoto H, Nojima M, Hori M, Tateoka K, Nakata K, Takagi M, Saito M, Hirokawa N, Tokino T, et al. Relation between Ku80 and microRNA-99a expression and late rectal bleeding after radiotherapy for prostate cancer. Radiother Oncol. 2015;115(2):235–9.

137. Lodes MJ, Caraballo M, Suciu D, Munro S, Kumar A, Anderson B. Detection of cancer with serum miRNAs on an oligonucleotide microarray. PLoS ONE. 2009;4(7):e6229.

138. Leite KR, Tomiyama A, Reis ST, Sousa-Canavez JM, Sanudo A, Dall'Oglio MF, Camara-Lopes LH, Srougi M. MicroRNA-100 expression is independently related to biochemical recurrence of prostate cancer. J Urol. 2011;185(3): 1118–22.

139. Dip N, Reis ST, Abe DK, Viana NI, Morais DR, Moura CM, Katz B, Silva IA, Srougi M, Leite KR. Micro RNA expression and prognosis in low-grade non-invasive urothelial carcinoma. Int Braz J Urol. 2014;40(5):644–9.

13

Nadir PSA level and time to nadir PSA are prognostic factors in patients with metastatic prostate cancer

Atsushi Tomioka*, Nobumichi Tanaka, Motokiyo Yoshikawa, Makito Miyake, Satoshi Anai, Yoshitomo Chihara, Eijiro Okajima, Akihide Hirayama, Yoshihiko Hirao and Kiyohide Fujimoto

Abstract

Background: Primary androgen deprivation therapy (PADT) is the most effective systemic therapy for patients with metastatic prostate cancer. Nevertheless, once PSA progression develops, the prognosis is serious and mortal. We sought to identify factors that predicted the prognosis in a series of patients with metastatic prostate cancer.

Methods: Two-hundred eighty-six metastatic prostate cancer patients who received PADT from 1998 to 2005 in Nara Uro-Oncology Research Group were enrolled. The log-rank test and Cox's proportional hazards model were used to determine the predictive factors for prognosis; rate of castration-resistant prostate cancer (CRPC) and overall survival.

Results: The median age, follow-up period and PSA level at diagnosis were 73 years, 47 months and 174 ng/mL, respectively. The 5-year overall survival rate was 63.0%. The multivariable analysis showed that Gleason score (Hazard ratio [HR]:1.362; 95% confidence interval [C.I.], 1.023-1.813), nadir PSA (HR:6.332; 95% C.I., 4.006-9.861) and time from PADT to nadir (HR:4.408; 95% C.I., 3.099-6.271) were independent prognostic factors of the incidence of CRPC. The independent parameters in the multivariate analysis that predicted overall survival were nadir PSA (HR:5.221; 95% C.I., 2.757-9.889) and time from PADT to nadir (HR:4.008; 95% C.I., 2.137-7.517).

Conclusions: Nadir PSA and time from PADT to nadir were factors that affect both CRPC and overall survival in a cohort of patients with metastatic prostate cancer. Lower nadir PSA level and longer time from PADT to nadir were good for survival and progression.

Keywords: Prostate cancer, Metastasis, Risk factors

Background

Prostate cancer is the fourth most commonly diagnosed cancer and the ninth leading cause of cancer deaths among males in Japan [1]. At the moment, Japanese prostate cancer patients show higher risk characteristics compared with the patients in the United States, and the proportion of metastatic patients is still high [2,3]. Whereas primary androgen deprivation therapy (PADT) is standard for metastatic prostate cancer, most patients progress to castration-resistant prostate cancer (CRPC) at various intervals after PADT. Prostate specific antigen (PSA) is a biomarker for

diagnosis, risk classification, and monitoring of the disease. Most patients will experience a substantial decline in PSA levels, and their PSA levels may remain low or undetectable for years. Nevertheless, CRPC occurs frequently [4]. CRPC follows an androgen-independent state, which leads to widespread metastases. PSA progression in advanced prostate cancer indicates clinical progression in patients treated with PADT within a median of 6 months [5]. The substantial variability in the clinical course of metastatic prostate cancer has led to the evaluation of a number of prognostic factors with respect to their roles in determining the treatment strategy and ability to predict the response to therapy. In most clinical trials of prostate cancer, an improvement of 50% in the serum PSA is used as a marker of

* Correspondence: tomioka515@yahoo.co.jp
Department of Urology, Nara Medical University, 840 Shijo-cho, Kashihara, Nara 634-8522, Japan

response [6,7]. The criteria for disease progression when using changes in PSA is defined by the Prostate Cancer Clinical Trials Working Group (PCWG2) [6] and the Prostate-Specific Antigen Working Group (PSAWG) [7], and has been validated by the data-sets from two large Southwest Oncology Group Trials (SWOG 9346 and 9916) [8]. We endeavored to identify risk factors for prognosis in our series of patients with hormone naïve metastatic prostate cancer.

Methods

This study retrospectively evaluated 286 Japanese patients with metastatic prostate cancer who received PADT following diagnosis in the Nara Uro-Oncology Research Group (NUORG) between January 1998 and December 2005. The diagnosis was based on prostate biopsy. Abdominal computed tomography and/or bone scans were used in all cases with suspected metastases. All patients were treated with PADT using a luteinizing hormone-releasing hormone (LH-RH) agonist, surgical castration, anti-androgen monotherapy or combined androgen blockade (CAB).

Follow-up data were retrieved from the hospital medical records. Patients were followed every month for the first 3 months and every 3 months thereafter. The nadir PSA level was defined as the lowest PSA level after PADT. CRPC was defined as the first day when the PSA was increased for three consecutive times or when clear clinical radiological evidence of progressive disease was shown. This study analyzed the incidences of progression times to CRPC after the initiation of PADT and overall survival time. The progression rate to CRPC and overall survival rate were estimated and both univariate and multivariate analyses were carried out to determine the prognostic value of age (≤75 years vs. ≥76 years), TNM classification (UICC 2002 [9]), pathological Gleason score (6–8 vs. 9–10), PSA level at diagnosis (<100 ng/mL vs. 100–500 ng/mL vs. ≥500 ng/mL), nadir PSA level (<0.2 ng/mL vs. 0.2-4 ng/mL vs. ≥4 ng/mL), time from PADT to nadir (≥12 months vs. 6–12 months vs. <6 months) and time from PADT to CRPC (No occurrence of CRPC vs. ≥12 months vs. 6–12 months vs. <6 months).

Statistical analyses were carried out using the SPSS software package (SPSS Inc., Chicago, Illinois, version 17.0) and p < 0.05 was considered to be statistically significant. Overall survival was estimated by the Kaplan-Meier method. The log rank test was used to assess differences between groups. The Cox proportional hazards regression model was performed to analyze independent predictors of CRPC and overall survival. Only the variables that were found to be significant in the univariate analyses (p < 0.05) were entered into the multivariate analysis to determine the most significant factor for predicting disease outcome.

The Medical Ethics Committee of Nara Medical University approved this retrospective study, and it was exempted to obtain informed consent from the patients in consideration of the aim and methods of this study.

Results

The characteristics of the patients are shown in Table 1. The median age and PSA at diagnosis were 73 years (range 50 to 92) and 174 ng/mL (range 5.7 to 21864), respectively. The median follow-up was 47 months (range 2 to 128) and the treatment of PADT was CAB in 92.0% of the patients. There were no differences in the progression time to CRPC and overall survival between PADTs (LH-RH agonist, surgical castration, anti-androgen monotherapy or CAB) (Data are not shown). Most patients initially responded to PADT. The median nadir PSA level was 0.3 ng/mL (range 0.001 to 650) and 42.7% of patients reached a nadir PSA <0.2 ng/mL. The median time from PADT to nadir was 9.45 months (range 1 to 64). 72.4% of patients progressed to CRPC and the median time to progression after the initiation of treatment was 13 months (range 1 to 97). The 5-year overall survival rate was 63.0%, the median survival time from CRPC was 45 months, and 35.7% of patients died during the follow-up period, of which cancer deaths and other cause deaths were 27.6% and 8.0%, respectively.

T stage (T2 vs. T3, T4), Gleason score (6–8 vs. 9–10), PSA at diagnosis (<100 ng/mL vs. ≥500 ng/mL), nadir PSA (<0.2 ng/mL vs. 0.2-4 ng/mL) and time from PADT to nadir (≥12 months vs. 6–12 months vs. <6 months) were significantly associated with the progression time to CRPC (Table 1). A lower nadir PSA level and a longer time from PADT to nadir were associated with a lower proportion of patients with CRPC progression. The median progression time to CRPC of the patients with nadir PSA <0.2 ng/mL, 0.2-4 ng/mL and ≥4 ng/mL were 38 months, 13 months and 8 months, respectively (p < 0.005). The median progression time to CRPC of the patients whose time from PADT to nadir were ≥12 months, 6-12 months and <6 months, were 35 months, 13 months and 7 months, respectively (p < 0.005). The median nadir PSA level of the patients with time from PADT to nadir ≥12 months, 6–12 months and <6 months, were 0.1 ng/mL, 0.3 ng/mL and 1.18 ng/mL, respectively (p < 0.05: ≥12 months vs. <6 months). The univariate analysis showed that the Gleason score, PSA at diagnosis, nadir PSA and time from PADT to nadir were associated with progression to CRPC (Table 2). The multivariate analysis showed that Gleason score, nadir PSA and time from PADT to nadir were significant independent factors.

The log-rank test showed that overall survival was correlated with nadir PSA (<0.2 ng/mL vs. 0.2-4 ng/mL vs. ≥4 ng/mL), time from PADT to nadir (≥12 months

Table 1 Characteristics of patients and the results of the log-rank test of prognostic factors

		Median (range)	No. of patients	No. of CRPC	Median progression time (months)		No. of deaths	Median survival time (months)	
Total			286	207	19		102	113	
Age		73 (50–91)							
	≤75		179	132	19		69	85	
	≥76		107	75	18	n.s.	33	none	n.s.
T	T1		4	2	57		0	all alive	
	T2		31	18	37	*(T2 vs. T3, T4)	9	111	
	T3		162	114	19		60	83	
	T4		89	73	14		33	77	n.s.
N	N0		164	116	19		59	79	
	N1		122	91	19	n.s.	43	99	n.s.
M	M0		50	31	26		9	99	
	M1		236	176	18	n.s.	93	83	n.s.
Gleason score	6-8		181	83	21	*	63	115	
	9-10		105	124	14		39	85	n.s.
PSA at diagnosis		174 (5.7-21864)							
	<100		105	64	23		31	85	
	100-500		97	73	16	*(<100 vs. ≥500)	36	113	
	≥500		84	70	15		35	none	n.s.
Nadir PSA level		0.3 (0.001-650)							
	<0.2		122	71	38		26	115	
	0.2-4		112	86	13	**	44	62	***
	≥4		52	50	8		32	25	
Time from PADT to Nadir		9.45 (1–64)							
	≥12		114	74	35		23	113	
	6-12		83	62	13	**	39	79	***
	<6		89	71	7		40	28	
Time from PADT to CRPC		13 (1–97)							
	No CRPC		79				14	none	
	≥12		112				32	113	***
	6-12		63				34	35	
	<6		32				22	21	

*P<0.005, **all P<0.001, ***P<0.001 without No CRPC vs. ≥12
PADT: primary androgen deprivation therapy.
CRPC: castration resistant prostate cancer.

vs. 6–12 months vs. <6 months) and time from PADT to CRPC (≥12 months vs. 6–12 months vs. <6 months) (Table 1). The multivariate analysis showed that nadir PSA and time from PADT to nadir were independent factors associated with overall survival (Table 3).

Discussion

A PSA test provides useful information, not only for the screening of prostate cancer but also for monitoring following treatment. Moreover, PSA monitoring before and after PADT are useful to evaluate the response to treatment in patients with prostate cancer. PSA concentrations decrease by 80% in approximately 80% of patients in the first month following PADT [10], and normalize in 95% of cases within 3–6 months [11]. Rising PSA after the nadir value under PADT represents the first objective sign of CRPC. PSA recurrence usually predates clinical progression of metastatic prostatic cancer after PADT [6,12]. Most of the patients in the current series initially responded to PADT; 43.2% of patients reached a nadir PSA <0.2 ng/mL,

Table 2 Hazards ratio estimate and confidence intervals from proportional hazards modeling of progression to CRPC

		Univariate analysis			Multivariate analysis		
		Hazard ratio	95% C.I.	P value	Hazard ratio	95% C.I.	P value
Age		0.993	0.975-1.011	0.425	0.990	0.972-1.007	0.248
T	T1	1					
	T2	1.359	0.315-5.867	0.681			
	T3	2.142	0.528-8.691	0.286			
	T4	3.336	0.816-13.647	0.094			
Gleason score	6-8	1			1		
	9-10	1.518	1.148-2.009	0.003	1.362	1.023-1.813	0.034
PSA at diagnosis	<100	1			1		
	100-500	1.374	0.981-1.923	0.064	0.990	0.691-1.417	0.955
	≥500	1.616	1.149-2.271	0.006	1.099	0.682-1.492	0.965
Nadir PSA level	<0.2	1			1		
	0.2-4	2.778	2.011-3.836	<0.001	2.794	1.984-3.936	<0.001
	≥4	6.339	4.315-9.313	<0.001	6.332	4.066-9.861	<0.001
Time from PADT to nadir	≥12	1			1		
	6-12	2.091	1.480-2.953	<0.001	2.245	1.559-3.232	<0.001
	<6	4.131	2.956-5.774	<0.001	4.408	3.099-6.271	<0.001

95% CI.: 95% confidence interval.
PADT: primary androgen deprivation therapy.
CRPC: castration resistant prostate cancer.

72.4% had progression to CRPC and the median time from PADT to CRPC was 13 months.

We sought to identify risk factors for the prognosis of a series of patients with metastatic prostate cancer before or during PADT. We believe that it could be useful to decide on the best treatment strategy to predict which patients are more likely to develop early progression to CRPC. There are many views about the prognostic value of the PSA level at diagnosis. Several PSA-related parameters have been reported, including PSA at diagnosis, pattern of PSA decrease after treatment, time to nadir PSA and percentage of PSA decrease. Some authors found that the PSA level at diagnosis did not predict the time to progression [5,13]. However, others have proposed that PSA at diagnosis predicts the disease response to androgen suppression [14-16]. Early normalization of PSA delays the time to progression, and in combination with the Gleason score, PSA is an important prognostic factor to predict the

Table 3 Hazards ratio estimate and confidence intervals from proportional hazards modeling of overall survival

		Univariate analysis			Multivariate analysis		
		Hazard ratio	95% C.I.	P value	Hazard ratio	95% C.I.	P value
Age		0.987	0.962-1.013	0.324	0.994	0.967-1.021	0.647
Nadir PSA level	<0.2	1			1		
	0.2-4	3.038	1.852-4.982	<0.001	2.329	1.342-4.040	0.003
	≥4	7	4.109-11.925	<0.001	5.221	2.757-9.889	<0.001
Time from PADT to nadir	≥12	1			1		
	6-12	2.544	1.473-4.393	0.001	1.483	0.789-2.789	0.221
	<6	6.918	4.174-11.467	<0.001	4.008	2.137-7.517	<0.001
Time from PADT to CRPC	No CRPC	1			1		
	≥12	0.963	0.509-1.822	0.907	0.718	0.367-1.407	0.335
	6-12	4.323	2.310-8.089	<0.001	1.419	0.664-3.031	0.367
	<6	9.021	4.570-17.808	<0.001	1.712	0.731-4.005	0.215

95% CI.: 95% confidence interval.
PADT: primary androgen deprivation therapy.
CRPC: castration resistant prostate cancer.

efficacy of the therapy [17]. The decline of PSA to <4 ng/mL after the initiation of PADT within 3 months is thought to be more important than the Gleason score in determining the time to progression [17].

Nadir PSA after PADT is usually evaluated in relation to progression to CRPC [13,16,18-21]. The ability to achieve an undetectable PSA level as nadir is the most significant predictor of the time to CRPC for metastatic and advanced prostatic cancer and the time to nadir PSA is significantly and positively correlated with the PSA progression-free survival [13]. Failure to attain a nadir PSA of <1 ng/mL after treatment predicts early progression to CRPC [20,21]. In the current series, the median nadir PSA level was 0.3 ng/mL. We classify the nadir PSA level into <0.2 ng/mL, 0.2-4 ng/mL and ≥4 ng/mL, because PSA level <0.2 ng/mL is an undetectable PSA and the normal PSA value is less than 4 ng/mL. Then, nadir PSA (<0.2 ng/mL vs. 0.2-4 ng/mL vs. ≥4 ng/mL) was a significant independent factor that predicted the progression to CRPC after PADT.

Nadir PSA levels after PADT are usually evaluated in relationship to the overall survival time. A nadir PSA of >2 ng/mL predicts poorer overall survival [21]. By using the data of a randomized phase 3 trial, a PSA level of ≤4 ng/mL after 7 months of PADT was a strong independent predictor of improvement survival in metastatic hormone-sensitive prostate cancer [22]. Time to nadir < 6 months, Gleason score >7 and nadir PSA ≥0.2 ng/mL independently predicted shorter overall survival in patients with metastatic hormone-sensitive prostate cancer [18], which included patients who underwent definitive initial local therapy (radical prostatectomy or radiotherapy) and did not showed the factor of time to CRPC after initiation of PADT. Nadir PSA <0.2 ng/mL and longer time to nadir (>9 months) during PADT are the most important early predictors for survival in prostate cancer patients with bone metastasis [23]. The current study included the metastatic prostate cancer patients treated only with PADT, also predicts the factor of progression to CRPC and showed a nadir PSA (<0.2 ng/mL vs. 0.2-4 ng/mL vs. ≥4 ng/mL) and the time from PADT to nadir (≥12 months vs. 6−12 months vs. <6 months) were independent factors for overall survival. Nadir PSA and time from PADT to nadir are important factors associated with both CRPC and overall survival. This indicates that a simple measurement of PSA was strongly associated with time to CRPC and overall survival in metastatic CRPC, and the optimal cut-off point of the nadir PSA and the time from PADT to nadir predicts a short or long response of PADT.

Longer time to reach nadir PSA was associated with a lower nadir PSA level and this may simply indicate continued androgen sensitivity. The mechanisms responsible for the association of shorter time to nadir with a worse prognosis are not clear. A rapid decrease in the PSA level may be related to a transcriptional effect of PADT on PSA progression rather than prostate cancer cell death [20]. A rapid decrease in the PSA level after PADT may be due to ablation of the androgen receptor function, and quick suppression of androgen/androgen receptor during PADT may have a negative effect on disease progression, because the androgen receptor can act as a tumor suppressor for prostate cancer [24]. Another possibility is that a rapid removal of hormone-sensitive prostate cancer cells may induce an environment that allows the growth of hormone-resistant prostate cancer cells [23].

There are limitations to the current study. Firstly, some important factors, such as lactate dehydrogenase, alkaline phosphatase, albumin, testosterone, hemoglobin and performance status were not included in this analysis, because they were not routinely measured in the patients. Secondly, we only reported the outcomes of PADT but not evaluated the following results of second-line treatment such as chemotherapy. Thirdly, there may be interobserver variation of the Gleason score between general pathologists and uropathologists.

Conclusions

PSA progression and PSA decline provide clinically meaningful information early during the treatment course of patients with metastatic prostate cancer who are unlikely to benefit from standard PADT long before they develop CRPC. Further prospective data and external validation of independent datasets are needed to confirm these findings.

Lower nadir PSA value and longer time to nadir PSA after the initiation of PADT correlate with lower progression to CRPC and higher overall survival.

Abbreviations
PADT: Primary androgen deprivation therapy; CRPC: Castration-resistant prostate cancer; PSA: Prostate specific antigen; LH-RH: Hormone-releasing hormone; CAB: Combined androgen blockade.

Competing interests
The authors declare that they have no competing interests.

Authors' contributions
AT contributed to analysis and interpretation of data and was involved in drafting the manuscript. TN contributed to conception and helped to draft the manuscript. MY, MM, SA and YC contributed to acquisition of data. EO and AH contributed to acquisition of data and helped to draft the manuscript. YH and KF conceived and supervised the study, helped to draft the manuscript and was involved in revising it critically for important intellectual content. All authors read and approved the final manuscript.

Acknowledgments
The authors acknowledge the efforts of Nara Uro-Oncology Research Group (Nara Medical University Hospital, Nara Prefectural Nara Hospital, Nara Prefectural Mimuro Hospital, Nara City Hospital, Yamato Takada Municipal Hospital, Uda City Hospital, Saiseikai Nara Hospital, Saiseikai Chuwa Hospital, Takanohara Central Hospital, Takai Hospital, Hirao Hospital, Nara Yukoukai Hospital, Hanna Central Hospital, Hoshigaoka Koseinenkin Hospital, Osaka Gyoumeikan Hospital, Osaka Kaisei Hospital, Tane General Hospital, Okanami General Hospital and Matsusaka Chuo General Hospital) that registered the patient's data.

References

1. Matsuda A, Matsuda T, Shibata A, Katanoda K, Sobue T, Nishimoto H: Cancer Incidence and Incidence Rates in Japan in, A Study of 21 Population-based Cancer Registries for the Monitoring of Cancer Incidence in Japan (MCIJ) Project. *Jpn J Clin Oncol* 2007, 2013(43):328–336.

2. Tanaka N, Fujimoto K, Hirayama A, Yoneda T, Yoshida K, Hirao Y: Trends of the primary therapy for patients with prostate cancer in Nara uro-oncological research group (NUORG): a comparison between the CaPSURE data and the NUORG data. *Jpn J Clin Oncol* 2010, 40:588–592.

3. Tanaka N, Hirayama A, Yoneda T, Yoshida K, Shimada K, Konishi N, Fujimoto K: Trends of risk classification and primary therapy for Japanese patients with prostate cancer in Nara Uro-Oncological Research Group (NUORG)-a comparison between 2004–2006 and 2007–2009. *BMC Cancer* 2013, 10:588.

4. D'Amico AV, Chen MH, Roehl KA, Catalona WJ: Preoperative PSA velocity and the risk of death from prostate cancer after radical prostatectomy. *N Engl J Med* 2004, 351:125–135.

5. Miller JI, Ahmann FR, Drach GW, Emerson SS, Bottaccini MR: The clinical usefulness of serum prostate specific antigen after hormonal therapy of metastatic prostate cancer. *J Urol* 1992, 147:956–961.

6. Scher HI, Halabi S, Tannock I, Morris M, Stemberg CN, Carducci MA, Eisenberger MA, Higano C, Bubley GJ, Dreicer R, Petrylak D, Kantoff P, Basch E, Kelly WK, Figg WD, Small EJ, Beer TM, Wilding G, Martin A, Hussain M: Prostate Cancer Clinical Trials Working Group: Design and end points of clinical trials for patients with progressive prostate cancer and castrate levels of testosterone: recommendations of the Prostate Cancer Clinical Trials Working Group. *J Clin Oncol* 2008, 26:1148–1159.

7. Bubley GJ, Carducci M, Dahut W, Dawson N, Daliani D, Eisenberger M, Figg WD, Freidlin B, Halabi S, Hudes G, Hussain M, Kaplan R, Myers C, Oh W, Petrylak DP, Reed E, Roth B, Sartor O, Scher H, Simons J, Sinibaldi V, Small EJ, Smith MR, Trump DL, Wilding G: Eligibility and response guidelines for phase II clinical trials in androgen-independent prostate cancer: recommendations from the Prostate-Specific Antigen Working Group. *J Clin Oncol* 1999, 17:3461–3467.

8. Hussain M, Goldman B, Tangen C, Higano CS, Petrylak DP, Wilding G, Akdas AM, Small EJ, Donnelly BJ, Sundram SK, Burch PA, Dipaola RS, Crawford ED: Prostate-specific antigen progression predicts overall survival in patients with metastatic prostate cancer: data from Southwest Oncology Group Trials 9346 (Intergroup Study 0162) and 9916. *J Clin Oncol* 2009, 27:2450–2456.

9. Sobin LH, Wittekind CH: *TNM Classification of Malignant Tumors.* 6th edition. New York: Wiley-Liss Inc.; 2002:184–187.

10. Arai Y, Yoshiki T, Yoshida O: Prognostic significance of prostate specific antigen in endocrine treatment for prostatic cancer. *J Urol* 1990, 144:1415–1419.

11. Matzkin H, Eber P, Todd B, van der Zwaag R, Soloway MS: Prognostic significance of changes in prostate-specific markers after endocrine treatment of stage D2 prostatic cancer. *Cancer* 1992, 70:2302–2309.

12. Newling DW, Denis L, Vermeylen K: Orchiectomy versus goserelin and flutamide in the treatment of newly diagnosed metastatic prostate cancer. Analysis of the criteria of evaluation used in the European Organization for Research and Treatment of Cancer–Genitourinary Group Study 30853. *Cancer* 1993, 72:3793–3798.

13. Benaim EA, Pace CM, Lam PM, Roehrborn CG: Nadir prostate-specific antigen as a predictor of progression to androgen-independent prostate cancer. *Urology* 2002, 59:73–78.

14. Cooper EH: Prostate specific antigen in diagnosis, staging, and follow-up of prostate cancer. *Prostate Suppl* 1992, 4:125–128.

15. Dijkman GA, Janknegt RA, De Reijke TM, Debruyne FM: Long-term efficacy and safety of nilutamide plus castration in advanced prostate cancer, and the significance of early prostate specific antigen normalization. International Anandron Study Group. *J Urol* 1997, 158:160–163.

16. Morote J, Trilla E, Esquena S, Abascal JM, Reventos J: Nadir prostate-specific antigen best predicts the progression to androgen-independent prostate cancer. *Int J Cancer* 2004, 108:877–881.

17. Kiper A, Yigitbasi O, Imamoglu A, Tuygun C, Turan C: The prognostic importance of prostate specific antigen in the monitorisation of patients undergoing maximum androgen blockade for metastatic prostate cancer. *Int Urol Nephrol* 2006, 38:571–576.

18. Choueiri TK, Xie W, D'Amico AV, Ross EW, Hu JC, Pomerantz M, Regan MM, Taplin ME, Kantoff PW, Sartor O, Oh WK: Time to prostate-specific antigen nadir independently predicts overall survival in patients who have metastatic hormone-sensitive prostate cancer treated with androgen-deprivation therapy. *Cancer* 2009, 115:981–987.

19. Kwak C, Jeong SJ, Park MS, Lee E, Lee SE: Prognostic significance of the nadir prostate specific antigen level after hormone therapy for prostate cancer. *J Urol* 2002, 168:995–1000.

20. Park SC, Rim JS, Choi HY, Kim CS, Hong SJ, Kim WJ, Lee SE, Song JM, Yoon JH: Failing to achieve a nadir prostate-specific antigen after combined androgen blockade: predictive factors. *Int J Urol* 2009, 16:670–675.

21. Sim HG, Lau WK, Cheng CW: Predictors of androgen independence in metastatic prostate cancer. *BJU Int* 2004, 93:1221–1224.

22. Hussain M, Tangen CM, Higano C, Schelhammer PF, Faulkner J, Crawford ED, Wilding G, Akdas A, Small EJ, Donnelly B, MacVicar G, Raghavan D: Southwest Oncology Group Trial 9346 (INT-0162): Absolute prostate-specific antigen value after androgen deprivation is a strong independent predictor of survival in new metastatic prostate cancer: data from Southwest Oncology Group Trial 9346 (INT-0162). *J Clin Oncol* 2006, 24:3984–3989.

23. Sasaki T, Ohnishi T, Hoshina A: Nadir PSA level and time to PSA nadir following primary androgen deprivation therapy are the early survival predictors for prostate cancer patients with bone metastasis. *Prostate Cancer Prostatic dis* 2011, 14:248–252.

24. Huang SP, Bao BY, Wu MT, Choueiri TK, Goggins WB, Huang CY, Pu YS, Yu CC, Huang CH: Impact of prostate-specific antigen (PSA) nadir and time to PSA nadir on disease progression in prostate cancer treated with androgen-deprivation therapy. *Prostate* 2011, 71:1189–1197.

14

Clinical intervals and diagnostic characteristics in a cohort of prostate cancer patients in Spain

Xavier Bonfill[1,2,3,4], María José Martinez-Zapata[1,2,3*], Robin WM Vernooij[2], María José Sánchez[1,5], María Morales Suárez-Varela[1,6], Javier de la Cruz[1,7], José Ignacio Emparanza[1,8], Montserrat Ferrer[1,9], José Ignacio Pijoán[1,10], Juan M. Ramos-Goñi[11], Joan Palou[3,12], Stefanie Schmidt[13], Víctor Abraira[1,14], Javier Zamora[1,14] and on behalf of the EMPARO-CU study group

Abstract

Background: Little is known about the healthcare process for patients with prostate cancer, mainly because hospital-based data are not routinely published. The main objective of this study was to determine the clinical characteristics of prostate cancer patients, the, diagnostic process and the factors that might influence intervals from consultation to diagnosis and from diagnosis to treatment.

Methods: We conducted a multicentre, cohort study in seven hospitals in Spain. Patients' characteristics and diagnostic and therapeutic variables were obtained from hospital records and patients' structured interviews from October 2010 to September 2011. We used a multilevel logistic regression model to examine the association between patient care intervals and various variables influencing these intervals (age, BMI, educational level, ECOG, first specialist consultation, tumour stage, PSA, Gleason score, and presence of symptoms) and calculated the odds ratio (OR) and the interquartile range (IQR). To estimate the random inter-hospital variability, we used the median odds ratio (MOR).

Results: 470 patients with prostate cancer were included. Mean age was 67.8 (SD: 7.6) years and 75.4 % were physically active. Tumour size was classified as T1 in 41.0 % and as T2 in 40 % of patients, their median Gleason score was 6.0 (IQR:1.0), and 36.1 % had low risk cancer according to the D'Amico classification. The median interval between first consultation and diagnosis was 89 days (IQR:123.5) with no statistically significant variability between centres. Presence of symptoms was associated with a significantly longer interval between first consultation and diagnosis than no symptoms (OR:1.93, 95%CI 1.29–2.89). The median time between diagnosis and first treatment (therapeutic interval) was 75.0 days (IQR:78.0) and significant variability between centres was found (MOR:2.16, 95%CI 1.45–4.87). This interval was shorter in patients with a high PSA value ($p = 0.012$) and a high Gleason score ($p = 0.026$).

Conclusions: Most incident prostate cancer patients in Spain are diagnosed at an early stage of an adenocarcinoma. The period to complete the diagnostic process is approximately three months whereas the therapeutic intervals vary among centres and are shorter for patients with a worse prognosis. The presence of prostatic symptoms, PSA level, and Gleason score influence all the clinical intervals differently.

Keywords: Prostatic neoplasms, Male urogenital diseases, Multicentre study, Cohort study, Prospective study

* Correspondence: mmartinezz@santpau.cat
[1]CIBER de Epidemiología y Salud Pública (CIBERESP), Madrid, Spain
[2]Institute of Biomedical Research (IIB Sant Pau), Iberoamerican Cochrane Centre, Barcelona, Spain
Full list of author information is available at the end of the article

Background

Prostate cancer is the most frequently diagnosed cancer among Spanish men. With an incidence of 65.2 per 100 000 persons per year (27 853 new cases yearly 21.7 % of the total cancer in men), it is overall the second most frequent cancer in Spain [1]. Worldwide, it is the second most frequently diagnosed cancer among men (1 111 689 new cases, 15.0 % of all cancers in men) and overall the fourth most common cancer [1]. The incidence of prostate cancer has increased over the last decades, partly due to the more frequent use of diagnostic tools such as prostate-specific antigen (PSA) testing and needle biopsies in asymptomatic men [2–4]. The impact on mortality is high. Mortality rates in Spain showed a slight increase between 1980 and 1998 but have since decreased [5, 6]. In 2012, the estimated mortality associated with prostate cancer was 5481 in Spain and 307 471 worldwide, making it the third leading cause of death due to cancer for men in Spain (8.6 % of the total) and the sixth leading cause worldwide (6.6 % of the total) [1]. Furthermore, prostate cancer reduces the quality of life of patients [7, 8].

The economic burden of prostate cancer is one of the largest among malignant tumours due to the high incidence of the disease and increasing survival rates [9]. It is estimated to cost 11.85 billion USD annually in the USA [9]. Total costs for diagnosing, treating, and monitoring patients with prostate cancer for five years have been estimated to be approximately £7294.2 per patient and £92.74 million overall in the United Kingdom [10].

The Spanish Health System is funded by taxes. It offers universal coverage and is managed regionally within each of the 17 autonomous communities. Healthcare is divided into two broad areas, primary care and hospital care. Prostate cancer is generally detected in primary care centres, where patients might undergo some diagnostic tests. For confirmatory tests, however, such as a prostate biopsy, the patient is referred to a hospital for specialised healthcare. Direct access to specialised healthcare may also occur through the hospital emergency services, but this is less frequent.

Several international initiatives have been launched to obtain detailed and reliable information regarding the healthcare process for prostate cancer patients. This information includes the time intervals between first consultation to diagnosis, and first treatment. Such projects include The European Cancer Registry-based Study of Survival and Care of Cancer Patients (EUROCARE) [11], the Patient Outcome Research Teams (PORTS) [12], and the Cancer of the Prostate Strategic Urologic Research Endeavour (CAPSURE) [13]. Information can also be obtained from databases containing regional and national incidence and mortality statistics, from hospital minimum data sets, and from hospital-based cancer registries that allow a description and generic comparison of hospital healthcare [14, 15]. These sources of information, however, do not include the type of data needed to identify the diagnostic processes, therapeutic approaches, and prognostic factors in prostate cancer. Recently, one study regarding prostate cancer has been conducted in Spain, with the objective to estimate prostate cancer incidence and profile the newly-diagnosed cases using a nationwide hospital-based registry [16, 17]. However, this study fails to examine the diagnosis and therapeutic processes and possible factors influencing these time intervals. The objective of the EMPARO-CU study is to examine the clinical care process and health outcomes of patients with urologic tumours during the first year from the histopathological prostate cancer confirmation. In this paper we describe the patients' baseline characteristics at hospital entry and the time intervals between the first consultation and diagnosis, and between diagnosis and start of treatment and possible factors influencing these intervals.

Methods

The EMPARO-CU study is a multicentre, cohort study of bladder and prostate cancer, conducted in seven tertiary hospitals in Spain: *Fundació Puigvert-Hospital de la Santa Creu i Sant Pau* (coordinating centre) and *Hospital del Mar* in Barcelona, *Hospital Universitario 12 de Octubre* and *Hospital Universitario Ramón y Cajal* in Madrid, *Hospital Universitario Donostia* in Donostia-San Sebastián, *Hospital General Universitario de Valencia* in Valencia, and *Hospital Universitario Virgen de las Nieves* in Granada (list of participants in Appendix). The protocol was approved by the research ethics committees at each participating centre (Table 1). Patients were enrolled from October 2010 to September 2011. Consecutive patients were selected from the urologic and oncology departments at each centre. Inclusion criteria were: 1) diagnosis of prostate cancer during the study period, independently of the tumour stage; 2) diagnosis and treatment at one of the participating hospitals; and 3) agreement to participate and signed informed consent.

Table 1 List of ethic committees that approval the study

Hospital de la Santa Creu i Sant Pau (Barcelona)
Fundación Puigvert (Barcelona)
Hospital 12 de Octubre (Madrid)
Hospital Ramón y Cajal (Madrid)
Autonómico del País Vasco
Hospital Donosti (San Sebastián)
Hospital General Universitario de Valencia
Hospital Nuestra Señora del Mar (Barcelona)
Hospital Virgen de las Nieves (Granada)

The EMPARO-CU study focuses on the clinical care process and health outcomes of patients with urologic tumours. In this paper we describe the patients' baseline characteristics at hospital entry and the intervals between the first consultation and diagnosis, and between diagnosis and start of treatment. Information regarding patient status before the diagnosis (such as symptoms at first visit) was collected retrospectively. Study data were collected from the medical records and from structured interviews with individual patients. Variables of interest were: socio-demographic data, body mass index (BMI), Charlson index, ECOG WHO score, first specialist consulted, diagnostic tests performed to establish a diagnosis of prostate cancer, pathological results of prostate biopsy [18], PSA values, total Gleason scores, clinical stages, time from first symptom to first consultation, and time from first consultation to primary diagnosis and first treatment (Fig. 1). Time from first symptom to first consultation was defined as the date on which the patients experienced the first symptoms related to prostate cancer. The date of first consultation was considered the date on which the patient first consulted a healthcare professional for the symptoms that led to prostate cancer screening. For asymptomatic patients, the first consultation was considered the date on which the physician performed prostate screening. We considered the first histological confirmation as the confirmatory diagnosis of the disease. The reference date to calculate intervals was the date of biopsy that confirmed the histological diagnosis of prostate cancer. The time interval between the first consultation and biopsy was considered the diagnostic interval. The time between the biopsy and first treatment was considered the therapeutic interval.

Categorical variables are described using relative frequency, and continuous variables are described using mean and standard deviation (SD) or median and interquartile range (IQR) for skewed distribution variables. The frequency of missing values is reported for each variable.

The association between time variables and potential predictors was assessed using multilevel (patients at first level and hospitals at second level) logistic regression models. The variables included as potential predictors in both models were age, BMI, education level, ECOG WHO score, specialist at first consultation, primary tumour clinical stage, PSA value, Gleason score, and presence of prostate cancer symptoms. Continuous time variables were transformed into dichotomous variables. In agreement with previous studies, cut-offs chosen were an interval of 100 days between first consultation and diagnosis and 30 days between diagnosis and treatment [19, 20]. These intervals were based on recommendations about optimal diagnostic and therapeutic intervals [21, 22]. We first fitted an empty model that considered only the random effect of the hospital on the variability

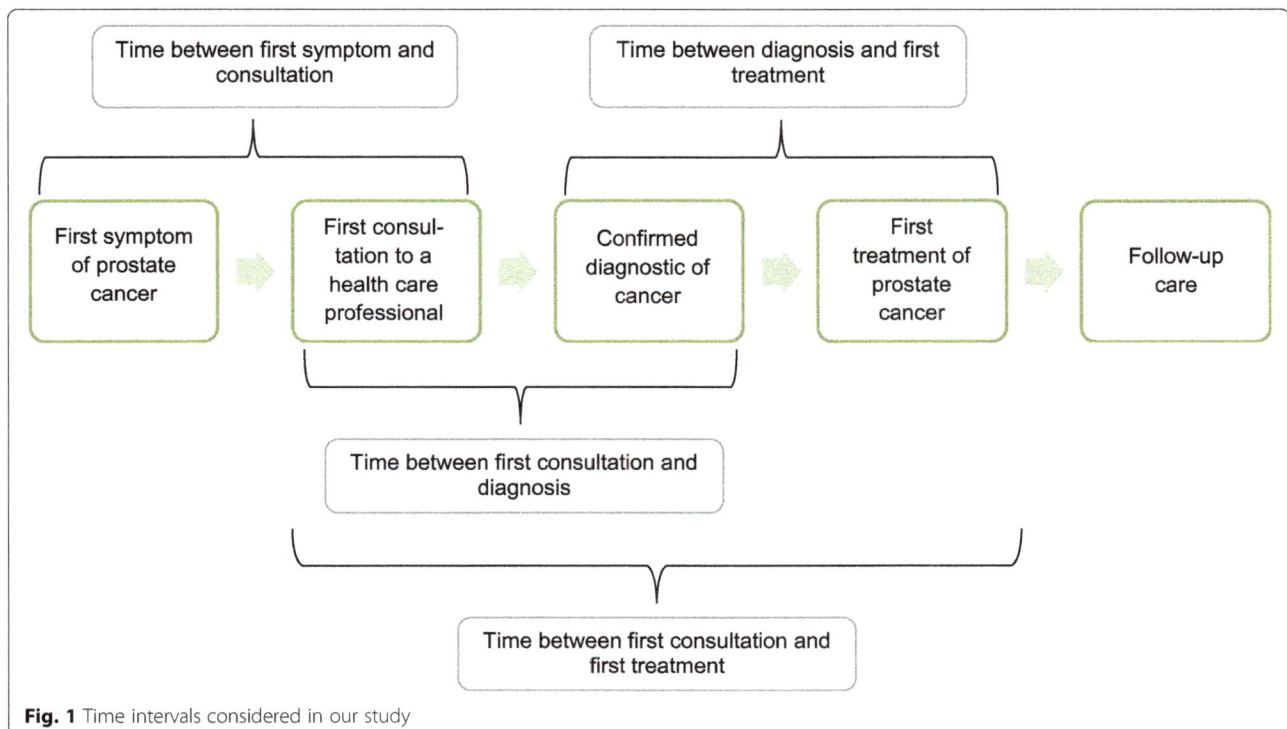

Fig. 1 Time intervals considered in our study

Table 2 Characteristics of prostate cancer patients

Variables	N = 470
	n (%)
Mean age ± SD	67.8 ± 7.6
Missing (%):	2.3
Mean BMI ± SD	28.1 ± 4.5
Missing (%)	3.8
Working status	
Active	83 (17.7)
Sick leave	15 (3.1)
Retired	347 (73.8)
Unemployed	17 (3.6)
Other	4 (0.9)
Missing	4 (0.9)
Education (%)	
No education	47 (10.2)
Incomplete primary education	80 (17.2)
Primary education	109 (23.5)
Graduate school	99 (21.3)
Upper secondary studies	62 (13.4)
University	67 (14.5)
Missing	6 (1.2)
Setting first consultation (%)	
Primary care	355 (75.5)
Hospital	86 (18.5)
Other	23 (5.0)
Missing	6 (1.2)
Symptoms (%)	
No symptoms or discomfort	251 (53.4)
One or more symptoms	170 (36.2)
Missing	49 (10.4)
Start of first symptoms including patients with discomfort (%)	
Since one month	55 (11.7)
Between one month and one year	242 (51.4)
Later than a year	56 (12.0)
No symptoms	68 (14.5)
Missing	49 (10.4)
ECOG WHO (%)	
Fully active:	356 (75.7)
Restricted or worse:	105 (22.3)
Missing:	9 (2.0)
Charlson index (%)	
1:	358 (75.8)
2:	68 (14.4)
3:	26 (5.5)

Table 2 Characteristics of prostate cancer patients *(Continued)*

4:	13 (2.8)
≥5:	5 (1.5)
Median PSA (ng/mL) ± IQR	7.6 ± 7.8
Missing (%):	3.4
Total Gleason (%)	
2-6:	262 (55.6)
7:	127 (26.9)
>7:	74 (15.6)
Missing:	7 (1.9)
Median total Gleason ± IQR	6.0 ± 1.0
Primary tumour clinical stage (T) (%)	
Tx:	1 (0.2)
T1a-c:	194 (41.0)
T2a-c:	189 (40.1)
T3a-b :	74 (15.7)
T4:	8 (1.7)
Missing:	4 (1.3)
Regional lymph nodes clinical stage (N) (%)	
Nx-N0:	460 (97.7)
N1:	10 (2.3)
Missing:	0 (0.0)
Distance metastasis clinical stage (M) (%)	
Mx-M0:	460 (97.9)
M1a-c:	10 (2.1)
Missing:	0 (0.0)
D'Amico Classification (%)	
Low risk:	170 (36.1)
Medium risk:	115 (24.5)
High risk:	185 (39.4)
Missing:	0 (0.0)
Median time between first consultation and diagnosis in days ± IQR	89.0 ± 123.5
Missing (%):	4.0
Median time between diagnosis and first treatment in days ± IQR	75.0 ± 78.0
Missing (%):	3.2
Median time between first consultation and first treatment in days ± IQR	176.0 ± 151.0
Missing (%):	6.6

of the two outcomes investigated. We then fitted univariate models with each potential predictor. The final model was fitted through a backward selection procedure based on Wald tests results. Both the empty model and the final multilevel models were estimated by maximum likelihood based on Gaussian quadrature points [23].

To estimate the random inter-hospital variability, we used the intra-cluster correlation coefficient (ICC) and the median odds ratio (MOR). The ICC indicates the fraction of the total outcome variability that is attributable to the area level (in our case, hospital level) and provides a measure of the within-hospital homogeneity. A lower ICC indicates a lower likelihood of patients' sharing hospital experiences. However, because the ICC can be difficult to interpret because of binary outcomes, the partition of variance between different levels does not have the intuitive interpretation of the linear model. We therefore also calculated the MOR, defined as the median value of the odds ratio between the hospital at highest risk (longest time interval) and the hospital at lowest risk when randomly picking out two hospitals. The MOR can be conceptualised as the increased risk (in median) that a patient would have if moved to a hospital with a higher risk [24]. The measure of fixed effect was the odds ratio (OR) with 95 % confidence intervals. A p-value lower than 0.05 was considered statistically significant for all statistical analyses. Data analyses were performed using SPSS statistical software, version 20.0 (SPSS INC., Chicago, IL, USA) and Stata v12 (StataCorp. 2011. Stata Statistical Software: Release 12. College Station, TX: StataCorp LP).

Results

Of the 502 patients recruited, 32 were excluded because they did not meet the inclusion criteria. The study group was therefore composed of 470 patients. Mean age was 67.8 years (SD:7.6), 337 (71.9 %) had completed at least primary studies, and 347 (73.8 %) were retired (Table 2). The mean BMI was 28.1 (SD:4.5) and 354 (75.4 %) had no physical limitations according to the ECOG WHO performance status. The Charlson comorbidity index was between one and three for 451 participants (96.2 %). Prostate screening was performed in primary care settings for 355 of the 470 patients (75.5 %), and in hospital settings for 86 of these participants (18.3 %). In 53.4 % of patients, the disease was identified during a routine visit or during consultation for another cause because no symptoms or only discomfort caused by prostate cancer had been noted. The median PSA value for the patients without symptoms was 7.2 (IQR: 6.9). From the total group, 36.2 % were symptomatic; 48.1 % of these patients had lower urinary tract symptoms such as increased frequency of urination (16.3 %), and 7.6 % had symptoms related to the tumour. The time from the first symptom to first consultation was between one month and one year for 50.8 % of participants. The clinical stage of the primary tumour was T1a-c in 41.0 % cases and T2 a-c in 40 % cases; 2.3 % had regional lymph nodes (N1) and 2.3 % had distant metastases (M1). The median PSA value was 7.6 (IQR: 7.8) ng/mL and the total Gleason score was between two and six for 55.6 % of participants. According to the D'Amico classification, 36.1 % of patients had low-risk cancer and 39.4 % had high-risk cancer (Table 2).

All patients had a prostate biopsy and 82.9 % underwent a prostate ultrasound study. A renal ultrasonography was performed in 23.8 % of patients and a bladder ultrasonography in 22.5 % (Table 3). Table 4 shows the patients' characteristics for each participating hospital. The median diagnostic interval was 89.0 days (IQR: 123.5). No statistically significant differences were found between hospitals for this interval (MOR: 1.00). Patients with one or more symptoms had an OR of 1.93 (95 % CI 1.29–2.89, P = 0.001) of having an interval between first consultation and diagnosis of more than 100 days (Table 5). No significant differences were found for groups of patients differing in age, BMI, education level, ECOG WHO score, the specialist at first consultation, primary tumour stage, PSA, or total Gleason scores.

The median therapeutic interval was 75 days (IQR: 78.0) (Table 5). No statistically significant association was found between groups for this interval regarding age, BMI, education level, specialist at first consultation, or primary tumour stage (Table 6). A higher PSA value and a higher Gleason score shortened the interval between diagnosis and treatment. Patients with a PSA value higher than 10 or a total Gleason score higher than 7 had an OR of 0.5 (95 % CI 0.29–0.86, P = 0.012) and 0.53 (95 % CI 0.30–0.93, P = 0.026), respectively, to

Table 3 Diagnostic variables of prostate cancer patients

Diagnostic test	N = 470
	n (%)
Ultrasound (%)	
Prostate ultrasound:	390 (82.9)
Renal ultrasound:	112 (23.8)
Bladder ultrasound:	106 (22.5)
Puncture (%)	
Biopsy:	464 (98.7)
Aspiration:	32 (6.8)
Scintigraphy (%)	63 (13.4)
Nuclear magnetic resonance (%)	
Abdominal:	66 (14.0)
Thoracic:	1 (0.2)
Cranial:	1 (0.2)
CT scan (%)	
Abdominal:	30 (6.4)
Abdominothoracic:	33 (7.0)
Toracic:	14 (3.0)
Cranial:	3 (0.6)

Table 4 Characteristics of prostate cancer patients by hospitals

Centres	A (n = 48)	B (n = 91)	C (n = 37)	D (n = 78)	E (n = 112)	F (n = 33)	G (n = 75)
Mean age ± SD	72.6 ± 6.1	66.9 ± 7.7	67.3 ± 5.6	67.8 ± 6.7	67.1 ± 7.8	66.2 ± 6.9	67.6 ± 9.2
Missing (%):	0.0	2.2	0.0	5.1	0.0	6.1	4.1
Mean BMI ± SD	28.2 ± 5.7	27.3 ± 3.5	27.6 ± 3.8	28.8 ± 6.4	28.9 ± 4.1	27.6 ± 4.3	27.2 ± 2.9
Missing (%):	0.0	4.4	0.0	3.8	0.9	21.2	4.1
Median PSA (ng/mL) ± IQR	10.4 ± 15.5	5.7 ± 3.4	6.7 ± 3.7	7.8 ± 7.7	8.6 ± 12.2	7.0 ± 3.8	8.7 ± 8.2
Missing (%):	2.1	8.8	0.0	6.4	0.0	3.0	1.4
ECOG WHO (%)							
Fully active:	72.9	84.6	91.9	71.8	69.6	63.6	75.3
Restricted or worse:	25.0	15.4	8.1	23.1	30.4	33.3	17.8
Missing:	2.1	0.0	0.0	5.1	0.0	3.0	6.8
Primary tumour clinical stage (T) (%)							
Tx:	0.0	0.0	0.0	1.3	1.3	0.0	0.0
T1a-c	45.8	45.1	16.2	37.2	37.2	43.8	41.1
T2a-c:	43.8	39.6	56.8	37.2	37.2	33.0	19.3
T3a-b :	6.3	14.3	21.6	20.5	20.5	22.3	6.8
T4:	4.1	1.0	0.0	3.8	3.8	0.9	1.4
Missing:	0.0	0.0	5.4	0.0	0.0	0.0	1.4
Regional lymph nodes clinical stage (N) (%)							
Nx-N0:	100.0	98.9	100.0	92.3	100.0	100.0	97.3
N1:	0.0	1.1	0.0	7.7	0.0	0.0	2.7
Missing:	0.0	0.0	0.0	0.0	0.0	0.0	0.0
Distance metastasis clinical stage (M) (%)							
Mx-M0:	95.8	100.0	100.0	93.6	98.2	100.0	98.6
M1a-c:	4.2	0.0	0.0	6.4	1.8	0.0	1.4
Missing:	0.0	0.0	0.0	0.0	0.0	0.0	0.0
D'Amico Classification (%)							
Low risk:	14.6	50.5	54.1	32.1	39.3	36.4	21.9
Medium risk:	27.1	12.1	29.7	17.9	23.2	45.5	34.2
High risk:	58.3	37.4	16.2	50.0	37.5	18.1	42.5
Missing:	0.0	0.0	0.0	0.0	0.0	0.0	1.4
Total Gleason (%)							
2-6:	16.7	73.6	64.9	68.0	66.9	36.4	31.5
7:	29.2	19.8	29.7	17.9	18.8	51.5	43.8
>7:	54.1	6.6	2.7	10.2	14.3	9.1	19.2
Missing:	0.0	0.0	2.7	3.9	0.0	3.0	5.5
Median total Gleason ± IQR	8.0 ± 1.0	6.0 ± 1.0	6.0 ± 1.0	6.0 ± 2.0	6.0 ± 1.0	7.0 ± 1.0	7.0 ± 1.0
Median time between first consultation and diagnosis in days ± IQR	99.5 ± 139.0	79.0 ± 211.0	110.0 ± 117.0	78.5 ± 107.3	92.0 ± 99.0	133.0 ± 195.0	76.5 ± 100.0
Missing (%):	0.0	3.3	5.4	7.7	4.5	6.1	1.4
Median time between diagnosis and first treatment in days ± IQR	30.5 ± 127.5	78.0 ± 62.0	83.0 ± 72.0	104.0 ± 70.5	55.0 ± 66.5	73.5 ± 84.5	70.0 ± 95.0
Missing (%):	0.0	4.4	0.0	1.3	6.3	3.0	2.7
Median time between first consultation and first treatment in days ± IQR	164.0 ± 232.0	154.0 ± 207.0	212.0 ± 165.0	200.0 ± 130.0	166.0 ± 112.8	203.0 ± 149.8	165.0 ± 128.5
Missing (%):	0.0	6.6	5.4	9.0	8.9	9.1	4.1

Table 5 Time interval between first consultancy and diagnosis and potential determinant (Univariate regression)

	Median (days)	IQR (days)	ICC/MOR / OR >100 days	95 % CI MOR / 95 % CI OR	P-value
Hospital random effect			0.00		
Empty model			1.00	1.00–1.00	1.000
Age					
<65 years	84.0	182.0	1		
≥65 years	91.0	105.5	0.96	0.64–1.43	0.830
BMI					
<25	102.0	163.0	1		
≥25	86.0	110.3	0.64	0.40–1.01	0.057
Education level					
Primary education or lower	90.5	108.5	1		
Graduate school or higher	86.0	139.0	1.00	0.69–1.45	0.992
ECOG WHO Score					
Fully active	87.5	126.8	1		
Restrictive or worse	95.0	129.0	1.18	0.76–1.83	0.474
Specialist first consultation					
Primary care	91.0	139.5	1		
Hospital or specialist	79.0	106.0	0.78	0.50–1.22	0.277
Primary tumour clinical stage (T)					
T1a–T1c	95.5	141.3	1		
T2a–T4	85.0	108.5	0.73	0.50–1.07	0.110
PSA value					
<10	95.0	135.5	1		
≥10	84.0	108.5	0.81	0.54–1.21	0.310
Total Gleason score					
<7	87.0	140.0	1		
≥7	91.0	111.5	0.87	0.60–1.27	0.464
Symptoms					
No symptoms or discomfort	83.0	110.0	1		
One or more symptoms	110.0	174.0	1.93	1.29–2.89	0.001

have an interval between diagnosis and treatment of more than 30 days. The MOR for the random effect of the hospital where the patient received care was 2.16 (95 % CI 1.45–4.87, $P = 0.000$).

Discussion

This multicentre cohort study aimed to describe the healthcare process in patients with prostate cancer in Spain. We focused on the characteristics of patients and tumours and we evaluated diagnosis and treatment delays in healthcare.

Our study included 470 patients diagnosed with prostate adenocarcinoma in a hospital care setting. Prostate biopsy and ultrasound were the most frequently performed diagnostic tests. The mean age of

our population, the proportion of asymptomatic low risk patients and the median Gleason grade were similar to those reported in previous studies in Spain and in other countries [16, 19, 25–29]. The percentage of localised tumours in our population (81 %) was similar to that in an earlier study (89.8 %) in Spain conducted by Cozar et al. but considerably higher than that in the European study of Gatta et al. These discordant findings might be explained by differences between countries and years regarding accesibility to health services and physicians' attitudes towards screening tests [30].

In our study, clinical symptoms were present in 36.2 % of all patients, the most common symptom being disorders of the lower urinary tract (48.1 %) and symptoms

Table 6 Time interval between diagnosis and first treatment and potential determinants

Characteristic	Univariate regression					Multivariate regression		
Hospital random effect			Empty model ICC/MOR	95 % CI MOR	P-value	FInal model ICC/MOR	95 % CI MOR	P-value
			0.18/2.22	1.52–4.58	0.000	0.17/2.16	1.45–4.87	0.000
	Median (days)	IQR (days)	OR >30 days	95 % CI OR		OR >30 days	95 % CI OR	
Age								
<65 years	78.0	74.0	1					
≥65 years	71.0	79.0	0.70	0.40–1.21	0.198			
BMI								
<25	75.0	76.0	1					
≥25	72.0	81.0	1.06	0.60–1.90	0.831			
Education level								
Primary education or lower	76.0	77.8	1					
Graduate school or higher	70.0	77.5	1.25	0.76–2.06	0.386			
ECOG WHO Score								
Fully active	77.0	74.8	1					
Restrictive or worse	54.0	77.0	0.55	0.32–0.95	0.033			
Specialist first consultation								
Primary care	76.0	77.0	1					
Hospital or specialist	74.0	79.5	0.86	0.48–1.56	0.621			
Primary tumour clinical stage (T)								
T1a–T1c	84.0	77.0	1					
T2a–T4	69.0	79.0	0.59	0.35–0.98	0.040			
PSA value								
<10	86.0	75.0	1					
≥10	50.0	81.0	0.41	0.24–0.68	0.001	0.50	0.29–0.86	0.012
Gleason score								
<7	85.5	68.8	1					
≥7	55.0	88.0	0.42	0.25–0.71	0.001	0.53	0.30–0.93	0.026
Symptoms								
No symptoms or discomfort	78.0	72.0	1					
One or more symptoms	73.5	80.3	0.62	0.37–1.05	0.073			

related with the tumour (7.6 %). These results are similar to those in the study of Cozar *et al.* where the frequency of lower urinary tract symptoms was 39.5 % of patients and the frequency of symptoms related to the tumour was 11.6 % [16]. In our study, the median interval between first consultation and diagnosis was 89.0 days, comparable to the 72 days in the study by Hansen et al. [31] and the 101 days reported by Torring et al. [32].

We did not find any variability in diagnostic interval between hospitals regarding age, BMI, education level, first visit with a specialist, tumour stage, PSA value, or Gleason score. However, the presence of symptoms lengthened this interval possibly because some symptoms of prostate cancer can be confused with benign prostatic hyperplasia.

Previous studies in Spain that determined the therapeutic intervals in cancer patients were generally conducted in a single hospital [33–35]. The most recently published multicentre study analysed this interval for six types of cancer, including prostate cancer [19], and found the mean therapeutic interval was longer than in our study (102.5 days (SD:71.6) vs. 80.4 days (SD:60.9)). However, we defined this interval as the time between the biopsy and the first oncological treatment, whereas the investigators in the previous study defined it as the time between the first diagnostic test of any kind and first oncological treatment. In contrast with the study by Perez *et al.* [19], our study was prospective, it had a larger number of cases, patients were from several different autonomous regions of the country, and information was obtained not only from medical records but also through patient interviews.

We observed that patients with a higher PSA value and a higher Gleason score had a shorter interval between diagnosis and first treatment than patients with lower values. Pérez et al. [19] reported similar findings in patients with advanced stages of prostate cancer. An explanation for this shorter interval could be that due to their worse prognosis, these patients usually receive hormonal therapy initially or exclusively, a treatment that is easier to administer than radiotherapy, chemotherapy, or surgery [36].

Our results show a statistically significant variability between centres in relation to the therapeutic interval. The heterogeneity in intervals could be associated with the wide diversity in population characteristics, healthcare organisation and clinical policies in the different regions in Spain.

One of the main strengths of our study is that our sample of patients is a representative sample of the approximately 28.000 yearly incident prostatic cancer patients diagnosed in Spain because they were recruited from seven hospitals in five autonomous regions. In addition, the study's prospective nature guarantees consistency and accuracy of the data collected, surpassing the common shortcomings of a retrospective collection of information. The study may have limitations, however, such as information bias. Given that it is based exclusively on information obtained in a hospital setting, outpatient factors such as those related to consultation at a primary level, could not have been taken into consideration. Nevertheless, as urologic cancer care is mainly provided in the hospital setting, in our view this limitation has little practical relevance.

Conclusions

Most incident prostate cancer patients in Spain are diagnosed at an early stage of an adenocarcinoma. The period to complete the diagnostic process is approximately three months whereas the therapeutic intervals vary among centres and are shorter for patients with a worse prognosis. The presence of prostatic symptoms, PSA level, and Gleason score influence the clinical intervals differently.

Appendix
EMPARO study group
Coordinating investigator: Xavier Bonfill Cosp (Iberoamerican Cochrane Centre. Public Health and Clinical Epidemiology Service. Hospital de la Santa Creu i Sant Pau, IIB Sant Pau, Barcelona, Spain).

Project manager: Mª José Martínez Zapata (Iberoamerican Cochrane Centre. IIBSant Pau, Barcelona, Spain).

Clinical research assistants: Alborada Martínez (Universidad de Valencia); Enrique Morales Olivera (Escuela Andaluza de Salud Pública, Granada, Spain); Esther Canovas, Laura Muñoz, Gemma Mas, René Acosta, Ekaterina Popova (Iberoamerican Cochrane Centre. IIBSant Pau, Barcelona, Spain); Irma Ospina (Hospital 12 de Octubre, Madrid, Spain); Mª José Velázquez (Hospital Donostia, Donostia, Spain); Tamara Ruiz Merlo (Hospital Ramón y Cajal, Madrid, Spain); Gael Combarros Herman, Judit Tirado Muñoz (IMIM, Barcelona, Spain).

Statistical analysis: Robin Vernooij (Iberoamerican Cochrane Centre. IIBSant Pau, Barcelona, Spain); Victor Abraira (Unidad de Bioestadística Clínica. Hospital Universitario Ramón y Cajal. IRYCIS, Madrid, Spain).

Co-investigators:

Barcelona, Spain
Virginia Becerra Bachito, Montserrat Ferrer Fores, Stefanie Schmidt, Olatz Garin, Yolanda Pardo (IMIM - Hospital del Mar Medical Research Institute-); Albert Frances (Hospital del Mar); Carola Orrego Villagran, Rosa Suñol (Instituto U. Avedis Donabedian); Dimelza Osorio, Gemma Sancho Pardo, Ignasi Bolívar, José Pablo Maroto, Mª Jesús Quintana, Martin Lorente, Cristina (Hospital de la Santa Creu i Sant Pau); Ferran Algaba, Palou Redorta, Salvador Esquena (Fundació Puigvert); Jordi Bachs (Fundació Privada Hospital de la Santa Creu i Sant Pau); Mª José Martínez Zapata (Iberoamerican Cochrane Centre. IIBSant Pau).

Bilbao, Spain
Amaia Martínez Galarza, José Ignacio Pijoán Zubizarreta, Lorea Martínez (Hospital Universitario Cruces-BioCruces Health Research Institute).

Tenerife, Spain
David Manuel Castro Diaz, Juan Manuel Ramos Goñi, Julio López Bastida (HTA Unit of the Canary Islands Health Service).

Granada, Spain
Armando Suárez Pacheco, Cesar García López, Jose Manuel Cozar Olmo (Hospital Universitario Virgen de las Nieves); Carmen Martínez, Daysy Chang Chan, Mª Jose Sanchez Perez (Escuela Andaluza de Salud Pública).

Madrid, Spain
Ana Isabel Díaz Moratinos, Angel Montero Luis, Asunción Hervás, Carmen Vallejo Ocaña, Costantino Varona, Javier Burgos, Javier Zamora, Jose Alfredo Polo Rubio, Luis López-Fando Lavalle, Miguel Angel Jiménez Cidre, Muriel Garcia, Alfonso, Nieves Plana Farras, Rosa Morera López, Sonsoles Sancho Garcia, Víctor Abraira,

Victoria Gómez Dos Santos (Hospital Ramón y Cajal); Agustín Gómez de la Cámara, Javier de la Cruz, Juan Passas Martínez, Humberto García Muñoz, Mª Ángeles Cabeza Rodríguez (Hospital 12 de Octubre).

San Sebastián, Spain
Irune Ruiz Díaz, José Ignacio Emparanza, Juan Pablo Sanz Jaka (Hospital Universitario Donostia).

Valencia, Spain
Agustín LLopis González, María Morales (Universidad de Valencia); Carlos Camps, Cristina Caballero Díaz, Emilio Marqués Vidal, Francisco Sánchez Ballester, Joaquín Ulises Juan Escudero, Jorge Pastor Peidro, José López Torrecilla, Mª Macarena Ramos Campos, Miguel Martorell Cebollada (Consorcio Hospital General Universitario de Valencia).

Abbreviations
PSA: Prostate-specific antigen; SD: Standard deviation; IQR: Interquartile range; BMI: Body mass index; OR: Odds ratio; ICC: Intra-cluster correlation coefficient; MOR: Median odds ratio.

Competing interests
The authors declare that they have no competing interest.

Authors' contributions
Study concepts: XB. Study design: XB, MJM. Data acquisition: All authors. Quality control of data and algorithms: MJM, RV. Data analysis and interpretation: XB, MJM, RV. Statistical analysis: RV, VA. Manuscript preparation: XB MJM, RV. Manuscript editing: All authors. Manuscript review: All authors. All authors read and approved the final manuscript.

Acknowledgements
We would like to thank Andrea Cervera Alepuz for the English review and editing of the manuscript. Funding: Instituto Carlos III: Fondo de Investigación Sanitaria PS09/01204. Spain.

Author details
[1]CIBER de Epidemiología y Salud Pública (CIBERESP), Madrid, Spain. [2]Institute of Biomedical Research (IIB Sant Pau), Iberoamerican Cochrane Centre, Barcelona, Spain. [3]Universitat Autònoma de Barcelona, Barcelona, Spain. [4]Public Health and Clinical Epidemiology Service, Hospital de la Santa Creu i Sant Pau, Barcelona, Spain. [5]Instituto de Investigación Biosanitaria de Granada, Escuela Andaluza de Salud Pública, Granada, Spain. [6]Department of Preventive Medicine, Unit of Public Health and Environmental Care, University of Valencia, Center for Public Health Research (CSISP), Valencia, Spain. [7]Hospital 12 de Octubre, Madrid, Spain. [8]Clinical Epidemiology Unit, Hospital Universitario Donostia, BioDonostia, San Sebastian, Spain. [9]IMIM (Hospital del Mar Medical Research Institute), Health Services Research Group, Barcelona, Spain. [10]Unidad de Epidemiología Clínica y Soporte Metodológico, UICEC de BioCruces-SCReN, Barakaldo, Spain. [11]Health Services Research on Chronic Patients Network (REDISSEC), HTA Unit of the Canary Islands Health Service (SESCS), S/C de Tenerife, La Laguna, Spain. [12]Fundació Puigvert, Barcelona, Spain. [13]Department of Experimental and Health Sciences, Universidad Pompeu Fabra (UPF), Barcelona, Spain. [14]Unidad de Bioestadística Clínica, Hospital Universitario Ramón y Cajal, IRYCIS, Madrid, Spain.

References
1. Ferlay J, Soerjomataram I, Ervik M, Dikshit R, Eser S, Mathers C, et al. GLOBOCAN 2012 v1.0, Cancer incidence and mortality worldwide: IARC CancerBase No. 11. Lyon, France: International Agency for Research on Cancer; 2013. [http://globocan.iarc.fr]. Accessed 14 Apr 2014.
2. Eastham JA, Riedel E, Scardino PT, Shike M, Fleisher M, Schatzkin A, et al. Variation of serum prostate-specific antigen levels: an evaluation of year-to-year fluctuations. JAMA. 2003;289(20):2695–700.
3. Penson DF, Rossignol M, Sartor AO, Scardino PT, Abenhaim LL. Prostate cancer: epidemiology and health-related quality of life. Urology. 2008;72(6 Suppl):S3–11.
4. Stamey TA, Caldwell M, McNeal JE, Nolley R, Hemenez M, Downs J. The prostate specific antigen era in the United States is over for prostate cancer: what happened in the last 20 years? J Urol. 2004;172(4):1297–301.
5. Sánchez MJ, Payer T, De Angelis R, Larrañaga N, Capocaccia R, Martinez C. CIBERESP working group cancer incidence and mortality in Spain: estimates and projections for the period 1981–2012. Ann Oncol. 2010;21(3):30–6.
6. Larrañaga N, Galceran J, Ardanaz E, Franch P, Navarro C, Sánchez MJ, et al. Prostate cancer incidence trends in Spain before and during the prostate-specific antigen era: impact on mortality. Ann Oncol. 2010;21 Suppl 3:83–9.
7. Mickevičienė A, Vanagas G, Ulys A, Jievaltas M, Smailytė G, Padaiga Ž. Factors affecting health-related quality of life in prostate cancer patients. Scand J Urol Nephrol. 2012;46(3):180–7.
8. Litwin MS, Hays RD, Fink A, Ganz PA, Leake B, Leach GE, et al. Quality-of-life outcomes in men treated for localized prostate cancer. JAMA. 1995;273(2):129–35.
9. Mariotto AB, Yabroff KR, Shao Y, Feuer EJ, Brown ML. Projections of the cost of cancer care in the United States: 2010–2020. J Natl Cancer Inst. 2011;103:117–28.
10. Sangar VK, Ragavan N, Matanhelia SS, Watson MW, Blades RA. The economic consequences of prostate and bladder cancer in the UK. BJU Int. 2005;95(1):59–63.
11. Sant M, Allemani C, Santaquilani M, Knijn A, Marchesi F, Capocaccia R, et al. EUROCARE-4. Survival of cancer patients diagnosed in 1995–1999. Results and commentary. Eur J Cancer. 2009;45(6):931–91.
12. Salive ME, Mayfield JA, Weissman NW. Patient outcomes research teams and the agency for health care policy and research. Health Serv Res. 1990;25(5):697–708.
13. Lubeck DP, Litwin MS, Henning JM, Stier DM, Mazonson P, Fisk R, et al. The CaPSURE database: a methodology for clinical practice and research in prostate cancer. CaPSURE Research Panel. Cancer of the Prostate Strategic Urologic Research Endeavor. Urology. 1996;48(5):773–7.
14. Navarro C, Martos C, Ardanaz E, Galceran J, Izarzugaza I, Peris-Bonet R, et al. Population-based cancer registries in Spain and their role in cancer control. Ann Oncol. 2010;21 suppl 3:iii3–13.
15. Calle JE, Saturno PJ, Parra P, Rodenas J, Pérez MJ, Eustaquio FS, et al. Quality of the information contained in the minimum basic data set: Results from an evaluation in eight hospitals. Eur J Epidemiol. 2000;16(11):1073–80.
16. Cózar JM, Miñana B, Gómez-Veiga F, Rodríguez-Antolín A, Villavicencio H, Cantalapiedra A, et al. Registro nacional de cáncer de próstata 2010 en España [National prostate cancer registry 2010 in Spain]. Actas Urol Esp. 2013;37(1):12–9.
17. Cózar JM, Miñana B, Gómez-Veiga F, Rodríguez-Antolín A, Villavicencio H, 25 Urology Units, Asociación Española de Urología, et al. Prostate cancer incidence and newly diagnosed patient profile in Spain in 2010. BJU Int. 2012;110(11 Pt B):E701–6.
18. American Joint Committee on Cancer. AJCC cancer staging manual. 6th ed. New York, NY: Springer; 2002. p. 335–40.
19. Pérez G, Porta M, Borrell C, Casamitjana M, Bonfill X, Bolibar I, et al. Interval from diagnosis to treatment onset for six major cancers in Catalonia, Spain. Cancer Detect Prev. 2008;32(3):267–75.
20. Kawakami J, Hopman WM, Smith-Tryon R, Siemens DR. Measurement of surgical wait times in a universal health care system. Can Urol Assoc J. 2008;2(6):597–603.
21. Saad F, Finelli A, Dranitsaris G, Goldenberg L, Bagnell S, Gleave M, et al. Canadian surgical wait times (SWAT) initiative. Does prolonging the time to prostate cancer surgery impact long-term cancer control: a systematic review of the literature. Can J Urol. 2006;13 Suppl 3:16–24.
22. Fleshner N, Dranitsaris G, Finelli A, Tsihlias J, Bell D, Gleave M. Canadian surgical wait times (SWAT) initiative. Surgical wait times for patients with urological cancers: a survey of Canadian surgeons. Can J Urol. 2006;13 Suppl 3:3–13.

23. Rabe-Hesketh S, Skrondal A. Multilevel and longitudinal modeling using stata. College Station, TX: Stata Press; 2008.

24. Merlo J, Chaix B, Ohlsson H, Beckman A, Johnell K, Hjerpe P, et al. A brief conceptual tutorial of multilevel analysis in social epidemiology: using measures of clustering in multilevel logistic regression to investigate contextual phenomena. J Epidemiol Community Health. 2006;60(4):290–7.

25. Gatta G, Zigon G, Buemi A, Coebergh JW, Colonna M, Contiero P, et al. Prostate cancer in Europe at the end of 1990s. Acta Oncol. 2009;48(6):867–73.

26. Andrén O, Fall K, Franzén L, Andersson S-O, Johansson J-E, Rubin MA. How well does the Gleason score predict prostate cancer death? a 20-year followup of a population based cohort in Sweden. J Urol. 2006;175:1337–40.

27. Bill-Axelson A, Garmo H, Lambe M, Bratt O, Adolfsson J, Nyberg U, et al. Suicide risk in men with prostate-specific antigen–detected early prostate cancer: a nationwide population-based cohort study from PCBaSe Sweden. Eur Urol. 2010;57:390–5.

28. Holmstrom B, Johansson M, Bergh A, Stenman U-H, Hallmans G, Stattin P. Prostate specific antigen for early detection of prostate cancer: longitudinal study. BMJ. 2009;339:b3537.

29. Smith DP, King MT, Egger S, Berry MP, Stricker PD, Cozzi P, et al. Quality of life three years after diagnosis of localised prostate cancer: population based cohort study. BMJ. 2009;339:b4817.

30. Salinas M, López-Garrigós M, Miralles F, Chinchilla V, Ortuño M, Aguado C, et al. Evaluation of PSA testing by general practitioners: regional study in the autonomic Community of Valencia. Arch Esp Urol. 2011;64(5):435–40.

31. Hansen RP, Vedsted P, Sokolowski I, Søndergaard J, Olesen F. Time intervals from first symptom to treatment of cancer: a cohort study of 2,212 newly diagnosed cancer patients. BMC Health Serv Res. 2011;11:284.

32. Tørring ML, Frydenberg M, Hansen RP, Olesen F, Vedsted P. Evidence of increasing mortality with longer diagnostic intervals for five common cancers: a cohort study in primary care. Eur J Cancer. 2013;49(9):2187–98.

33. Porta M, Gallén M, Malats N, Planas J. The influence of diagnostic delay upon cancer survival. An analysis of five tumour sites. J Epidemiol Community Health. 1991;45:225–30.

34. Maguire A, Porta M, Malats N, Gallén M, Piñol JL, Fernández E. Cancer survival and the duration of symptoms. An analysis of possible forms of the risk function. Eur J Cancer. 1994;30:785–92.

35. Fernández E, Porta M, Malats N, Belloc J, Gallén M. Symptom to diagnosis interval and survival in cancers of the digestive tract. Dig Dis Sci. 2002;47:2434–40.

36. NCCN Clinical Practice Guidelines in Oncology (NCCN Guidelines®). Prostate cancer. Version 1. 2014. NCCN.org

15

The struggle towards 'the New Normal': a qualitative insight into psychosexual adjustment to prostate cancer

Narelle Hanly[1], Shab Mireskandari[2*] and Ilona Juraskova[2]

Abstract

Background: Despite the growing body of literature which highlights the potential for significant and enduring side-effects of prostate cancer treatment, there is limited research exploring the experience of living with the treatment-induced side-effects such as sexual dysfunction, and their repercussions for men and their partners. The aim of this qualitative study was to explore factors influencing psychosexual adjustment, self-perception, and unmet information and support needs of prostate cancer patients and their partners.

Methods: Twenty-one men, recruited via a prostate cancer support group newsletter, participated in face-to-face semi-structured interviews, which were subjected to thematic analysis.

Results: The qualitative analysis revealed three inter-connected main themes which contributed to men's psychosexual adjustment: i) Psychosexual impact, ii) Communication and support, and iii) Integration process. Men reported distressing sexual and urinary difficulties, tainted self-perception and altered intimate relationships. Receiving adequate information and support, and having good communication with their doctors and partners facilitated better adjustment to prostate cancer treatment. Coming to terms with the significant impact of treatment had involved making lifestyle changes, coping with emotional struggles and striving to accept and integrate their post-treatment "new normal" self and sexual life.

Conclusions: The importance of adequate communication with health professionals and partners, especially regarding treatment effects on sexual function and rehabilitation options, was highlighted as a key factor facilitating the adjustment process. Prostate cancer patients would benefit from improved access to timely and tailored information and decision-making resources, ongoing multidisciplinary care, and support groups, as well as appropriate referrals for sexual and psychological counselling.

Keywords: Prostate cancer, Sexual function, Self-perception, Qualitative research

Background

In 2009, 19,438 cases of prostate cancer (PC) were diagnosed in Australia [1], with a five-year survival rate of 92% [2]. Following diagnosis, men are presented with a number of treatment options, including: i) observation without invasive treatment, with a view to intervene in the event of disease progression (i.e. active surveillance or watchful waiting); ii) removal of the prostate (RP – radical prostatectomy, nerve sparing or non-nerve sparing, delivered via open, laparoscopic, or robot-assisted surgery); or, iii) radiotherapy (RT – external radiation or brachytherapy). In addition, hormone therapy (ADT – androgen deprivation therapy) may also be offered alongside another mode of treatment for prostate cancer as adjuvant therapy [3]. Survival rates are similar across treatment options [4].

At 3 years post-treatment, urinary dysfunction (e.g. urinary incontinence) is more common amongst men treated with radical prostatectomy (up to 15%), and bowel problems (e.g. faecal incontinence and bleeding from the bowel) are more commonly reported by men treated with radiotherapy (up to 15%). Sexual dysfunction three years post-treatment is common across all modalities (nerve

* Correspondence: shab.mireskandari@sydney.edu.au
[2]Centre for Medical Psychology & Evidence-based Decision-making (CeMPED), School of Psychology, The University of Sydney, Level 6, Chris O'Brien Lifehouse (C39Z), Sydney, NSW 2006, Australia
Full list of author information is available at the end of the article

sparing RP 68%, non-nerve sparing RP 87%, external RT 68%, brachytherapy 36%, ADT 98%) [4]. Treatment-induced changes in sexual function include erectile dysfunction (ED), absent or diminished ejaculate, changed orgasmic sensation, urine loss during arousal or orgasm (climacturia), decreased libido and penile shortening [5-7]. In addition to these physical side-effects, men also report impaired body image and self-esteem [4,8,9]. ADT may also result in fatigue, weight gain, loss of muscle mass and body hair, hot flushes, sexual dysfunction, diminished genitalia size, depression, mood swings and reduced cognitive function with associated decline in quality of life [10]. Given the high survival rate, the majority of men diagnosed with PC are living with these physical and psychological consequences of treatment which have persistent effect on their quality of life [4].

Until recent years, how men felt about the impact of treatment side-effects was not addressed in any detail [11]. Sexual function was usually evaluated quantitatively, in terms of erections and the ability to achieve vaginal penetration, with much less emphasis on diminished desire and intimacy [12], and the impact of sexual problems on relationships [13]. Current research which recognises the broader psychosexual impact of treatment-related functional changes has found that many men report a negative association between physical side-effects and their intimate relationships [14,15], and self-perception [16], including reduced quality of sexual intimacy, decreased sexual desire and sexual confidence, impaired feelings of masculinity, lower self-esteem and poorer body image [16,17].

It is not surprising then that post-treatment side-effects have been found to increase anxiety and depression [4,8,9,18] which can impact on already reduced sexual function [19,20]. Men may also grieve for their diminished sexual quality of life, decreased libido and lost sexual fantasy life, as a result of their decreased self-worth and a depleted view of their masculinity [21].

Studies have shown that after PC treatment, men express unmet needs related to sexuality. Smith et al. [22] found that 47% of participants in their study described unmet needs related to changes in sexual feelings and the associated impact on relationships. In contrast, men who believe they received adequate information to enable informed treatment decision-making have been found to be less likely to report being unhappy with their doctor or distressed about side-effects [23,24].

Further investigations of men's experiences of treatment-induced side-effects is required to gain a better understanding of the issues underlying the complex post-treatment changes in the men's lives. Such deeper understanding can then inform the development of much needed tailored interventions to assist men in coping with post-treatment changes in sexual function and activity, as well as self-

identity. The aim of the current study was to further explore the experiences of men treated for PC and their psychosexual adjustment, as well as identifying unmet information and support needs.

Methods

This study was approved by the ethics committees at the University of Sydney and Concord Repatriation General Hospital. An advertisement was placed in the Concord Hospital Prostate Cancer Support Group newsletter inviting men who had been diagnosed and treated for PC in the past 5 years to participate. Men younger than 18 years, with insufficient English to understand and give informed consent and participate in the interview, or who had concurrent malignancy (of another type) and/or psychiatric disorder, were excluded from participating in the study. Phone screening for eligibility was conducted for self-selected men who responded to the study advertisement.

All eligible men participated in an individual, face-to-face, semi-structured interview with the first author (NH). On average, the interviews lasted approximately 1.5 hour (range = 50 minutes to 2 hours). An *aide-memoire* was used to structure the interview, outlining the major questions and topics to be covered during the interview, whilst leaving the wording and sequencing of questions open. Questions were designed with detailed probes targeting patient experiences in a number of areas which covered: pre-treatment knowledge of potential treatment-related side effects, including discussion of side effects with clinicians; experience of sex and sexual activity pre-treatment and at the time of interview, changes in sexual life since treatment, management of changes in sexual life post treatment, effects of treatment on quality of life, impact on existing relationship or on ability of single men to seek a relationship, coping strategies and information provision prior to treatment. These broad areas were chosen on the basis of a review of the literature and the consensus among the authors based on their extensive expertise. All participants provided written informed consent with guarantees of confidentiality.

The interviews were audio-taped, transcribed and subjected to thematic analysis in accordance with Braun and Clark's [25] methodology: i) familiarisation with the data, ii) code generation, iii) searching for themes, iv) reviewing themes, v) defining and naming themes, and vi) producing the report. Through the first stage of open coding, the data was grouped into smaller segments with a descriptor or 'code' attached to each segment; followed by axial coding, which entailed the codes being grouped into similar categories. These features were checked for emerging patterns, variability and consistency and commonality across participants until saturation (i.e. when analysis produced no new themes or categories) was reached. Throughout the iterative analysis, researchers (NH and IJ) discussed the key features of the data, enhancing researcher sensitivity and overcoming selective inattention.

Results
Demographic and medical characteristics
Of the 30 men who responded to the advertising, 3 men did not meet the eligibility criteria as they were more than 5 years post-treatment. A further 6 men opted to withdraw from the study, citing: partner's reluctance for them to participate (n = 2), believing they could not provide any useful information (n = 1), and no reason given (n = 3), resulting in 21 completed interviews (response rate 78%).

Demographic and medical characteristics of participants are summarized in Table 1. About two-thirds of the participants were aged 60–69 years at the time of the interview (62%), and more than half were aged 50–59 years at the time of treatment (52%). The majority of participants were married (76%), heterosexual (95%), had post-school qualifications (62%) and approximately half worked full-time (52%).

All 21 participants had been initially diagnosed with localised prostate cancer amenable to treatment with curative intent. Nineteen participants (90%) underwent radical prostatectomy with a further 2 participants (10%) treated with high dose rate brachytherapy (HDRB) and ADT (one had completed ADT and one nearing completion). At the time of their interview, 4 (19%) participants had undergone further treatment for localised disease progression, with 1 undergoing RT, 1 RT and ADT; and 2 treated with ADT alone. Six (29%) men were within the first 12 months since initial treatment, 13 (62%) were less than 3 years, and 2 (9%) were less than 5 years since treatment.

Thematic analysis
Analysis of the participants' interviews revealed three main themes relating to men's post-treatment psychosexual adjustment: i) psychosexual impact, ii) communication and support, iii) integration process; with a number of sub-themes emerging in each main theme as illustrated in Figure 1.

Theme 1: psychosexual impact

Significant sexual and urinary difficulties Physical changes reported by participants included erectile dysfunction, urinary incontinence, urine leakage during arousal or at orgasm, reduced penile size, lack of or reduced ejaculate, change in intensity of orgasm, reduced desire and pain.

The inability to achieve and/or maintain an erection and therefore have penetrative intercourse precluded some

Table 1 Demographic and medical characteristics of participants (N = 21)

Current age (years)	n	%
50-59	8	38.1%
60-69	13	61.9%
Age at Treatment (years)		
<49	1	4.8%
50-59	11	52.4%
60-69	9	42.9%
Marital Status		
Married	16	76.2%
Single	2	9.5%
Divorced	2	9.5%
Relationship (not living together)	1	4.8%
Sexual Orientation		
Heterosexual	20	95.2%
Homosexual	1	4.8%
Education		
Year 10 or less	7	33.3%
Year 12	1	4.8%
>Year 12	13	61.9%
Employment		
Full-time	11	52.4%
Part-time	2	9.5%
Retired	7	33.3%
Unable to work	1	4.8%
Treatment		
Radical Prostatectomy	19	90.5%
High Dose Brachytherapy and ADT	2	9.5%
Radical prostatectomy		
Plus radiotherapy	1	4.7%
Plus radiotherapy and ADT	1	4.7%
Plus ADT	2	9.5%
Time Since Treatment		
≤ 5 months	2	9.5%
5-12 months	4	19%
≤2 years	7	33.3%
≤3 years	6	28.6%
≤5 years	2	9.5%

ADT – Androgen Deprivation Therapy.

participants from sexual intimacy, as many viewed sexual interaction as equating with penetrative intercourse.

"...minimal erections, so there's no penetration....The major issue has been around penetration and the inability to be able to get an erection." [age 65]

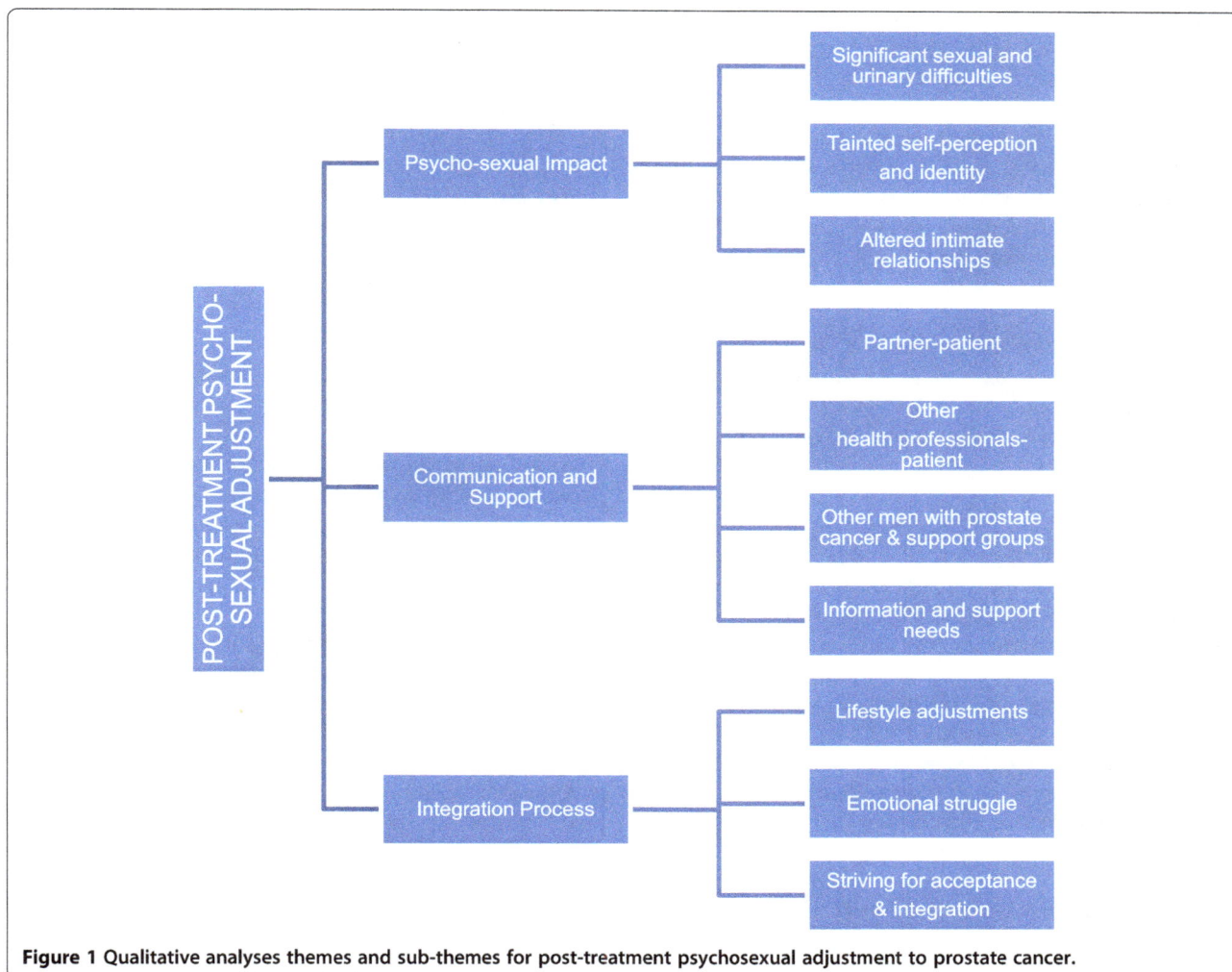

Figure 1 Qualitative analyses themes and sub-themes for post-treatment psychosexual adjustment to prostate cancer.

Some men noticed that, unlike previously when erections had been spontaneous, they now consciously thought about what was happening during arousal, thinking about how long their erection would last, what their partner was thinking and whether they could "perform" – all of which further negatively impacted arousal and sexual experience.

"You do think about it [erection]... and that probably takes away from the moment." [age 59]

"...when it does come to having, coming close to – whether it be penetration or just physical foreplay, I get very tense or just lose interest completely." [age 51]

Changes in orgasm including diminished intensity or even complete absence of orgasm, lack of or reduced ejaculate, negative changes in emotional experience of orgasm, and changes in libido and desire were also reported.

"I don't have sexual difficulties because I don't have any sexual urges. When I say that, my wife and I aren't intimate, we cuddle but that's about it, cuddle and kiss." [age 61]

"You feel a bit detached... It's a bit like doing it with someone else's dick... the feeling dies off quickly and there's no "afterglow" like there was before." [age 59]

Many men reported that the side effects of ED therapies, their cost and the effort required to use them were prohibitive. Additionally, ED therapies did not work for some men or were not an acceptable option (e.g. penile injections).

"With Viagra I can actually partly engorge my penis in a crouching position ... I bought a vacuum kit with the

rubber bands so I can achieve enough of an erection
to have penetrative sex ...it's a bit of a production."
[age 62]

Urinary incontinence and ongoing urine leakage was a
significant issue for a number of men. One participant
refused to use pads and wore dark clothes to disguise
wet patches, yet described leakage-related embarrassment. A participant explained how it affected his quality
of life:

"[Urinary incontinence] stopped me...before I used to
do a lot of walking. But one of the things it really
inhibited was going for a swim. Because you can't
swim with a pad on and you can't go to the beach
with your pants starting to get wet all the time."
[age 62]

Urine leakage during arousal and/or at orgasm was
found to be a difficult and embarrassing issue, sometimes leading to avoidance of physical intimacy for these
men and in some instances, for their wife/partner.

"...a couple of times it [urine leak] happened and [my
wife] got so angry, she jumped up and went and had a
shower and I felt terrible...she refused to even talk
about sex anymore...can't blame my wife and I
couldn't blame myself because you just can't control
it." [age 58]

Tainted self-perception and identity Several men reported PC and its related physical changes had significantly affected their self-perception and self-esteem.
Sexual difficulties resulted in feeling less confident,
particularly for single men some of whom chose not
to engage in new social interactions with potential for
intimacy. Men described feelings of inadequacy and
embarrassment due to urinary leakage, ED and smaller
genitalia.

"I think my impression of myself now as a man is a bit
lower than before I had that operation." [age 60]

"It's very hard to put it into words... it [being able
to have erections] is part of your self-image, your
self-confidence...when it [ED] happens it really does
change you." [age 54]

You're suddenly different, non-performing... you're
almost like ...the eunuchs ...you feel like you've been
neutered almost. A normal healthy, heterosexual male
as far as I know, feels that [erection] is a powerful
thing for him and to have it taken away, takes a bit
of you away." [age 54]

Impotence was found to have a deep impact on self-
perception, above and beyond sexual interactions. Low-
ered self-esteem due to impotence was reported by one
man as affecting his confidence to four-wheel drive in
the same pre-treatment "aggressive" manner.

"The self-esteem gnaws away at you in really unusual
situations...sexuality is important but self-esteem
and self-confidence tends to hang off that issue."
[age 62]

Men who reported a good response to medical therapy
to achieve erections reported the additional benefit of
restored confidence in themselves as males.

"Since having the needles it's given me a lot more
confidence...It's a lovely feeling, you feel very proud of
yourself. You put the needle in and everything's
working again. Being a selfish male and my ego...."
[age 58]

Altered intimate relationships In general, men described their partners as being supportive in terms of
diagnosis and treatment, even if issues related to treatment side-effects were problematic. Most married men
reported that their diagnosis and treatment had an impact on their relationship with their wife. In some cases,
men reported a positive impact of PC diagnosis on their
relationships:

"I do feel that I'm in a very loving relationship and I
am very well loved. I think that has always been the
case but it is probably more so after the operation."
[age 62]

"It is not just the sexual stuff, it's about your feelings
for each other. As a man, it's not just about
satisfying yourself but it's about making sure that
you're satisfying each other.... that's with the sexual
aspect, the emotional aspect, the communication.
I find myself cuddling my wife a lot more often.
I find myself being very considerate and watching
her and anticipating...I'm more in tune with maybe
how she's feeling or how she's responding now."
[age 53]

Some men worried about their partners and how they
were affected by the changes in their sexual functioning.

"... I thought that the fact that I couldn't make love
properly anymore had affected my wife. She says it
didn't but I know. She even asked her sister how many
times they make love... and I'm thinking, this was an
issue for her." [age 58]

For men who defined sexual intimacy as penetrative intercourse, lack of erections meant no sexual intimacy.

"It doesn't worry me not having sex - we've discussed it that there's nothing we can do, so there's no sex life in our place...there's no sexual intimacy." [age 61]

Some partners who were otherwise supportive were not always willing to try non-penetrative sexual activity, particularly if such activities had not previously been part of their sexual repertoire.

"I'm not comfortable with things like that [outer-course, manual stimulation or oral sex]...they are not an option for her and I." [age 61]

A gay participant's embarrassment due to ED and urine leakage led to reduced socializing and significant reduction in sexual encounters.

"You take headache tablets before the Caverject and have a wee...and have a towel in bed. It's always been spontaneous...pick someone up and go home with them...I can't go to their place, I've got to think of what I've got to do so they can't see what I'm doing." [age 67]

Understandably, couples who had pre-existing relationship and sexual issues appeared to face greater challenges adjusting to treatment side-effects.

Theme 2: communication and support
Men who reported they had good communication with their partner, doctor and other health professionals reported better adjustment to PC, especially regarding sexual outcomes.

Doctor-patient Men reported great trust in doctors who provided them with adequate information and ample opportunity to ask questions.

"I wrote all the questions and asked him [doctor] when I went in there and he said 'don't worry about the other people in the waiting area you're in here now and I will take the time to answer all your questions' and he did." [age 69]

Some men noted that they felt uncomfortable talking about sexual issues and if their doctor did not raise the subject, neither did they.

"He didn't tell me the [sexual] after effects and to be quite honest I didn't ask." [age 61]

A number of participants noted that their doctor raised the topic of sexual function often which was appreciated,

particularly if the man was uncomfortable having that particular conversation.

"Honestly, my urologist said 'why I keep bringing it up is because some people won't talk about it [sexual side-effects]' and I suppose that's right." [age 63]

A few men reported their urologist had failed to pick up on the emotional cues indicating emotional distress, and hence they sought help themselves elsewhere.

"With the resultant depression I became extremely distressed and morose and ... I asked my GP to refer me to a psychologist which he did." [age 69]

Partner-patient Communication difficulties which existed for some couples prior to diagnosis were compounded by problems associated with PC. Couples who had previously communicated well on difficult issues reported communicating similarly well about difficulties associated with treatment.

"Well, what you get afterwards is only a product of what's been going on beforehand isn't it?" [age 54]

Some men discussed hiding their need to use some ED treatments from their partners.

"I think my wife would be absolutely shocked if she knew. I think that deep down when she found out I was taking these tablets [Viagra], she wasn't happy with that, and I think if she found out I was having injections – geez. I haven't told her about the injections, I've sort of kept that one to myself." [age 60]

Some participants explained that while medical procedures were discussed with their partners, the possible impact on their sexual life had not been discussed.

"Even though I talked about the treatment, what I was going through, and wanting to find the doctor that could ensure erections after the operation, we didn't actually talk about what will happen after the operation. She [wife] knew what I was going through, she knew why I was going to see all these different doctors and all this, but we didn't actually sit down and say 'ok, when the operation takes place and whatever happens afterwards, what's it going to be like?' We didn't talk about that." [age 59]

Other health professionals-patient Out of 21 participants, nine had been referred to another health professional (such as specialised prostate cancer nurse, psychologist) for support at the time of diagnosis and all the men reported this as being very helpful.

"Talking to the nurse at the hospital and the staff from the Cancer Council Telephone Support Group, talking to the psychologist ...I got the message that 'there is light at the end of the tunnel, there is hope'." [age 53]

Other men with prostate cancer and support groups Men who had attended a support group described it as a reliable source of information and a confidential and safe opportunity to discuss their concerns.

"Those meetings are pretty good. I understood more about things...I learned a lot really. And it's good to hear other people's problems and what they had". [age 60]

Information and support needs Those who had access to adequate information, felt they were better prepared for treatment side-effects and found it easier to adapt to ongoing changes. Some participants felt they should have received more information about side-effects, the likelihood of their occurrence and available management strategies. A frequent comment was that in the early phase of their diagnosis men did not know enough about prostate cancer and its effects to know what questions to ask.

"I sat in the hospital and didn't know what was going to happen to me. It's alright to say 'oh, you're going to have an operation' but what does it mean." [age 61]

For some men potential sexual rehabilitation options were not discussed in any detail by their doctor and they felt uncomfortable initiating the discussion.

"It was just in passing one day [the doctor] said to me, 'Oh, why don't you try this drug. It's better than Viagra' and of course it had no effect. And then about a year later he said 'oh, why don't you try the Caverject'." [age 58]

Most men believed early referral for ongoing support from other health professionals other than their doctor (e.g. nurse, psychologist), would have reduced their anxiety and improved their understanding of treatment procedures, side-effects and management options.

"I think there probably does need to be an opportunity, away from the surgeon, for discussion about those physical details in more detail than I received." [age 62]

Some men commented that health professionals should provide men and their partners with information regarding feelings they may experience, and encourage and support couples to explore sexual activities other than penetrative intercourse.

Theme 3: integration process

Lifestyle adjustments To accommodate the functional changes resulting from treatment, many men reported making positive lifestyle changes such as improved diet and exercise which had lead to better overall general health.

"One of the big benefits that's come out of it is that I now really do look after myself." [age 63]

Men with post-treatment urinary incontinence discussed lifestyle changes such as reducing general fluid and alcohol intake, and planning activities and travel around availability and access to toilets.

Emotional struggles Living with the consequences of PC and its treatment was difficult for many of the participants who described experiencing emotions such as shock, anger, depression, disappointment and a sense of loss associated with ongoing changes in sexual function, penile shortening and loss of libido.

"And it's hard sometimes, some days it's very hard. And you get disappointed but you know, you've got no choice." [age 58]

"I don't have crying fits, I used to, but I don't now." [age 61]

In some instances struggling with PC had acted as a catalyst for psychological distress around issues unrelated to cancer diagnosis e.g. retirement. Men with progressive disease reported greater emotional impact and more difficulties adjusting to ED and incontinence.

Striving for acceptance and integration Not all the men felt they had successfully accepted the changes following treatment and reported believing that it is an ongoing process.

Men described using various coping strategies from the time of diagnosis to living with post-treatment side effects. Denial behaviour was discussed by some men such as not reading information provided, or leaving the room while doctors were providing information. Some men reported minimising the occurrence/impact of possible sexual side-effects, as they believed they would not suffer any side-effects, or they would not be significant and they would be able to adjust.

"I really didn't think about it [ED] then. I thought I was very strong and fit, would get through it and it wouldn't really affect me. I was very positive that 'well, I'll get over it and there won't be any problems with me and if they're minor, I'll adjust to them'." [age 58]

A few men engaged in unhelpful behaviours such as excessive alcohol intake despite the potential for embarrassing urinary leakage.

In contrast, a number of men discussed that their general positive attitude had helped them through the difficulties they had experienced.

"I guess it's a mindset that says 'today is going to be a new day'. I'm better than what I was before.... I have a positive aspiration." [age 53]

Some reported that talking to other men who have been through treatment and to experienced PC health professionals, helped in accepting the post-treatment changes and 'getting on' with their life after cancer.

Some men reported they had re-evaluated aspects of their life and this had helped them adjust to their new circumstances.

"When things finally settle down and you think 'this is what it's going to be like forever' then you accept it. I came across that [concept] on one of those health shows on TV, talking about people having to accept 'the new normal' and I thought that's a lovely phrase. I could relate it to me." [age 58]

Discussion

The aim of the current research was to explore men's experiences of PC and the impact of treatment-induced changes on men's sexual life, self-perception, as well as their intimate relationships. Three themes underlying the men's post-treatment adjustment were found: psychosexual impact, communication and support, and integration process, each of which was comprised of a number of sub-themes. Participants discussed significant physical, functional, psychological, emotional and relationship changes as a result of PC treatment which affected their sexual life, self-perception and relationship. The importance of receiving adequate information from treating doctors and having good communication with their doctors, partners and other health professionals were highlighted as major contributors to better adjustment for men in this study.

The significant sexual functioning issues reported by the participants reflect previous research findings (e.g. Dahn et al. [17]) emphasising the need for patients to be well-informed about treatments for erectile dysfunction and to be offered sexual counselling. Men in this study appeared to benefit from discussions and interventions for treatment side-effects, particularly those affecting sexual and urinary functioning. However, if both men and their treating doctors are uncomfortable discussing sexual function in any detail, men may be deprived of the opportunity to better understand and better manage their erectile dysfunction [26]. Hence, men with PC (and their partners) would benefit from access to multidisciplinary sources of care, including prostate nurse-led psychoeducational sessions and psychological care, as well as access to support groups. An important point was made by Wootten et al. [27] who found men's management techniques are more emotion-based in relation to sexual dysfunction and more problem-focused with regard to incontinence and suggest this may be a consequence of inadequate information being provided about the practical management of sexual dysfunction.

Participants discussed the impact of post-treatment changes in sexual function on their partners and intimate relationships. The level of concern of patients on their sexual function may not be shared to an equal degree by their partners [28]. Indeed, PC patients and their partners have been found to differ on sexual-related measures [29]. While patients express unease with the sexual side-effects of their cancer treatment and this is a significant area of concern, their female partners recognize decreased sexual desire in their partners post-treatment, but this is not considered a primary concern [30]. As greater sexual dissatisfaction has been found to be associated with poorer marital adjustment in couples who reported low levels of communication, psychosocial interventions that facilitate healthy spousal communication and address sexual rehabilitation needs of both the patients and their partners after PC treatment seem essential [31]. Hence, the partners' involvement in sexual rehabilitation is warranted.

In addition to addressing sexual functioning, understanding the impact of PC treatment on the masculine gender role may facilitate better understanding of men's adjustment following treatment [32]. Male sexual potency is seen as an important social masculine trait [32]. Hence, it is not surprising that for many men with PC, the loss of sexual function is associated with feelings of tremendous despair, as it may disrupt the identity of men who define masculinity through sexual performance [32]. Interventions may focus on promoting a more flexible gender schema such as a view of men's identity as not being limited to their sexual performance, to allow better adaption to diminished sexual function [33].

Steginga et al. [11] found that 25% of 206 men in their study who had been treated for PC continued to report moderate to high unmet needs for information related to investigations, treatment options, side-effects and their management. Receiving written information preoperatively, no matter how comprehensive, is not sufficient to foster the patient's management of all post-operative consequences of PC [34]. Personal follow-up support such as telephone follow-up calls has been found to facilitate better adjustment after surgery [34]. Christie et al. [35] found that discussions about treatment options with people from the patients' social networks, prior to beginning treatment, significantly contributed to improvements in affect for patients at1 and 6 months following treatment, while discussions with physicians predicted an increase in positive affect 1 month following treatment.

The limited research on psychosocial interventions for men with PC points to significant improvements in the men's psychosexual adjustment [36]. Group cognitive-behavioural and psycho-education interventions have been found to be helpful in promoting better psychological adjustment and quality of life (QOL) for patients; while coping skills training for couples has been found to improve QOL for partners [36]. A counseling intervention aimed at improving levels of sexual satisfaction and increasing successful utilization of medical treatment for ED for patients and their partners was found to significantly increase sexual function and satisfaction [37]. A computer-assisted, nurse-led intervention focusing on providing education and support resulted in long-term improvements in quality of life outcomes related to sexual functioning and cancer worry [38]. A randomized controlled trial of a 10-week group-based cognitive–behavioral stress management intervention with older men who had undergone a radical prostatectomy was found to be highly effective in promoting sexual recovery [39]. It is anticipated that the obtained findings will inform future research to identify the best practice model for the development of a psycho-educational intervention for men/couples from diagnosis through treatment, recovery and rehabilitation. It is hoped that provision of such an intervention early in the disease trajectory will lead to improved quality of care and quality of life of men affected by PC and their partners/families.

Limitations

The study population was self-selected from a newsletter mailing list of a Prostate Cancer Support Group, coordinated by the researcher (NH). Therefore self-selection bias may characterise this sample. Since the sample consisted of men for localised or locally advanced PC and 19 of 21 participants underwent radical prostatectomy, the findings may not reflect experiences of men with metastatic PC and those undergoing other treatment types. Further, the interviewer's female gender may have potentially affected participants' responses given the intimate nature of the subject matter. However,

participants' appeared candid when discussing the impact of side-effects on their QOL and their relationships. A final interview question asked whether anything would have made the men feel more comfortable during the interview and all responded they were comfortable. In addition, given that the interviewer was also the participants' support group coordinator, the impact of this on the participants' answers cannot be known. Some participants explained that they preferred to be interviewed by the coordinator whom they knew rather than a stranger.

Conclusions

A timely provision of information and ongoing multidisciplinary support to men diagnosed with prostate cancer and their partners will afford them a better understanding of the potential impact of side-effects, particularly related to sexual function, on their personal and social relationships, their body image, self-esteem and sexuality. By identifying potential issues early and providing relevant information and support, men will be better prepared to accept and adjust to the post-treatment changes in their sexual function. Future research is recommended to examine a nurse-led information and psychosocial support role and to confirm the benefits reported by participants in this study and identify other potential benefits or otherwise. It should also identify appropriate content, optimum timing and duration of a nurse-led information and psychosocial intervention to develop the best practice model of care for tailoring interventions for men with PC, thereby providing long-term benefits to men and their partners adjusting to changed sexual function after treatment. A multidisciplinary approach to PC care whereby clinicians, nurses, allied health professionals as well as peers work together to provide appropriate information and support over time seems needed in order to adequately address the complex adjustment process of men with PC and their partners.

Abbreviations
PC: Prostate cancer; RP: Radical prostatectomy; RT: Radiation therapy; ADT: Androgen deprivation therapy; ED: Erectile dysfunction; QOL: Quality of life.

Competing interests
Narelle Hanly, Shab Mireskandari and Ilona Juraskova declare that they have no conflict of interest or competing interests.

Authors' contributions
NH conceived and coordinated the study, conducted the interviews, analysed the data and drafted the manuscript. SM helped to draft the results and the manuscript. IJ supervised the study, helped with the analysis and write up of the results and the manuscript. All authors have read and approved the final manuscript.

Acknowledgements
The authors would like to express their gratitude to the men who participated in this study and without whose frank and honest discussions, this research would not have been possible.

Author details

[1]Faculty of Health Sciences, The University of Sydney, Sydney, NSW, Australia. [2]Centre for Medical Psychology & Evidence-based Decision-making (CeMPED), School of Psychology, The University of Sydney, Level 6, Chris O'Brien Lifehouse (C39Z), Sydney, NSW 2006, Australia.

References

1. Australian Institute of Health and Welfare & Australasian Association of Cancer Registries: **Cancer in Australia: an overview, 2012. Cancer series no. 74 Cat. no. CAN 70.** In *Cancer series no 74 Cat no CAN 70*, Cancer series no. 74 Cat. no. CAN 70. Canberra: AIHW; 2012.

2. Australian Institute of Health and Welfare 2012, Australian Institute of Health and Welfare: **Cancer survival and prevalence in Australia: period estimates from 1982 to 2010. Cancer Series no. 69. Cat. no. CAN 65.** Canberra: AIHW; 2012.

3. Soloway CT, Soloway MS, Kim SS, Kava BR: **Sexual, psychological and dyadic qualities of the prostate cancer 'couple'.** *BJU Int* 2005, **95**(6):780–785.

4. Smith DP, King MT, Egger S, Berry MP, Stricker PD, Cozzi P, Ward J, O'Connell DL, Armstrong BK: **Quality of life three years after diagnosis of localised prostate cancer: population based cohort study.** *BMJ* 2009, **339**:b4817.

5. Savoie M, Kim SS, Soloway MS: **A prospective study measuring penile length in Men treated with radical prostatectomy for prostate cancer.** *J Urol* 2003, **169**:1462–1464.

6. Munding MD, Wessells HB, Dalkin BL: **Pilot study of changes in stretched penile length 3 months after radical retropubic prostatectomy.** *J Urol* 2001, **58**:567–569.

7. Benson JS, Abern MR, Levine LA: **Penile shortening after radical prostatectomy and Peyronie's surgery.** *Curr Urol Rep* 2009, **10**:468–474.

8. Fischer M, Visser A, Voerman B, Garssen B, van Andel G, Bensing J: **Treatment decision making in prostate cancer: Patients' participation in complex decisions.** *Patient Educ Couns* 2006, **3**:308–313.

9. Wei J, Dunn R, Sandler H: **Comprehensive comparison of health-related quality of life after contemporary therapies for localized prostate cancer.** *J Clin Oncol* 2002, **20**:557–566.

10. Elliott S, Latini DM, Walker LM, Wasssersug R, Robinson JW: **Androgen deprivation therapy for prostate cancer: recommendations to improve patient and partner quality of life.** *J Sex Med* 2010, **7**(9):2996–3010.

11. Steginga SK, Occhipinti S, Dunn J, Gardiner RA, Heathcote P, Yaxley J: **The supportive care needs of men with prostate cancer 2000.** *Psychooncology* 2001, **10**:66–75.

12. Schover LR, Fouladi RT, Warneke CL, Neese L, Klein EA, Zippe C, Kupelian PA: **The Use of treatments for erectile dysfunction among survivors of prostate carcinoma.** *Cancer* 2002, **95**(11):2397–2407.

13. Wittman D, Northouse L, Foly S, Gilbert S, Wood DP Jr, Balon R, Montie JE: **The psychosocial aspects of sexual recovery after prostate cancer treatment.** *Int J Impotence Res J Sex Med* 2009, **21**(2):99–106.

14. Pereira RF, Daibs YS, Tobias-Machado M, Pompeo ACL: **Quality of life, behavioral problems, and marital adjustment in the first year after radical prostatectomy.** *Clin Genitourin Cancer* 2011, **9**(1):53–58.

15. Green HJ, Wells DJN, Laakso L: **Coping in men with prostate cancer and their partners: a quantitative and qualitative study.** *Eur J Cancer Care (Engl)* 2011, **20**(2):237–247.

16. Clark JA, Inui TS, Silliman RA, Bokhour BG, Krasnow SH, Robinson RA, Spaulding M, Talcott JA: **Patients' perceptions of quality of life after treatment for early prostate cancer.** *J Clin Oncol* 2003, **21**(20):3777–3784.

17. Dahn J, Penedo F, Gonzalez J, Esquiabro M, Antoni M, Roos B, Schneiderman N: **Sexual functioning and quality of life after prostate cancer treatment: considering sexual desire.** *Urology* 2004, **63**(2):273–277.

18. Couper JW, Love AW, Duchesne GM, Bloch S, Macvean M, Dunai JV, Scealy M, Costello A, Kissane DW: **Predictors of psychosocial distress 12 months after diagnosis with early and advanced prostate cancer.** *Med J Aust* 2010, **193**(5 Suppl):S58–S61.

19. Laumann EO, Paik A, Rosen RC: **Sexual dysfunction in the United States, prevalence and predictors.** *JAMA* 1999, **281**:537–544.

20. Roesch SC, Adams L, Hines A, Palmores A, Vyas P, Tran C, Pekin S, Vaughn AA: **Coping with prostate cancer: a meta-analytic review.** *J Behav Med* 2005, **28**(3):281–293.

21. Hedestig O, Sandman PO, Tomic R, Widmark A: **Living after radical prostatectomy for localized prostate cancer: a qualitative analysis of patient narratives.** *Acta Oncol* 2005, **44**(7):679–686.

22. Smith JF, Caan BJ, Sternfeld B, Haque R, Quesenberry CP Jr, Quinn VP, Shan J, Walsh TJ, Lue TF, Jacobsen SJ, Van Den Eeden SK: **Racial disparities in erectile dysfunction among participants in the California Men's Health Study.** *J Sex Med* 2009, **6**(12):3433–3439.

23. Folkman S, Lazarus RS: **An analysis of coping in a middle-aged community sample.** *J Health Social Behav* 1980, **21**:219–239.

24. Cassileth BR, Volckmar D, Goodman RL: **The effect of experience on radiation therapy patients' desire for information.** *Int J Radiat Oncol Biol Phys* 1980, **6**:493–496.

25. Braun V, Clark V: **Using thematic analysis in psychology.** *Qual Res Psychol* 2006, **3**:77–101.

26. Incrocci I: **Sexual function after external beam radiotherapy for prostate cancer: What do we know?** *Oncology/Haematology* 2006, **57**:165–173.

27. Wootten AC, Burney S, Foroudi F, Frydenberg M, Coleman G, Ng KT: **Psychological adjustment of survivors of localised prostate cancer: investigating the role of dyadic adjustment, cognitive appraisal and coping style.** *Psychooncology* 2007, **16**(11):994–1002.

28. Couper J, Bloch S, Love A, Macvean M, Duchesne GM, Kissane D: **Psychosocial adjustment of female partners of men with prostate cancer: a review of the literature.** *Psychooncology* 2006, **15**(11):937–953.

29. Garos S, Kluck A, Aronoff D: **Prostate cancer patients and their partners: differences in satisfaction indices and psychological variables.** *J Sex Med* 2007, **4**(5):1394–1403.

30. Rivers BM, August EM, Gwede CK, Hart A Jr, Donovan KA, Pow-Sang JM, Quinn GP: **Psychosocial issues related to sexual functioning among African-American prostate cancer survivors and their spouses.** *Psychooncology* 2011, **20**(1):106–110.

31. Badr H, Taylor CLC: **Sexual dysfunction and spousal communication in couples coping with prostate cancer.** *Psychooncology* 2009, **18**(7):735–746.

32. Burns SM, Mahalik JR: **Understanding how masculine gender scripts may contribute to men's adjustment following treatment for prostate cancer.** *Am J* 2007, **1**(4):250–261.

33. Gray RE, Fitch MI, Mykhalovskiy E, Church K: **Hegemonic masculinity and the experience of prostate cancer: A narrative approach.** *J Aging Identity* 2002, **7**:43–62.

34. Burt J, Caelli K, Moore K, Anderson M: **Radical prostatectomy: men's experiences and postoperative needs.** *J Clin Nurs* 2005, **14**(7):883–890.

35. Christie KM, Meyerowitz BE, Giedzinska-Simons A, Gross M, Agus DB: **Predictors of affect following treatment decision-making for prostate cancer: conversations, cognitive processing, and coping.** *Psychooncology* 2009, **18**(5):508–514.

36. Chambers SK, Pinnock C, Lepore SJ, Hughes S, O'Connell DL: **A systematic review of psychosocial interventions for men with prostate cancer and their partners.** *Patient Educ Couns* 2011, **85**(2):e75–e88.

37. Canada AL, Neese LE, Sui D, Schover LR: **Pilot intervention to enhance sexual rehabilitation for couples after treatment for localized prostate carcinoma.** *Cancer* 2005, **104**(12):2689–2700.

38. Giesler RB, Given B, Given CW, Rawl S, Monahan P, Burns D, Azzouz F, Reuille KM, Weinrich S, Koch M, Champion V: **Improving the quality of life of patients with prostate carcinoma: a randomized trial testing the efficacy of a nurse-driven intervention.** *Cancer* 2005, **104**(4):752–762.

39. Molton IR, Siegel SD, Penedo FJ, Dahn JR, Kisinger DNTL, Carver CS, Shen B, Kumar M, Schneiderman N, Antoni MH: **Promoting recovery of sexual functioning after radical prostatectomy with group-based stress management: The role of interpersonal sensitivity.** *J Psychosom Res* 2008, **64**:527–536.

16

Chromosomal abnormalities and Y chromosome microdeletions in infertile men from Morocco

Yassine Naasse[1,3], Hicham Charoute[1], Brahim El Houate[1], Chadli Elbekkay[2], Lunda Razoki[2], Abderrahim Malki[3], Abdelhamid Barakat[1*] and Hassan Rouba[1]

Abstract

Background: Male infertility is responsible for 50 % of infertile couples. Thirty percent of male infertility is due to cytogenetic and genetic abnormalities. In Arab and North African populations, several studies have shown the association of these chromosomal abnormalities with male infertility. Our objective is to evaluate the frequency of chromosomal abnormalities and Y chromosome microdeletions in infertile men from Morocco.

Methods: A total of 573 Moroccan infertile men (444 azoospermic and 129 oligozoospermic men) referred for cytogenetic analysis to the Department of Cytogenetics of the Pasteur Institute of Morocco, were screened for the presence of chromosomal abnormalities and Y chromosome microdeletions.

Results: Chromosomal abnormalities accounted for approximately 10.5 % (60/573). Fifty six cases among them have sex chromosome abnormalities (93.34 %), including Klinefelter's syndrome in 41 patients (68.34 %). Autosomal chromosome abnormalities (6.66 %) were observed in 4 patients. Chromosomal abnormalities were more prevalent in azoospermic men (13.06 %) than in oligospermic men (1.55 %). Y microdeletions were detected in 16 of 85 patients (AZFc: 14.12 %, AZFbc: 4.70 %), most of them where azoospermic men with no chromosomal abnormality.

Conclusions: These results highlighted the need for efficient molecular genetic testing in male infertility diagnosis. In addition, a genetic screening should be performed in infertile men before starting assisted reproductive treatments.

Keywords: Male infertility, Chromosomal abnormalities, Y microdeletions, Severe oligozoospermia, Azoospermia

Background

Infertility is a public health problem; approximately 15 % of couples have difficulty or are unable to conceive [1]. Whereas, from 30 % to 50 % of infertility cases are due to a male factor [2]. There are many and diverse causes of male infertility, including accidental causes, congenital birth defects, functional impairments, environmental pollutants, or genetic factors. The latter represents between 10 % and 15 % of severe male infertility [3, 4].

Chromosomal anomalies are considered as one of the most important causes of male infertility [5–7]. Their incidence is higher in infertile men than the general population

(about 10 times) [8]. Chromosomal abnormalities (structural or numerical) are often detected in azoospermia and severe oligospermia [9], at frequencies ranging from 10 % to 23.62 % and from 1.10 % to 13.33 %, respectively [8, 10–14].

Chromosomal abnormalities are not the only genetic causes of male infertility. Deletion of the Y chromosome region containing the azoospermia factor (AZF) is considered the most common genetic cause of male infertility [15]. Three regions on Y chromosome long arm (AZFa, AZFb and AZFc) are recurrently deleted in men with severe spermatogenic failure [16]. The frequency of these microdeletions in azoospermic and severe oligospermic men is between 1 % and 50 % [16–18].

This study aimed to assess the different types of Y chromosome abnormalities and microdeletions, and their frequency in a Moroccan group of infertile men. In addition, we conducted several comparisons between

* Correspondence: hamid.barakat@pasteur.ma
[1]Laboratoire de Génétique Moléculaire Humaine, Département de la Recherche Scientifique, Institut Pasteur du Maroc, 1 Place Louis Pasteur, 20360 Casablanca, Morocco
Full list of author information is available at the end of the article

frequencies found in the current study and frequencies reported in other populations.

Methods

Patients

A group of 573 Moroccan infertile men were involved in this retrospective study. These patients with azoospermia or severe oligozoospermia were recruited at the Pasteur Institute of Morocco from 1998 to 2013. Patients with azoospermia or severe oligozoospermia resulting from endocrine or obstructive causes were excluded. The average age was 38.70 ± 7.00 years. The Karyotype was performed for all patients, while the screening for Y-chromosomal microdeletions was conducted in 85 patients for whom DNA samples were available.

Ethics statement

We obtained written informed consent from each subject and the study protocol was approved by the local committee on research ethics of the Pasteur Institute of Morocco.

Chromosomal analysis

Peripheral blood was collected in heparinized vacutainers. The cells were harvested and cultured in the laboratory of cytogenetics. Samples were incubated in an RPMI-1640 solution in the presence of phytohemagglutinin (PHA-E) for 72 h at 37 °C. 2 h before the end of the culture, colchicine was added. After centrifugation, the pellet recovered was treated with a hypotonic solution (0.075 M KCl). The samples were fixed by Carnoy fixative (acetic acid/methanol 1/3 acid). Fixed cell suspensions were spread on glass slides using a Pasteur pipette. These slides were immersed in the fixative Berger. The slides were immersed in the denaturing medium Earle. Then they undergone a Giemsa staining, and finally reading slides by G-banding technique using a microscope connected to a computer through a camera. At least 20 metaphases were counted for each sample.

Y-microdeletions studies

The genomic DNA extraction was carried out using the Phenol Chloroform standard conventional protocol in the laboratory of Human Molecular Genetics at the Pasteur Institute of Morocco. The samples were lysed by incubation of erythrocytes in Tris-EDTA (TE 20/5) followed by centrifugation. Once the pellet was white, it has undergone lysis of leukocytes by incubation in a solution containing Tris-EDTA (TE 10/5), 20 % SDS and Proteinase K overnight at 56 °C. Phenol was added and the tube centrifuged. After recovery of the upper aqueous phase, the Chloroform-Isoamyl Alcohol (24/1) was added. After centrifugation, the upper aqueous phase was recovered. Absolute Ethanol was added for DNA precipitation. Once recovered and dried, the DNA was

resuspended in Tris-EDTA (TE 10/1) 2 to 3 days and then diluted and stored at 4 °C before analysis.

Conventional microdeletions in the long arm of the Y chromosome (Yq) were detected by the polymerase chain reaction (PCR). 6 pairs of oligonucleotide primers were used to amplify the specific Y chromosome STS, which correspond to different loci of the azoospermia factors (AZF). Two sets of multiplex PCR reactions were performed for each patient. The primer pair that amplifies specific STS SRY gene was used as positive control.

The volume of the reaction mixture used in the multiplex PCR was 25 µl, containing 5 µl of DNA (25 ng/µl), 2.5 µl of $MgCl_2$ buffer (10X), 2 µl of dNTP (2.5 mM) 0.9 µl of $MgCl_2$ (25 mM), 0.2 µl of Taq DNA polymerase (5 units) and 0.8 µl of each primer (10 pM). On thermocycling, the Touch-Down PCR method was used to increase the specificity and reproducibility of the PCR by avoiding the presence of non-specific bands. The program used an initial denaturation of 5 min at 94 °C, followed by 5 cycles of 40 s at 94 °C, 45 s at 60 °C and 50 s at 72 °C, followed by 30 cycles of 35 s at 94 °C, 35 s at 58 °C and 40 s at 72 °C, and finally a final elongation of 7 min at 72 °C. Electrophoresis was performed on 3 % agarose gels containing Ethidium Bromide (EtBr) was performed for the control of the PCR products, using a size marker 100 bp. The gel was visualized under ultraviolet light.

Results

This study was performed on a sample of 573 infertile men, which were separated into two groups: men with non-obstructive azoospermia ($n = 444$; 77.48 %), and men with severe oligospermia ($n = 129$; 22.52 %) (Table 1). The average age is 38.70 ± 7.00 years. Cytogenetic analysis showed that among the 573 patients included in the study, 513 men (89.5 %) had a normal karyotype (46; XY), and 60 men (10.5 %) had various chromosomal abnormalities. Frequencies of these chromosomal abnormalities in patients with non-obstructive azoospermia and severe oligozoospermia, are 10.12 % ($n = 58$) and 0.35 % ($n = 2$), respectively. Among the 60 patients with chromosomal abnormalities, four (0.7 %) had an abnormality of autosomal chromosomes: Inversion 46; XY, inv 9 (p11; p13), and 56 men (9.8 %) had sex chromosome abnormalities: two mosaic forms 46; XY/47; XXY, one patient with 47; XYY, three patients with 45; X (15 %)/46; XY (85 %), three patients with 46; X, del Yq11, six patients with 46; XX, and the most frequent is Klinefelter syndrome (KFS) 47; XXY, it was found in 41

Table 1 Distribution of different types of infertility

Type of infertility	% (No. of men/Total No.)
Non obstructive Azoospermia	77.48 (444/573)
Oligozoospermia Severe	22.52 (129/573)

Table 2 Type and frequency of chromosomal anomalies in 573 Moroccan infertile men

	Non-obstructive Azoospermia	Severe Oligospermia	Overall those with counts < 5 million/ml
Sex Chromosome Aberrations			
47 ; XXY	8.79 % (39/444)	1.55 % (2/129)	7.16 % (41/573)
Mosaic 46 ;XY/47 ;XXY	0.46 % (2/444)	0 % (0/129)	0.35 % (2/573)
47 ;XYY	0.23 % (1/444)	0 % (0/129)	0.18 % (1/573)
45 ;X(15 %)/46 ;XY(85 %)	0.68 % (3/444)	0 % (0/129)	0.53 % (3/573)
46 ;X, del Y q11	0.68 % (3/444)	0 % (0/129)	0.53 % (3/573)
XX males (46 ;XX)	1.36 % (6/444)	0 % (0/129)	1.05 % (6/573)
Subtotal	12.2 % (54/444)	1.55 % (2/129)	9.8 % (56/573)
Autosomal Chromosome Abnormalities			
Inversion	0.9 % (4/444)	0 % (0/129)	0.7 % (4/573)
46 ;XY, inv 9 (p11 ;p13)			
Total	13.06 % (58/444)	1.55 % (2/129)	10.47 % (60/573)

patients (39 azoospermic men, and two men with severe oligozoospermia) (Table 2).

Molecular analysis was performed to detect Y chromosome microdeletions in 85 patients. Among these patients, twelve had a deletion of AZFc (14.12 %), four cases had a deletion of AZFbc, and 69 cases had an intact Y chromosome (81.18 %). No patient with a deletion of AZFa, AZFb or AZFabc was observed (Table 3). The occurrence of AZFc locus deletion is identical among azoospermic and oligospermic (50 %), whereas the AZFbc deletion was found in 75 % of azoospermic and 25 % of oligozoospermic patients (Table 3).

All cases with AZFc or AZFbc locus deletion had a normal karyotype (46; XY). For patients with no deletion ($n = 69$), only one case had the Klinefelter syndrome (47; XXY). The remaining patients had a normal karyotype (Table 4).

Discussion

Numerical and structural chromosome abnormalities played a principal role in male infertility. The prevalence of these abnormalities remained poorly studied and little discussed in the literature, including their prevalence in the Moroccan population.

Studies performed in different populations showed that the incidence of chromosomal abnormalities in infertile men varies between 2.2 % and 19.6 % [19]. In the current study, the frequency of chromosomal abnormalities in infertile men (non-obstructive azoospermic and severe oligozoospermic men) was 10.5 %. This frequency is comparable with those reported in Table 5. It is well known that the sperm count is inversely related to the presence of chromosomal abnormalities [20]. The proportion of chromosomal abnormalities in azoospermic men (13.06 %) was significantly higher than in severe oligospermic men (1.55 %), these frequencies were consistent with those found in other studies [20].

According to the study conducted by Ferlin et al., Klinefelter's syndrome frequency in infertile men reached respectively 10 % and 5 % in azoospermic and severe oligospermic men [4]. In our patients, we found that the Klinefelter syndrome 47; XXY was the most common in azoospermic men (9.25 %) than in oligospermic severe men (1.55 %). In consistence with other studies [21, 22], the mosaic forms of Klinefelter syndrome was found only in two azoospermic patients. Most men with KS are azoospermic and their ability to conceive remained too low [23]. However, Klinefelter Syndrome patients may have their own children genetically using the technique of testicular sperm extraction (TESE) or micro-TESE followed by ICSI [24]. However, their offspring have an increased risk for chromosomal abnormalities [25].

Structural rearrangements of the Y chromosome, including deletions, ring chromosome and isochromosomes may

Table 3 Type and frequency of Y-microdeletions in 85 infetiles men evaluated

	Non-obstructive azoospermia	Severe oligospermia	Overall those with counts < 5 million/ml
Absence of Y-microdeletions	76.81 % (53/69)	23.19 % (16/69)	81.18 % (69/85)
AZFc microdeletion	50 % (6/12)	50 % (6/12)	14.12 % (12/85)
AZFbc microdeletion	75 % (3/4)	25 % (1/4)	4.70 % (4/85)

Table 4 Incidence of Y-microdeletions in men with normal karyotype and men with Klinefelter Syndrome

	46 ; XY	47 ; XXY
Absence of Y microdeletions	98.55 % (68/69)	1.45 % (1/69)
AZFc deletion	100 % (12/12)	0 % (0/12)
AZFbc deletion	100 % (4/4)	0 % (0/4)

lead to different phenotypes. In this study, we detected three patients with deletion of the Y chromosome long arm, which are all azoospermic men. In fact, the long arm of the Y chromosome plays a crucial role in the process of spermatogenesis. Partial or total loss of the arm means the loss of genes controlling spermatogenesis, leading to a defect in sperm production [26, 27].

Disorders of sex development (DSD) regroup the clinical situation where the development of the chromosomal, gonadal or anatomical sex is atypical [28]. Three form of the DSD sex caused by chromosome aneuploidy were observed in our sample: The XX male, 47; XYY and 45; X/46; XY.

The "XX Male Syndrome" is one of the sex chromosome abnormalities. Men with this syndrome can have phenotype similar to those with Klinefelter's syndrome with normal male external genitalia, but they are sterile [29]. Studies have shown that the frequency of XX males among azoospermic varies between 0.6 % [30] and 3.7 % [21, 22]. In our study, the frequency of this chromosomal abnormality was 1.36 %.

Three patient have the mosaic 45; X (15 %)/46; XY (85 %), and one patient have 47; XYY, all of them are azoospermic. The mosaic form 45; X (15 %)/46; XY (85 %) are described in many studies and the phenotype can range from female phenotype and ambiguous to male phenotype with infertility [30]. The 47; XYY

syndrome is associated with behavior difficulties and in some case with infertility. Most males born with these chromosome patterns will go through life without being karyotyped [31]. Until now, no association was found between increased frequency of infertility and this syndrome.

Autosomal abnormalities are less frequent than sex chromosome abnormalities: 0.7 % versus 9.8 %. On the other hand, autosomal chromosome abnormalities are detected only in azoospermic men (0.9 %). These results are not similar with those reported in other studies [12, 30, 32]; Amouri et al. reported that gonosomal abnormalities are more common in azoospermic men, while autosomal abnormalities are more common in severe oligospermic men [23].

We identified 4 cases of autosomal chromosome abnormalities (0.7 %), all of them have the inversion 46; XY, inv 9 (p11; p13). This inversion even balanced may be a factor of structural chromosome aberrations during meiosis, and by the way a cause of the disturbances of spermatogenesis.

After the Klinfeleter syndrome, Y chromosome micodeletion are the second most frequent genetic cause of infertility. The frequencies of Y chromosome microdeletions differ from one study to another, and this may be due to several factors such as the choice of inclusion criteria, the STS markers used, and/or ethnicity of the study population [33, 34]. In our study, sixteen patients among the 85 analyzed infertile men showed the presence of Y microdeletions (18.83 %). This frequency is in accordance to that found by Ghorbel et al. (17.1 %) [21], Fayez et al. (20.4 %) [22], Imken et al. (3.15 %) [35] and El Oualid et al. (3.83 %) [36], although our cohort of patients showed a higher frequency, and this may be due to the low number of patients ascertained as well as the

Table 5 Comparison of chromosomal anomalies between this study and other similar studies

Authors	Regions	No. of cases	Frequencies %	Prevalence of chromosomal aberration % (No. of men/total No.)	
				Non-obstructive Azoospermia	Severe Oligospermia Counts < 5 million/ml
Tuerlings et al., 1998 [45]	Netherlands	968	3.51	6.45 % (4/62)	3.47 % (30/865)
Nagvenkar et al., 2005 [11]	India	88	10.22	14.29 % (6/42)	6.52 % (3/46)
Mohammed et al., 2007 [33]	Kuwait	289	7.95	19.44 % (21/108)	1.10 % (2/181)
Ng et al., 2009 [12]	Hong Kong	295	5.08	21.10 % (5/71)	4.46 % (10/224)
Kosar et al., 2010 [5]	South of Turkey	115	4.34	5.43 % (5/92)	0 % (0/23)
Alkhalaf et al., 2010 [46]	Kuwait	142	18.30	data not available	data not available
Mafra et al., 2011 [34]	Brazil	143	6.29	11.62 % (5/43)	4 % (4/100)
Zhang et al., 2012 [32]	Northeast China	135	14.07	17.28 % (14/81)	9.26 % (5/54)
Cavkaytar et al., 2012 [47]	Turkey	332	7.23	11.22 % (22/196)	1.47 % (2/136)
Amouri et al., 2014 [30]	Tunisia	476	10.92	14.10 % (46/328)	4.05 % (6/148)
Our study	Morocco	573	10.47	13.06 % (58/444)	1.55 % (2/129)

No.: number

high number of patients with Y microdeletions, but higher than that found in the Chinese population (6.4 %; 8.5 %; 9.1 %) [12, 37, 38] or other Arab populations (Kuwait (2.6 %) [33], Tunisia (2.7 % and 6.85 %) [39, 40], Saudi Arabia (3.2 %) [41] and Egypt (4 %) [42]. However, the frequency found in this study was included in the range of frequencies of wide world (1–55 %) [17, 18]. These microdeletions are more common in azoospermic ($n = 9$) than severe oligospermic ($n = 7$), and this proportion was found in many reports [33, 35, 37–40, 42].

In this report, we identified only deletions of the AZFc and AZFbc region, while no case with deletion of AZFa and/or AZFb was identified. This result is similar to that described in Ng et al. [12] and Imken et al. [35] reports, but different to the results found in other reports [17, 34, 42, 43]. Several studies have shown that AZFc deletion was the most common [22, 39, 40], and these results are in accordance with ours (14.12 %). However, other studies showed conflicting results [33, 35, 42, 44].

In this study, we showed that sixteen cases with microdeletions (AZFc and AZFbc) have no chromosomal abnormalities (normal karyotype 46; XY) (Table 4). While Ng et al. showed that all patients with AZFc deletion had a normal karyotype 46; XY, while all patients with AZFbc deletion had chromosomal abnormalities [12].

Conclusion

The prevalence of chromosomal abnormalities and Y chromosome microdeletions are comparable to that found in different parts of the world (North Africa, Asia and Europe). Indeed, the analysis of these genetic factors (karyotype, Y microdeletions, etc. ...) is highly recommended, to identify the causes of infertility and to choose the appropriate assisted reproduction technique, and also to reduce the risk of transmission of these genetic defects to the future generations.

Abbreviations

AZF: Azoospermia Factor; dNTP: Triphosphate Deoxyribonucleotides; DSD: Disorders of Sex Development; EDTA: Ethylenediaminetetraacetic acid; BET: Ethidium Bromide; ICSI: Intracytoplasmic Sperm Injection; KCl: Potassium Chloride; KFS: Klinefelter Syndrome; PCR: Polymerase Chain Reaction; PHA-E: Phytohemagglutinin- Erythrocytes; RPMI: Roswell Park Memorial Institute medium; SDS: Sodium Dodecyl Sulfate; SRY: Sex-determining Region of Y chromosome; STS: Sequence-tagged site; TE: Tris-EDTA; TESE: Testicular Sperm Extraction.

Competing interests

The authors declare that they have no competing interests.

Authors' contributions

AB and HR conceived, designed and coordinated the study. YN performed the laboratory work. BE helped in the laboratory work. YN and HC carried out statistical analysis. YN wrote the paper. CE, LR and AM participated in interpretation of results. All authors read and approved the final manuscript.

Authors' information

Not applicable.

Acknowledgments

We thank all patients for their cooperation. This work was supported by Institut Pasteur du Maroc. The authors would also like to thank Dr. Kenneth McElreavey for his contribution to this work.

Funding

This work received no specific grant from any funding agency.

Author details

[1]Laboratoire de Génétique Moléculaire Humaine, Département de la Recherche Scientifique, Institut Pasteur du Maroc, 1 Place Louis Pasteur, 20360 Casablanca, Morocco. [2]Laboratoire de Cytogénétique, Département de la Recherche Scientifique, Institut Pasteur du Maroc, 1 Place Louis Pasteur, 20360 Casablanca, Morocco. [3]Laboratoire de Physiopathologie et Génétique Moléculaire, Faculté des Sciences Ben M'Sik, Université Hassan II, Casablanca, Morocco.

References

1. Van Assche E, Bonduelle M, Tournaye H, Joris H, Verheyen G, Devroey P, et al. Cytogenetics of infertile men. Hum Reprod. 1996;4:1–24.
2. Gurunath S, Pandian Z, Anderson RA, Bhattacharya S. Defining infertility – a systematic review of prevalence studies. Hum Reprod Update. 2011;17:575–88.
3. Kim ED, Lipshultz LI. Male subfertility: diagnostic and therapeutic advances. Br J Urol. 1997;80(4):633–41.
4. Ferlin A, Arredi B, Foresta C. Genetic causes of male infertility. Reprod Toxicol. 2006;22:133–41.
5. Kosar PA, Ozcelik N, Kosar A. Cytogenetic abnormalities detected in patients with non-obstructive azoospermia and severe oligozoospermia. J Assist Reprod Genet. 2010;27:17–21.
6. Dohle GR, Halley DJ, Van Hemel JO, van den Ouwel AM, Pieters MH, Weber RF, et al. Genetic risk factors in infertile men with severe oligozoospermia and azoospermia. Hum Reprod. 2002;17:13–6.
7. Martin RH. Cytogenetic determinants of male fertility. Hum Reprod Updat. 2008;14:379–90.
8. Ceylan GG, Ceylan C, Elyas H. Genetic anomalies in patients with severe oligozoospermia and azoospermia in eastern Turkey: a prospective study. Genet Mol Res. 2009;8:915–22.
9. Chandley A. Chromosome anomalies and Y chromosome microdeletions as casual factors in male infertility. Hum Reprod. 1998;13:45–50.
10. Balkan M, Tekes S, Gedik A. Cytogenetic and Y chromosome microdeletion screening studies in infertile males with oligozoospermia and azoospermia in Southeast Turkey. J Assist Reprod Genet. 2008;25:559–65.
11. Nagvenkar P, Desai K, Hinduja I, Zaveri K. Chromosomal studies in infertile men with oligozoospermia & non-obstructive azoospermia. Indian J Med Res. 2005;122:34–42.
12. Ng PP, Tang MH, Lau ET, Ng LK, Ng EH, Tam PC, et al. Chromosomal anomalies and Y-microdeletions among Chinese subfertile men in Hong Kong. Hong Kong Med J. 2009;15:31–8.
13. Chiang HS, Wei HJ, Chen YT. Genetic screening for patients with azoospermia and severe oligo-asthenospermia. Int J Androl. 2000;23:20–5.
14. Zhou-Cun A, Yang Y, Zhang SZ, Zhang W, Lin L. Chromosomal abnormality and Y chromosome microdeletion in Chinese patients with azoospermia or severe oligozoospermia. Yi Chuan Xue Bao. 2006;33:111–16.
15. Krausz C, Degl'Innocenti S. Y chromosome and male infertility: update. Front Biosci. 2006;11:3049–61.
16. Vogt PH, Edelmann A, Kirsch S, Henegariu O, Hirschmann P, Kiesewetter F, et al. Human Y chromosome azoospermia factors (AZF) mapped to different subregions in Yq11.1. Hum Mol Genet. 1996;5:933–44.
17. Foresta C, Ferlin A, Garolla A, Moro E, Pistorello M, Barbaux S, et al. High frequency of well-defined Y-chromosome deletions in idiopathic Sertoli cell-only syndrome. Hum Reprod. 1998;13(2):302–07.
18. van der Ven K, Montag M, Peschka B, Leygraaf J, Schwanitz G, Haidl G, et al. Combined cytogenetic and Y chromosome microdeletion screening in males undergoing intracytoplasmic sperm injection. Mol Hum Reprod. 1997;3:699–704.

19. Nakamura Y, Kitamura M, Nishimura K, Koga M, Kondoh N, Takeyama M, et al. Chromosomal variants among 1790 infertile men. Int J Urol. 2001;8:49–52.
20. Lissitsina J, Mikelsaar R, Punab M. Cytogenetic analyses in infertile men. Arch Androl. 2006;52:91–5.
21. Ghorbel M, Gargouri Baklouti S, Ben Abdallah F, Zribi N, Cherif M, Keskes R, et al. Chromosomal defects in infertile men with poor semen quality. J Assist Reprod Genet. 2012;29:451–56.
22. Fayez AG, El-Sayed AS, El-Desouky MA, Zarouk WA, Kamel AK, Fahmi IM, et al. Molecular Characterization of Some Genetic Factors Controlling Spermatogenesis in Egyptian Patients with Male Infertility. Int J Infertility Fetal Med. 2012;3:69–77.
23. Smyth CM, Bremner WJ. Klinefelter syndrome. Arch Intern Med. 1998;158:1309–14.
24. Krausz C. Male infertility: pathogenesis and clinical diagnosis. Best Pract Res Clin Endocrinol Metab. 2011;25:271–85.
25. Ron-El R, Strassburger D, Gelman-Kohan S, Friedler S, Raziel A, Appelman Z. A 47, XXY fetus conceived after ICSI of spermatozoa from a patient with non-mosaic Klinefelter's syndrome: case report. Hum Reprod. 2000;15(8):1804–06.
26. Valetto A, Bertini V, Rapalini E, Baldinotti F, Di Martino D, Simi P. Molecular and cytogenetic characterization of a structural rearrangement of the Y chromosome in an azoospermic man. Fertil Steril. 2004;81:1388–90.
27. Siffroi JP, Chantot-Bastaraud S, Ravel C. Genetic origin of spermatogenesis impairments: clinical aspects and relationships with mouse models of infertility. Gynecol Obstet Fertil. 2003;31:504–15.
28. Lee PA, Houk CP, Ahmed SF, Hughes IA. Consensus statement on management of intersex disorders. International Consensus Conference on Intersex. Pediatrics. 2006;118:488–500.
29. Boucekkine C, Toublanc JE, Abbas N, Chaabouni S, Ouahid S, Semrouni M, et al. Clinical and anatomical spectrum in XX sex reversed patients. Relationship to the presence of Y specific DNA-sequences. Clin Endocrirol (Oxford). 1994;40:733–42.
30. Amouri A, Hammami W, Kilani O, Bouzouita A, Ayed W, Ben Meftah M, et al. Chromosomal evaluation in a group of Tunisian patients with non-obstructive azoospermia and severe oligozoospermia attending a Tunisian cytogenetic department. C R Biologies. 2014;337:223–28.
31. Abramsky L, Chapple J. 47, XXY (Klinefelter syndrome) and 47, XYY: estimated rates of and indication for postnatal diagnosis with implications for prenatal counseling. Prenat Diagn. 1997;17:363–68.
32. Zhang ZB, Jiang YT, Yun X, Yang X, Wang RX, Dai RL, et al. Male infertility in Northeast China: a cytogenetic study of 135 patients with non-obstructive azoospermia and severe oligozoospermia. J Assist Reprod Genet. 2012;29:83–7.
33. Mohammed F, Al-Yatama F, Al-Bader M, Tayel SM, Gouda S, Naguib KK. Primary male infertility in Kuwait: a cytogenetic and molecular study of 289 infertile Kuwaiti patients. Andrologia. 2007;39:87–92.
34. Mafra FA, Christofolini DM, Bianco B, Gava MM, Glina S, Belangero SI, et al. Chromosomal and molecular abnormalities in a group of Brazilian infertile men with severe oligozoospermia or non-obstructive azoospermia attending an infertility service. Int Braz J Urol. 2011;37:244–50.
35. Imken L, El Houate B, Chafik A, Nahili H, Boulouiz R, Abidi O, et al. AZF microdeletions and partial deletions of AZFc region on the Y chromosome in Moroccan men. Asian J Androl. 2007;9:674–78.
36. Eloualid A, Rhaissi H, Reguig A, Bounaceur S, El Houate B, Abidi O, et al. Association of spermatogenic failure with the b2/b3 partial AZFc deletion. PLoS One. 2012;7:e34902.
37. Tse JY, Yeung WS, Ng EH, Zhu HB, Teng XM, Liu YK, et al. A comparative study of Y chromosome microdeletions in infertile males from two Chinese populations. J Assist Reprod Genet. 2002;19:376–83.
38. Tse JY, Yeung WS, Lau EY, Ng EH, So WW, Ho PC. Deletions within the azoospermia factor subregions of the Y chromosome in Hong Kong Chinese men with severe malefactor infertility: controlled clinical study. Hong Kong Med J. 2000;6:143–46.
39. Hammami W, Kilani O, Ben Khelifa M, Ayed W, Abdelhak S, Bouzouita A, et al. Prevalence of Y chromosome microdeletions in infertile Tunisian men. Ann Biol Clin (Paris). 2014;72:331–6.
40. Rejeb I, M'rad R, Maazoul F, Trabelsi M, Ben Jemaa L, Chaabouni M, et al. Y chromosome microdeletions in Tunisian infertile males. PatBio. 2008;56:111–5.
41. Hellani A, Al-Hassan S, Iqbal M, Coskun S. Y chromosome microdeletions in infertile men with idiopathic oligo or azoospermia. J Exp Clin Assist Reprod. 2006;3:1–6.
42. Nowier SR, El-sheikh MM, Rasool HAA, Ismail S. Prevalence of Y Chromosome Microdeletion in Males with Azospermia And Severe Oligospermia in Egypt. Res J Med Medical Sci. 2009;4:189.
43. Simoni M, Bakker E, Krausz C. EAA/EMQN best practice guidelines for molecular diagnosis of Y-chromosomal microdeletions. State of art 2004. Int J Androl. 2004;27:240–49.
44. Elhawary NA, Seif-Eldin NS, Zaki M, Diab H. Azoospermia factor microdeletions: common tag STSs in infertile men with azoospermia and sever oligospermia from Egypt. BMC Genomics. 2014;15:25.
45. Tuerlings J, de France HF, Hamers A, Hordijk R, Van Hemel JO, Hansson K, et al. Chromosome studies in 1792 males prior to intracytoplasmic sperm injection: the Dutch experience. Eur J Hum Genet. 1998;6:194–200.
46. Alkhalaf M, Al-Shoumer K. Cytogenetic abnormalities and azoospermia factor (AZF) microdeletions in infertile men from Kuwait. J Mol Genet Med. 2010;26:232–34.
47. Cavkaytar S, Batioglu S, Gunel M, Ceylaner S, Karaer A. Genetic evaluation of severe male factor infertility in Turkey: a cross-sectional study. Hum Fertil. 2012;15:100–06.9.

17

Transperineal template-guided saturation biopsy aimed at sampling one core for each milliliter of prostate volume: 103 cases requiring repeat prostate biopsy

Yasushi Nakai[1] (iD), Nobumichi Tanaka[1*], Satoshi Anai[1], Makito Miyake[1], Shunta Hori[1], Yoshihiro Tatsumi[1], Yosuke Morizawa[1], Tomomi Fujii[2], Noboru Konishi[2] and Kiyohide Fujimoto[1]

Abstract

Background: We evaluated the cancer detection rate of prostate cancer using transperineal template-guided saturation biopsy aimed at sampling one core for each milliliter of prostate volume for patients requiring repeated prostate biopsies.

Methods: In total, 103 consecutive patients with repeated prostate biopsies were enrolled in this retrospective study. The number of biopsy cores was defined by prostate volume. In principle, one biopsy core covered 1 mL of prostate volume. We used a prostate brachytherapy template with a 5-mm grid and adopted a transperineal needle biopsy.

Results: The median age, prostate-specific antigen level, and prostate volume were 69 (range, 37–83) years, 9.2 (range, 1.9–107) ng/mL, and 34.7 (range, 18–76.7) mL, respectively. The median number of biopsy cores was 37 (range, 18–75 cores). Fifty-three patients (51.5%) were diagnosed with prostate cancer. The Gleason score was 6, 7, and 8–10 in 24.5, 64.2 and 11.3% patients, respectively. Forty-two patients (79.2%) were diagnosed with clinically significant PCa. Acute urinary retention was detected in 2 patients (1.9%).

Conclusions: Transperineal template-guided saturation biopsy with one core per milliliter of prostate volume helped achieve a high cancer detection rate and high significant cancer detection rate with acceptable biopsy-associated adverse events.

Keywords: Repeated prostate biopsy, Saturation biopsy, Transperineal template-guided biopsy

Background

Prostate-specific antigen (PSA) testing has been widely used for prostate cancer (PCa) screening, and transrectal ultrasound (TRUS)-guided biopsies have been widely performed [1, 2]. However, even with contemporary use of laterally directed extended TRUS-guided biopsies, the false-negative rate remains high [3]. Patients with negative diagnosis by TRUS-guided biopsy may need repeat biopsy if the following findings are present: increased PSA levels; abnormal findings on digital rectal examination (DRE), TRUS, and MRI; and previous biopsy showing high-grade

prostatic intraepithelial neoplasia (HGPIN) and/or atypical small acinar proliferation (ASAP). Cancer detection rates with TRUS-guided repeat biopsy have been reported to range from 10 to 21% [4–6]. These results indicate that patients continue to be under persistent clinical suspicion of PCa despite several repeated biopsies. To resolve this problem, several investigators have reported the use of saturation biopsy [7–12].

Prostate saturation biopsy was initially introduced by Borborogle et al. [7]; it consisted at least 20 biopsy cores. Saturation biopsy is performed via transrectal or transperineal routes, with similarly high detection rates [8–13]. Recently, the transperineal approach has been preferred because of sampling accuracy, particularly for the anterior prostate region [8–10]. Although the technique of transperineal

* Correspondence: sendo@naramed-u.ac.jp
[1]Department of Urology, Nara Medical University, 840 Shijo-cho, Kashihara-shi, Nara 634-8522, Japan
Full list of author information is available at the end of the article

saturation biopsy has varied among reports, the cancer detection rate has been reported to be between 40 and 60% in repeated biopsies [8–10, 14, 15]. Previous studies on saturation repeat biopsy showed higher detection rates than those on TRUS-guided repeat biopsy. However, the optimal number of biopsy cores remains in dispute. Buskirk et al. [16] showed that the number of needle incursions was the only prognostic factor of acute urinary retention (AUR). The incidence of AUR has been reported to be 10–39% [10, 17–19]. To prevent AUR, Ekwueme et al. [9] demonstrated the efficacy of transperineal saturation biopsy to avoid a needle incursion in the periurethral region, and AUR rate was found to be only 5.2%. Furthermore, McNeal and Chen et al. reported that PCa is rarely detected in the periurethral region [20, 21].

Under these circumstances, we conducted a study to evaluate the efficacy and safety of transperineal template-guided saturation biopsy (TTSB) aimed at sampling one core for each milliliter of prostate volume for patients who had undergone at least one negative TRUS-guided biopsy and requiring repeated prostate biopsy for increased PSA levels, abnormal findings on DRE, TRUS, and MRI, previous biopsy showing HGPIN, or ASAP.

Methods

Patient selection

From January 2008 to July 2014, we offered transperineal TTSB for patients considered to need prostate repeat biopsy when the following clinical factors were present: increased PSA levels; abnormal findings on DRE, TRUS, or MRI; and a previous biopsy showing HGPIN and/or ASAP. The number of previous TRUS-guided biopsies from TTSB showed 1–5 negative biopsies (median: 1). A total of 103 consecutive patients who received TTSB repeated prostate biopsy were enrolled in this study. Then we retrospectively analyzed the data. The institutional review board of the Nara Medical University approved this study.

Procedure of TTSB

All procedures were performed in the operating room. TTSB was performed in the dorsal lithotomy position under either general or spinal anesthesia; a 14-French urethral catheter was inserted before the procedure. Every patient received premedication with a single dose of 1 g cefazolin by intravenous infusion for preventing infection caused by TTSB. DRE was performed, and a transrectal probe (Toshiba Medical, Tochigi, Japan) attached to a brachytherapy stepping unit (AccuSeed, Bedfordshire, UK) was then inserted into the rectum. The low-echoic area was estimated and prostate volume was calculated using the following formula: length × width × height × 0.5236 [22]. The number of biopsy cores was estimated using the widest transverse section (Fig. 1). The interval between biopsy cores in a row was uniformly 5 mm in rows from right to left in the longitudinal view, except for

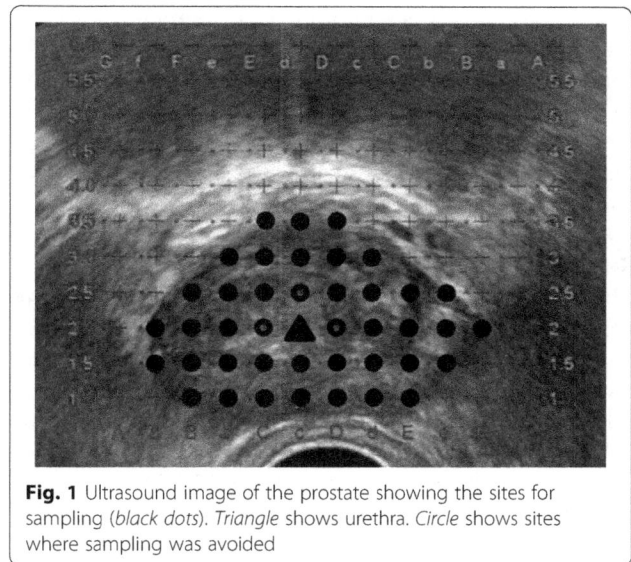

Fig. 1 Ultrasound image of the prostate showing the sites for sampling (*black dots*). *Triangle* shows urethra. *Circle* shows sites where sampling was avoided

the area nearest to and around the urethra. At a point where sufficient sample was not taken from the apex of the bladder, an additional core was considered to take the sample from a point near the bladder. The number of additional cores taken was determined by the calculated prostate volume, and the number of biopsy cores was determined based on prostate volume. To achieve a "saturation biopsy," one biopsy core per milliliter of prostate volume was required. The biopsy procedure was performed using an 18-gauge, 25-cm-long biopsy gun (Bard, Covington, GA, USA).

After TTSB, patients were monitored in the hospital until the next day noon. The next morning, the urethral catheter was removed. Patients were discharged once they could void successfully.

PSA density (PSAD) was calculated by dividing PSA by prostate volume. PSA velocity (PSAV) was defined as absolute increase in PSA level per year following the initial biopsy until the second biopsy. For patients with multiple PSA measurements prior to a saturation biopsy, we used the most recent value before the saturation biopsy date. Insignificant cancer was defined as a clinically insignificant Gleason score of 3, maximum tumor length of <4.5 mm, and total tumor length of <5.5 mm based on the report by Epstein [23].

Statistical analysis

Statistical analysis was performed with SPSS for Windows (version 20.0; IBM, Armonk, NY, USA). Pearson's correlation was calculated between pairs of variables. A Mann-Whitney U test was used for continuous variables and a chi-square test for categorical variables. Binary logistic regression analysis was used to estimate the independent parameter of positive TTSB.

The cutoff value was determined as the point closest to the upper left-hand corner in the receiver operating characteristic curve. Univariate analysis was first applied to isolate variables with a significant value of $P < 0.05$. Variables predictive of PCa by univariate analysis were included in multivariate analysis. A P value <0.05 was considered statistically significant.

Results

The median age, median PSA level, and median prostate volume were 69 (range, 37–83) years, 9.2 (range, 1.9–107) ng/mL, and 34.7 (range, 18–76.7) mL, respectively. The median number of previous TRUS biopsies sets was 1 (range, 1–5) and that of cores obtained by previous TRUS-guided biopsies was 12 (range, 8–13). TTSB resulted in a median of 37 cores (range, 18–75). Of the 103 patients, PCa was detected in 53 (51.5%). In 57 patients with gray-zone PSA (4–10 ng/ml), PCa was detected in 25 (43.9%). Patient age with positive biopsy was significantly higher than that with negative biopsy ($P < 0.01$), and PSAD of positive biopsy patients was significantly higher than that of negative biopsy patients ($P = 0.02$). Free PSA ratio of positive was significantly lower than that of negative biopsy patients ($P = 0.04$), abnormal findings on DRE were found more in positive biopsy patients than in negative ($P = 0.03$), and prostate volume of positive biopsy patients was significantly smaller than that of negative biopsy patients ($P < 0.01$). MRI was performed for 14 patients between the previous TRUS-guided biopsy and TTSB, and 9 patients underwent saturation biopsy because of abnormal findings on MRI. Six of nine patients (66.7%) were diagnosed with PCa on TTSB (Table 1)

Table 2 summarizes the number of positive cores and Gleason biopsy score. The distribution of positive cores was the most heavily weighted in those patients with 2–5 positive cores (50.1%). Gleason score distribution ranged from 6 to 9 with the vast majority 7 (64.2%). Eleven patients (20.8%) were diagnosed with clinically insignificant PCa.

In the cores taken from the posterior and anterior regions of the prostate, PCa was detected in 33/53 (62.2%) and 44/53 (83%) cases, respectively. The incidence of PCa in the anterior region of the prostate was significantly higher than that in the posterior ($P = 0.01$). GS ≥ 7 PCa was found in 24/53 (45.2%) and 31/53 (58.5%) cases in the cores taken from the posterior and anterior regions of the prostate, respectively. There was no significant difference ($P = 0.14$) in the incidence of GS ≥ 7 PCa between the posterior and anterior regions.

Age, free PSA ratio, PSA density, abnormal findings on DRE, and prostate volume were the significant factors in univariate analysis. In multivariate analysis, prostate volume was a negative predictor of positive PCa by TTSB (≤ 34.1 vs. > 34.1 mL, $P = 0.03$) and age was a positive predictor of positive PCa by TTSB (≤ 70.3 vs. > 70.3 years, $P < 0.01$) (Table 3).

There was no case of urosepsis and urinary tract infection. Only 2 of 103 (1.9%) patients needed catheterization after removal of the catheter. From one patient the urethral catheter could be removed after 6 days and from

Table 1 The clinical and pathological features of patients

Variables Median (range) or n (%)	Total $n = 103$	Prostate cancer $n = 53$	No prostate cancer $n = 50$	P
Age, years	69 (37–83)	71 (48–79)	67 (37–83)	<0.01[†]
No. of TRUS biopsies	1 (1–5)	1 (1–5)	1 (1–3)	0.48[†]
No. of cores obtained pre-TRUSBs	12 (8–13)	12 (8–13)	12 (8–12)	0.89[†]
PSA, ng/mL	9.2 (1.9–107)	10.7 (1.9–42.1)	8.8 (4.5–107)	0.33[†]
Free-PSA ratio, %	15.3 (1.3–67.1)	12.9 (4.3–25.7)	16.9 (1.3–67.1)	0.04[†]
PSA density, ng/mL/mL	0.26 (0.06–1.9)	0.33 (0.06–1.3)	0.23 (0.07–1.9)	0.02[†]
PSA velocity, ng/mL/year	1.12 (−29–129)	1.39 (−29–26)	0.75 (−8.8–129)	0.66
DRE, abnormal findings	17 (16.5)	13 (24.5)	4 (8.0)	0.03[‡]
TRUS, abnormal findings	21 (20.3)	14 (26.4)	7 (14.0)	0.13[‡]
MRI, abnormal findings ($n = 14$)	9/14 (64.2)	6/9 (66.7)	3/5 (60.0)	0.93[‡]
Prostate volume, mL	34.7 (18–76.7)	30.8 (18–65.1)	39.4 (20.1–76.7)	<0.01[†]
HGPIN on previous biopsy	13 (12.6)	7 (13.2)	6 (12.0)	0.88[‡]
ASAP on previous biopsy	10 (9.7)	8 (15.1)	2 (4.0)	0.06[‡]
No of cores obtained by TTSB	37 (18–75)	32 (22–66)	41.5 (18–75)	<0.01[†]
Core/volume, cores/mL	1.05 (0.80–1.77)	1.05 (0.80–1.31)	1.05 (0.80–1.77)	0.07[†]

[†]Mann-Whitney U test, [‡]Chi-squared test
TRUS transrectal ultrasound, PSA prostate specific antigen, DRE digital rectal examination, HGPIN high grade prostatic intraepithelial neoplasia, ASAP atypical small acinar proliferation, TTSB transperineal template-guided sasturation biopsy, Core/volume number of cores per unit volume of prostate

Table 2 The number of positive cores and cancer grade

	Count n (%) n = 53
No. of positive cores	
1	11 (20.8)
2–5	27 (50.1)
6–9	9 (17.0)
≥ 10	4 (7.5)
Gleason score	
6	13 (24.5)
7	34 (64.2)
8	4 (7.5)
9	2 (3.8)

Table 3 Univariate and multivariate analysis of factors that predict positive for prostate cancer

Variables	Univariate analysis		Multivariate analysis	
Categories	Odds ratio (95% CI)	P	Odds ratio (95% CI)	P
Age				
≤ 70.3	(Ref)		(Ref)	
> 70.3	3.80 (1.68–8.61)	<0.01	4.96 (1.67–14.7)	<0.01
No. of TURSBs				
≤ 1	(Ref)			
> 1	0.70 (0.31–1.60)	0.78		
No. cores obtained by pre-TURSBs				
≤ 10	(Ref)			
> 10	1.01 (0.87–1.16)	0.91		
PSA				
≤ 9.3	(Ref)			
> 9.3	1.85 (0.83–4.07)	0.12		
Free PSA ratio				
≤ 13.6	(Ref)		(Ref)	
> 13.6	0.33 (0.14–0.78)	0.01	0.45 (0.13–1.60)	0.22
PSA density				
≤ 0.27	(Ref)		(Ref)	
> 0.27	2.69 (1.20–6.01)	0.02	2.03 (0.468–6.01)	0.20
PSA velocity				
≤ 1.2	(Ref)			
> 1.2	1.91 (0.86–4.25)	0.11		
DRE				
Benign	(Ref)		(Ref)	
Suspicious	3.73 (1.12–12.3)	0.03	2.87 (0.72–11.5)	0.13
TRUS				
Benign	(Ref)			
Suspicious	2.20 (0.81–6.03)	0.12		
Prostate volume				
≤ 34.1	(Ref)		(Ref)	
> 34.1	0.24 (0.11–0.55)	<0.01	0.28 (0.09–0.90)	0.03
HGPIN on previous biopsy				
Absent	(Ref)			
Present	1.11 (0.35–3.58)	0.85		
ASAP on previous biopsy				
Absent	(Ref)			
Present	4.23 (0.86–21.2)	0.08		
Core/volume				
≤ 1.05	(Ref)			
> 1.05	3.28 (0.41–24.5)	0.26		

TRUSB transrectal ultrasound -guided biopsy, *PSA* prostate specific antigen, *DRE* digital rectal examination, *TRUS* transrectal ultrasound, *HGPIN* high grade prostatic intraepithelial neoplasia, *ASAP* atypical small acinar proliferation, *TTSB* transperineal template-guided sasturation biopsy

another after 10 days. Prostate volumes of the two patients were 73.1 and 46.0 mL. One patient had habitually used an alpha-1 adrenogenic receptor antagonist for benign prostatic hyperplasia.

Discussion

The overall cancer detection rate of the present study was 51.5%; this was comparable to that reported in the previous studies (26–68%) [8–10, 15, 18, 22, 24–29]. Studies including more than 100 cases have reported detection rates of 35.6–54.8% [9, 10, 18, 22, 28, 29]. Although the technique of TTSB and the number of biopsy cores varied among these studies, the cancer detection rate in repeated biopsy patients was almost similar.

Significant cancer by saturation biopsy was defined by Epstein et al. as follows: (a) Gleason score less than 7 and the number of positive cores as three or fewer or (b) Gleason score less than 7 and the maximal millimeters of cancer in one core less than 4.5 mm, with the total millimeters of cancer for all cores not exceeding 5.5 mm [23]. Previous studies have found that incidence rates of clinically significant cancer were 85.1 and 86.7% based on the Epstein's criteria [9, 24]. The present result (79.8%) was lower than those of these previous studies. Although increasing the number of cores may contribute to the high detection rate of insignificant cancer, the rate of detection of significant cancer in the present study was still high. Based on these results, TTSB should be considered for patients with persistent clinical suspicion of PCa without a negative previous biopsy.

In the present study, prostate volume showed a strong correlation with number of biopsy cores, and the mean number of biopsy cores per unit prostate volume was 1.06. This number is the highest in reports about TTSB [8–10, 13, 15, 18, 24–27]. However, the rate of detection of PCa was almost the same as that in other reports. This finding indicates that it is not necessary to sample as many cores as in our methods for detecting PCa. Subsequently, the number of cores may be reduced than that in our method. However, the optimal number of cores for saturation biopsy should be evaluated in the future.

Prostate volume has been considered a negative predictor of positive PCa by transperineal prostate biopsy in other reports [10, 28]. Merrick et al. used a 24-region technique with a median (mean, range) of 50.0 (51.1, 24–66) biopsy cores for patients whose mean prostate volume was 78.6 ml [10]. Symons et al. used a 14-region technique with a median (mean, range) of 15 (19.2, 4–47) biopsy cores for patients whose mean prostate volume was 45.8 ml [28]. In the present study, larger prostate volume predicted negative for PCa [odds ratio (OR), 0.29; 95%CI, 0.09–0.90] with a median (mean, range) of 37 (40.2, 18–75) biopsy cores for patients whose mean prostate volume was 38.5 ml. Even with this high number of biopsy cores per volume, large prostate volume was a negative predictor. This finding means that patients who have large prostates do not tend to have PCa. Based on these results and the detection rate with the high number of cores per volume in the present study, we can omit repeat biopsy for patients requiring repeated biopsy with large prostate. However, the positive predictive factors in the population of patients with large prostate should be determined in the future.

Multivariate analysis showed that age was a predictor of positive PCa. The median age of the patients (70 years) was higher than that in other reports [8–10]. It is believed [29] that the detection rate of PCa is higher in elderly than in younger men.

The reported incidence of AUR from TTSB ranged from 10 to 39% [10, 16–19] and obtaining more biopsy cores appears to have led to a high risk of AUR. In a previous study, Buskirk et al. [15] showed the relationship between needle trauma and AUR after TTSB. To prevent AUR, Ekwueme et al. [9] showed the safety of TTSB at 10-mm intervals by avoiding the periurethral region and reported the incidence of AUR as 5.9%. We obtained a low AUR rate of 1.9% by performing TTSB as described by Ekwueme et al., although we obtained more biopsy cores. Possible reasons for low rate of AUR are as follows: (a), catheterization overnight for all patients (b), smaller prostate volume in the patient population than other reports of saturation biopsy, and (c) avoiding insertion of needle to the periurethral region. In other studies, all patients were not catheterized overnight. [10, 11, 17–19] Prostate volume is a predictive factor for AUR [9]. AUR rate may rise in patient groups that include patients with larger prostates. However, in the present study, the mean prostate volume was smaller than that in other reports.

The present study had several limitations. First, it was retrospective study. Second, the median prostate volume in this study was smaller than that in other reports from Western countries. Indeed, the prostate volume of Japanese patients is smaller than that in Western populations [30]. Third, a control group of standard re-biopsy was lacking. The final limitation was the small cohort size.

Conclusions

We demonstrated the feasibility of TTSB aimed at sampling one core for each milliliter of prostate volume for patients with persistent clinical suspicion of PCa who had undergone at least one negative TRUS biopsy. A relatively high cancer detection rate (51.5%) and significant cancer detection rate (79.8%) could be achieved with a low AUR rate (1.9%).

Abbreviations
ASAP: Atypical small acinar proliferation; AUR: Acute urinary retention; DRE: Digital rectal examination; PCa: Prostate cancer; PSA: Prostate-specific antigen; PSAD: Prostate-specific antigen density; PSAV: Prostate-specific antigen velocity; TRUS: Transrectal ultrasound; TTSB: Transperineal template-guided saturation biopsy

Acknowledgements
None.

Funding
No funding was obtained for the present study.

Authors' contributions
YN interpreted the data and drafted the manuscript. NT conceived the study, participated in the study design, and revised the manuscript. SA, MM, SH, YT, and YM collected the data and proceeded biopsy. TF and NK collected the data and performed pathologic diagnosis. KF gave the final approval of the version to be published. All the authors have read and approved the final manuscript.

Competing interests
The authors declare that they have no competing interests.

Author details
[1]Department of Urology, Nara Medical University, 840 Shijo-cho, Kashihara-shi, Nara 634-8522, Japan. [2]Department of Pathology, Nara Medical University, 840 Shijo-cho, Kashihara-shi, Nara 634-8522, Japan.

References
1. Barry MJ. Clinical practice. Prostate-specific-antigen testing for early diagnosis of prostate cancer. N Engl J Med. 2001;344:1373–7.
2. Tanaka N, Shimada K, Nakagawa Y, et al. The optimal number of initial prostate biopsy cores in daily practice: a prospective study using the Nara Urological Research and Treatment Group nomogram. BMC Res Notes. 2015;8:689. doi:10.1186/s13104-015-1668-9.
3. Kawakami S, Okuno T, Yonese J, et al. Optimal sampling sites for repeat prostate biopsy: a recursive partitioning analysis of three-dimensional 26-core systemic biopsy. Eur Urol. 2007;51:675–83.
4. Keetch DW, Catalona WJ, Smith DS. Serial prostate biopsies in men with persistently elevated serum prostate specific antigen levels. J Urol. 1994;151:1571–4.
5. Djavan B, Zlotta A, Remzi M, et al. Optimal predictors of prostate cancer on repeat prostate biopsy: a prospective study of 1,051 men. J Urol. 2000;163:1144–8.
6. Park SJ, Miyake H, Hara I, et al. Predictors of prostate cancer on repeat transrectal ultrasound-guided systematic prostate biopsy. Int J Urol. 2003;10:68–71.
7. Borboroglu PG, Comer SW, Riffenburgh RH, et al. Extensive repeat transrectal ultrasound guided prostate biopsy in patients with previous benign sextant biopsies. J Urol. 2000;163:158–62.
8. Pal RP, Elmussareh M, Chanawani M, et al. The role of a standardized 36 core template-assisted transperineal prostate biopsy technique in patients

with previously negative transrectal ultrasonography-guided prostate biopsies. BJU Int. 2011;109:367–71.

9. Ekwueme K, Simpson H, Zakhour H, et al. Transperineal template-guided saturation biopsy using a modified technique: outcome of 270 cases requiring repeat prostate biopsy. BJU Int. 2013;111:E365–73.

10. Merrick GS, Gutman S, Andreini H, et al. Prostate cancer distribution in patients diagnosed by transperineal template-guided saturation biopsy. Eur Urol. 2007;52:715–24.

11. Stewart CS, Leibovich BC, Weaver AL, et al. Prostate cancer diagnosis using a saturation needle biopsy technique after previous negative sextant biopsies. J Urol. 2001;166:86–91.

12. Scattoni V, Zlotta A, Montorni R, et al. Extended and saturation prostatic biopsy in the diagnosis and characterization of prostate cancer: a critical analysis of the literature. Eur Urol. 2007;52:1309–22.

13. Abdollah F, Novara G, Briganti A, et al. Trans-rectal versus trans-perineal saturation rebiopsy of the prostate: is there a difference in cancer detection rate? Urology. 2011;77(4):921–5.

14. Zaytoun OM, Stephenson AJ, Fareed K, et al. When serial prostate biopsy is recommended: most cancers detected are clinically insignificant. BJU Int. 2012;110:987–92.

15. Mabjeesh NJ, Lidawi G, Chen J, et al. High detection rate of significant prostate tumors in anterior zones using transperineal ultrasound-guided template saturation biopsy. BJU Int. 2012;110:993–7.

16. Buskirk SJ, Pinkstadd DM, Petrou SP, et al. Acute urinary retention after transperineal template-guided prostate biopsy. Int J Radiat Oncol Biol Phys. 2004;59:1360–6.

17. Merrick GS, Taubenslag W, Andreini H, et al. The morbidity of transperineal template-guided prostate mapping biopsy. BJU Int. 2008;101:1524–9.

18. Pinkstaff DM, Igel TC, Petrou SP, et al. Systematic transperineal ultrasound-guided template biopsy of the prostate: three-year experience. Urology. 2005;65:735–9.

19. Moran BJ, Braccioforte MH, Conterato DJ. Re-biopsy of the prostate using a stereotactic transperineal technique. J Urol. 2006;176:1376–81.

20. McNeal JE. Origin and development of carcinoma in the prostate. Cancer. 1969;23:24–34.

21. Chen ME, Johnston DA, Tang K, et al. Detailed mapping of prostate carcinoma foci: biopsy strategy implications. Cancer. 2000;89:1800–9.

22. Terris MK. Determination of prostate volume by transrectal ultrasound. J Urol. 1991;145:984–7.

23. Epstein JI, Sanderson H, Carter HB. Utility of saturation biopsy to predict insignificant cancer at radical prostatectomy. Urology. 2005;66:356–60.

24. Bittner N, Merrick GS, Butler WM, et al. Incidence and pathological features of prostate cancer detected on transperineal template guided mapping biopsy after negative transrectal ultrasound biopsy. J Urol. 2013;190:509–14.

25. Demura T, Hioka T, Furuno T. Differences in tumor core distribution between palpable and nonpalpable prostate tumors in patients diagnosed using extensive transperineal ultrasound-guided template prostate biopsy. Cancer. 2005;103:1826–32.

26. Furuno T, Demura T, Kaneta T. Difference of cancer core distribution between first and repeat biopsy: In patients diagnosed by extensive transperineal ultrasound guided template prostate biopsy. Prostate. 2004;58:76–81.

27. Bott SR, Henderson A, Halls JE. Extensive transperineal template biopsies of prostate: modified technique and results. Urology. 2006;68:1037–41.

28. Symons JL, Huo A, Yuen CL, et al. Outcomes of transperineal template-guided prostate biopsy in 409 patients. BJU Int. 2013;112:585–93.

29. Castello-Porcar A, García-Morata F, Martinez-Jabaloyas JM. Prostate cancer detection rate at second and third biopsy. Predictive factors and risk groups for cancer diagnosis. Arch Esp Urol. 2014;67:605–14.

30. Masumoir N, Tsukamoto T, Kumamoto Y, et al. Japanese men have smaller prostate volumes but comparable urinary flow rates relative to American men: results of community based studies in 2 countries. J Urol. 1996;155:1324–7.

18

Evaluation of a rapid quantitative determination method of PSA concentration with gold immunochromatographic strips

Cheng-Ching Wu[1,6], Hung-Yu Lin[2], Chao-Ping Wang[6,7], Li-Fen Lu[3], Teng-Hung Yu[6], Wei-Chin Hung[6], Jer-Yiing Houng[4], Fu-Mei Chung[6], Yau-Jiunn Lee[5] and Jin-Jia Hu[1*]

Abstract

Background: Prostate cancer remains the most common cancer in men. Qualitative or semi-quantitative immunochromatographic measurements of prostate specific antigen (PSA) have been shown to be simple, noninvasive and feasible. The aim of this study was to evaluate an optimized gold immunochromatographic strip device for the detection of PSA, in which the results can be analysed using a Chromogenic Rapid Test Reader to quantitatively assess the test results.

Methods: This reader measures the reflectance of the signal line via a charge-coupled device camera. For quantitative analysis, PSA concentration was computed via a calibration equation. Capillary blood samples from 305 men were evaluated, and two independent observers interpreted the test results after 12 min. Blood samples were also collected and tested with a conventional quantitative assay.

Results: Sensitivity, specificity, positive and negative predictive values, and accuracy of the PSA rapid quantitative test system were 100, 96.6, 89.5, 100, and 97.4 %, respectively. Reproducibility of the test was 99.2, and interobserver variation was 8 % with a false positive rate of 3.4 %. The correlation coefficient between the ordinary quantitative assay and the rapid quantitative test was 0.960.

Conclusions: The PSA rapid quantitative test system provided results quickly and was easy to use, so that tests using this system can be easily performed at outpatient clinics or elsewhere. This system may also be useful for initial cancer screening and for point-of-care testing, because results can be obtained within 12 min and at a cost lower than that of conventional quantitative assays.

Keywords: Prostate specific antigen, Prostate cancer, Chromogenic rapid test reader, Gold immunochromatographic strip

Background

Measuring prostate specific antigen (PSA) levels is widely used to identify men with an increased risk of prostate cancer. The serum- or plasma-based immunoassays currently available are associated with time consuming sample processing and the need for sophisticated technical equipment. Therefore, various strip tests for the qualitative and semi-quantitative determination of PSA based on immunochromatographic measurements of serum [1–7] or whole blood [8] have been developed.

Visual assessment of the currently available whole blood assays allows for a yes or no decision without definite information regarding the concentration of PSA in the blood. Although this kind of qualitative assay is sufficient for clinical decision making, prognostic information inherent to the concentration of circulating PSA is lost. Furthermore, inter-individual variability of visual

* Correspondence: maxvic24@gmail.com
[1]Institute of Biomedical Engineering, National Cheng Kung University, Tainan 70101, Taiwan
Full list of author information is available at the end of the article

assessment of the test strip at the detection limit of the assay may cause lead to substantial analytical errors [9].

In this study, we evaluated an improved assay for PSA and a newly developed reader to overcome the limitations of previous tests and to enable reliable quantitative and rapid testing for PSA. This tool may be useful for initial cancer screening and may be applied in point-of-care testing.

Methods

Patients and serum samples

From June 2014 to May 2015, 305 male patients (mean age 67 years, range 40–98 years), with or without prostate disease were analysed. All of the men were evaluated at E-Da Hospital in Taiwan.

Control method

For comparative purposes, a blood sample from each patient was collected immediately before the test for use in the standard laboratory method, a chemiluminescent microparticle immunoassay (CMIA), to determine the concentration of PSA. The blood samples were allowed to clot for 1 h at room temperature before being centrifuged. The sera were then immediately analysed using an ABBOTT ARCHITECT *i* System analyzer PSA assay according to the manufacturer's instructions. The study protocol was approved by the Human Research Ethics Committee of the E-Da hospital, and written informed consent was obtained from each participant before enrolment.

Principles of the PSA rapid quantitative test system

The PSA rapid quantitative test system includes a special cassette (C.J. Biotec Corp. Pingtung, Taiwan) and a Chromogenic Test Reader (KAIWOOD Technology Co. Ltd., Tainan, Taiwan). The special cassette consists of two different regions: the sample well and the test area. The PSA test strip included the sample pad, conjugated pad, nitrocellulose membrane, absorption pad, and a backing card. The anti-PSA antibody and goat anti-mouse immunoglobulin G antibody defined as the test line and control line were immobilized on the nitrocellulose membrane. The anti-PSA antibody-colloidal gold conjugates were immobilized on the conjugated pad, which was defined as the mixture area. After the sample solution including the PSA antigen in the serum was dropped into the sample pad, the PSA antigen first bonded with the anti-PSA antibody-colloidal gold conjugates and then bonded with the anti-PSA antibody. When the PSA concentration was increased, larger volumes of the colloid gold were aggregated in the test line and this deepens the color of the test line. In addition, excess labeled antibody conjugate will be captured at control line and a second red colored line was also observed of the

membrane, indicating the proper test performance. The colored band must be visualized on the control line, so the test could be considered as invalid if there is no color line present in the control region.

The Chromogenic Test Reader mainly consists of an Advanced RISC Machine (ARM) processors, a complementary metal-oxide semiconductor (CMOS) sensor carrier, a set of LED lights, and a test strip carrier. The control and test lines of the PSA strip are captured by the Chromogenic Test Reader (Fig. 1). The test and control lines in the detection zone are recognized by an evaluation algorithm. The intensity of the test line, determined by measuring its reflectance, is directly proportional to the concentration of PSA. The top image in Fig. 2 shows the gold immunochromatographic assay (GICA) strip with PSA concentrations of 20 ng/mL and 60 ng/mL. The bottom image shows the corresponding curve of the GICA strip signal corresponding. The left peak of the strip is the test line, and the other is the control lines. The figure shows that the higher the PSA concentration the higher the peak of the test line. The acquired digital signal after pre-filtering was then processed by the ARM processors. In order to quantitatively analyse the GICA strip, the curve of the strip signal was first segment using the fuzzy C-means algorithm [10, 11] to obtain the location of the test line and control line. In addition, to establish a standard calibration curve for the Chromogenic Test Reader, we used serum samples with various PSA concentrations (60, 30, 20, 15, 10, 7.5, 3.25, 1 ng/mL) were injected into the PSA test strip. The serum samples were prepared by the high PSA concentration (60 ng/mL) of the antigen. The color intensity of test line analyzed by Chromogenic Test Reader was converted via the standard calibration curve and interpolation method into a PSA concentration.

Test procedure

The PSA test cassette is provided with droppers and a buffer solution. The patient's fingertip should be swabbed with alcohol and then allowed to dry for 30 s. The fingertip is then pricked with a sterile lancet to obtain one drop of blood, and the droppers are used to draw the blood sample and then transfer it to the sample well on the PSA cassette. After 2 min, two drops of a buffer solution are added to the sample well to allow the blood to migrate. If visible migration across the test area does not start, an additional drop of buffer solution can be added to the sample well. When PSA concentration levels are ≥ 4 ng/mL, a burgundy-coloured band should develop on the test line. For quantitative analysis and to reduce errors, the Chromogenic Test Reader is used to measure the colour signals of the test line, as shown in Fig. 1. Interpretation of the test must be done after 10 min.

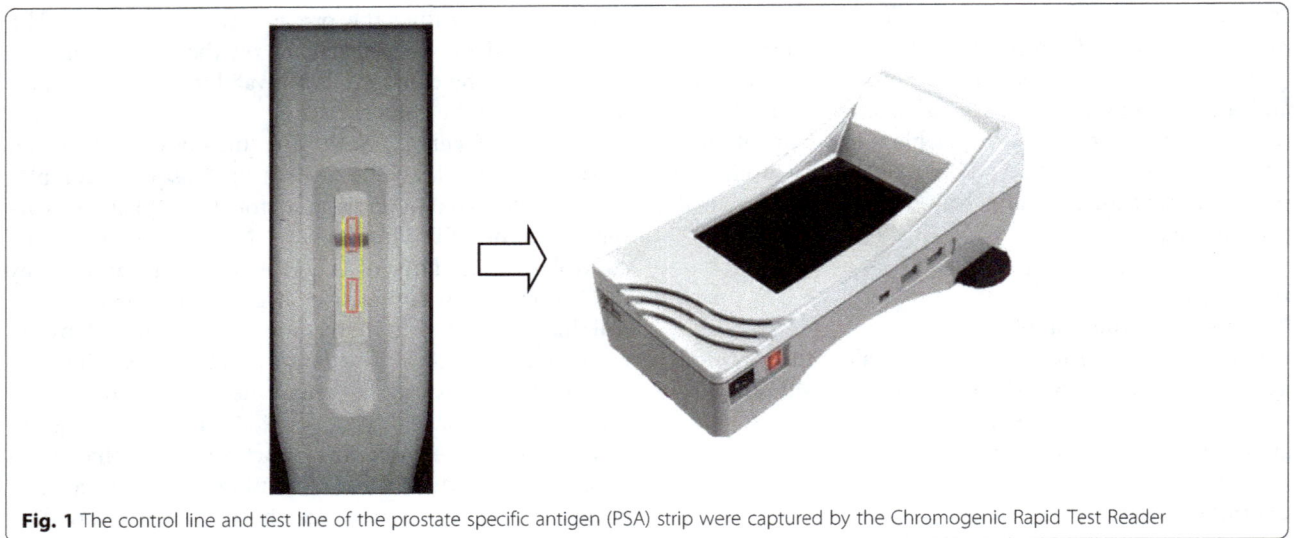

Fig. 1 The control line and test line of the prostate specific antigen (PSA) strip were captured by the Chromogenic Rapid Test Reader

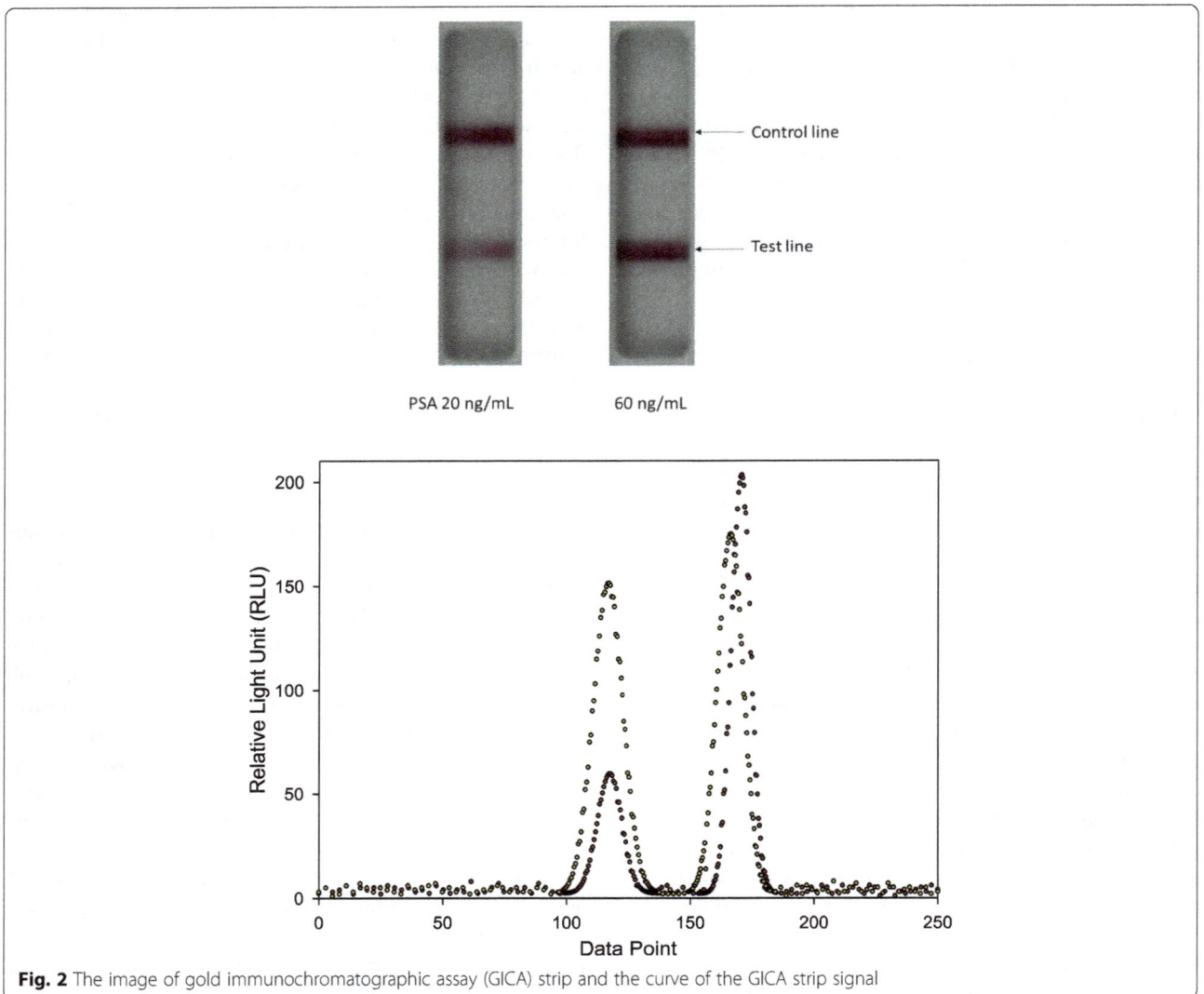

Fig. 2 The image of gold immunochromatographic assay (GICA) strip and the curve of the GICA strip signal

Evaluation of a rapid quantitative determination method of PSA concentration with gold...

139

Evaluation procedure

Two urologists who were unaware of the measured PSA values interpreted the tests independently from one another to avoid bias. The observers were also unaware that the two different tests were being performed on the same patients to avoid bias. Positive and negative results of each test were classified as true positive or negative and false negative or positive by comparing them with the quantitative PSA results as measured by the AB-BOTT ARCHITECT *i* System analyzer PSA assay, using the threshold value of 4 ng/ml.

Statistical analysis

All statistical analyses were performed using the Statistical Package for Social Science (SPSS for Windows, version 10.0; SPSS Inc., Chicago, Ill). Sensitivity, specificity, accuracy, positive and negative predictive values of the quantitative PSA test was calculated. Sensitivity was defined as the ratio between the true positive results and the sum of the true positive and false negative results. Specificity was defined as the ratio between the true negative results and the sum of the true negative and false positive results. The positive predictive value was defined as the ratio between the true positive results and the sum of all positive results, and the negative predictive value was defined as the ratio between the true negative results and the sum of all negative results. Accuracy was defined as the ratio between the sum of the true observations (positive and negative) and the total observations. Relationships between GICA method and CMIA method were examined using Pearson's correlation analyses.

Results

The patients were divided into two groups on the basis of the conventional quantitative PSA value. Of the 305 patients, 229 (75.1 %) had a PSA value of < 4 ng/mL (median 0.79 ng/mL; range 0.05-3.98 ng/mL) and 76 (25 %) had a PSA value of > 4 ng/mL (median 7.59 ng/mL; range 4.01-169.10 ng/mL). When the patients were divided into two groups on the basis of the rapid quantitative PSA value, of the 305 patients, 221 (72.5) had a PSA value of < 4 ng/mL (median 1.03 ng/mL; range 0.40-4.07 ng/mL) and 84 (27.5 %) had a PSA value of > 4 ng/mL (median 6.33 ng/mL; range 4.10-112.11 ng/mL).

The within-run imprecision experiments ($n = 9$) with the PSA rapid assay yielded CVs between 4.4 and 13.1 % for PSA concentrations between 1.12 and 12.39 ng/mL. The CV for day-to-day imprecision, performed as 9 repetitive measurements on 9 subsequent days, was between 6.6 and 7.3 % (Table 1).

The positive and negative results obtained by the two methods are shown in Table 2. In the table, (tp) indicates that both methods classified the test sample as positive;

Table 1 Analytical performance of the PSA test strip reader

	PSA concentration ng/mL	CV (%)	Sample material
Within-run imprecision ($n = 9$)	1.12	4.4	Blood
	1.20	8.6	Blood
	4.32	4.5	Blood
	4.16	4.4	Blood
	12.39	13.1	Blood
	3	8.3	Control
	5	8.9	Control
Day-to-day imprecision ($n = 9$)	3	6.6	Control
	5	7.3	Control

(tn) indicates that both methods classified the test sample as negative; (fn) indicates that the CMIA method classified the test sample as positive but the GICA method classified the test sample as negative; and (fp) indicates that the CMIA method classified the test sample as negative but the GICA method classified the test sample as positive. Sensitivity, specificity, positive and negative predictive values, and accuracy of the PSA rapid quantitative test system were 100 %, 96.6 %, 89.5 %, 100 %, and 97.4 %, respectively. The GICA method had a false positive rate of 3.4 and a false negative rate of 0 % compared to the CMIA method. There was a high level of reproducibility of the GICA test (99.2 %), with an overall concordance rate between the observers of 98 %. The correlation coefficient between the two methods was 0.960 (Fig. 3). In addition, the results of the PSA rapid quantitative test are comparable with those of other PSA one-step tests described in the literature, using serum or capillary blood (Table 3).

Discussion

In this study, we introduce a rapid quantitative determination method to measure the concentration of PSA using a GICA strip based on the Chromogenic Rapid Test Reader. Comparing the GICA method and the CMIA method revealed a strong correlation coefficient

Table 2 Positive and negative results obtained by the two methods

Results of the GICA method	Results of the CMIA method (gold standard)		
	Positive	Negative	Total
Positive	68 (tp)	8 (fp)	76
Negative	0 (fn)	229 (tn)	229
Total	68	237	305

GICA gold immunochromatographic assay, *CMIA* chemiluminescent microparticle immunoassay

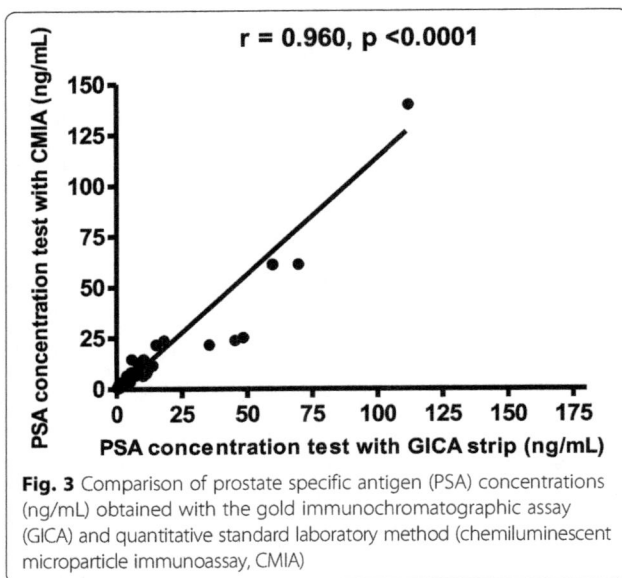

Fig. 3 Comparison of prostate specific antigen (PSA) concentrations (ng/mL) obtained with the gold immunochromatographic assay (GICA) and quantitative standard laboratory method (chemiluminescent microparticle immunoassay, CMIA)

Previously, the widespread use of PSA testing has been reported to be one of the factors that have led to a significant increase in the diagnosis of organ-confined tumours and a decline in prostate cancer mortality rates [16–19]. Furthermore, evaluation of serum PSA level at 45 years of salvage radiotherapy for biochemical relapses after prostatectomy may serve as a significant prognosticator for both biochemical and clinical disease-free outcomes [20]. McLeod DG suggested that PSA testing remains the most efficacious marker available, both to evaluate therapy and to use as a screening tool [21]. In the present study, we introduce an optical inspection system to measure PSA concentrations and a new detection model covering from qualitative to quantitative analysis. Of note, this system is very easy to use and it only needs an initial and brief training to interpret the test results correctly. In addition, it would be useful in the setting of both general practitioner and office urologist. Furthermore, it uses whole blood from a finger prick (30 µl) which is more patient-friendly than traditional venepuncture. In addition, other rapid PSA tests have been reported to require serum samples or capillary whole blood (approximately 80 µl) [1, 6, 22]. Using finger prick whole blood rather than a serum sample saves time (a standard laboratory process to obtain serum needs 1 h to allow for blood clotting after collection, and 10–15 min to separate serum from blood by centrifugation) and produces the final screening results in about 12 min. Another benefit of the PSA rapid quantitative test system is that the cost is significantly lower compared to a conventional quantitative serum PSA test in Taiwan, (about New Taiwan (NT) $300 vs. NT$400). Considering the number of people that could be

of 0.960 between these two methods. The results suggest that the GICA method may be applicable to quantitatively determine PSA concentrations.

The incidence rate of prostate cancer has increased remarkably. Since radical therapeutic methods are still limited, the early detection and treatment of prostate cancer is essential. Although screening for prostate cancer is still one of the most controversial issue in oncology, it is well recognized that a combination of a digital rectal examination or ultrasonography and a PSA test is the most useful and effective method to diagnose prostatic carcinoma [12–15].

Table 3 Performance of various PSA one-step tests reported in the literature

Author	PSA test	Sample	Time	Sensitivity	Specificity
Dok An et al [1]	One Step PSA™	Serum	15 min	100	90
Jung et al [3]	Chembio	Serum	10 min	67	87
Jung et al. [3]	Medpro	Serum	10 min	87	88
Jung et al. [3]	Syntron	Serum	10 min	93	93
Jung et al. [3]	Seratec	Serum	10 min	80	97
Lein et al. [4]	Tandem-E	Serum	12 min	63	92
Lein et al. [4]	IMx	Serum	12 min	68	95
Lein et al. [4]	LIA-mat	Serum	12 min	83	87
Madersbacher et al. [6]	Oncoscreen®	Serum	10 min	93	93
Berg et al. [8]	One-Step PSA	Serum	10 min	90.5	83.8
Fernández-Sánchez et al. [24]	CanAg	Serum	20 min	87	79
Fernández-Sánchez et al. [24]	Immulite	Serum	20 min	77	83
Berg et al. [8]	Urale®	Capillary whole blood	12 min	91	81
Miano et al. [23]	One-Step PSA	Capillary whole blood	20 min	97.6	90.4
Wu et al.	Quantitative	Capillary whole blood	12 min	100	96.6

involved in a screening programme for prostate cancer, the savings could be. Given the intended use of this test (initial prostate cancer screening programme), sensitivity is more important than specificity. The PSA rapid quantitative test system had a very high sensitivity (100 %), even near the cut-off value of PSA of 4 ng/ml. While the overall specificity was 96.6 %, the false-positive rate was 3.4 % with a PSA concentration in the range of 3–4 ng/ml. The accuracy was also very high (97.4 %). The results of the PSA rapid quantitative test are comparable with those of other PSA one-step tests described in the literature [1, 3, 4, 6, 8, 23,24], using serum or capillary blood (Table 3). Another advantage of the PSA rapid quantitative test is that the reader can be linked and send results directly to a hospital's or healthcare centre's data management system. As a result, it is now possible to measure highly specific and sensitive results of PSA concentration within 12 min without the need for a sophisticated clinical chemistry environment.

A previous study suggested that a semi-quantitative immunochromatographic test was difficult to perform and that interpretation was difficult. Furthermore, the rate of false strip test results was disappointing even for PSA values far from the cut-off value [25]. Various reasons, apart from the possible technical inferiority of the investigated product, may explain this finding. First, the colour stability of the test is particularly affected by variations in the reading time [3]. Second, the testing of whole blood instead of serum may be associated with less advantageous immunochromatographic properties. Third, well-known differences in the PSA methods [5, 26, 27] used for comparisons may influence the results such as: (1) Antibodies; affinity and specificity for various epitopes of PSA forms [28–30] or cross-reactivity to PSA homologous antigens [31]. (2) Calibration of the assay method. (3) Procedure of the assay; incubation time, equilibrium or kinetics [28, 32], adjuvants (e.g. stabilizing standard preparations, particularly albumin), "high-dose hook" effect. (4) Lot-to-Lot variations in assays [33]. (5) Interference; auto-anti-PSA- antibodies. Fourth, handling and interpretation of the strip tests was mostly performed by trained investigators in other studies. Ultimately, the performance of the test is highly dependent on the study population, particularly with regards to the distribution of PSA values and the prevalence and extent of PSA concentrations exceeding the cut-off value [25]. In the present study, the PSA rapid quantitative test had a higher sensitivity and specificity compared with previous studies [1, 3, 4, 6, 8, 22–24], which may be because the results were interpreted using technical signal detectors and a user with experience in handling and interpreting such detectors, which may overcome the problem that strip test are frequently difficult to read, since the colour reaction in the test field can be weak.

The main limitation of this test is that eight samples with values of less than 4 ng/mL showed false positive results in the range 3–4 ng/ml where the possibility of prostate cancer detection is still about 25 % [34]. The most important and most concerning cause of an elevated PSA is prostate cancer. However, prostate cancer is only one of many potential causes of an elevated PSA. Virtually anything that irritates the prostate will cause the PSA to rise, at least temporarily. The most common cause of PSA elevation includes benign prostatic hyperplasia (enlargement of the prostate, secondary to a noncancerous proliferation of prostate gland cells) and prostatitis (inflammation of the prostate). In fact, PSA elevation can also occur with prostate manipulation such as ejaculation, prostate examination, urinary retention or catheter placement, and prostate biopsy. Hence, elevated the specificity for this PSA rapid quantitative test system, ranging between 2 and 4 ng/mL, is need. Moreover, previous study indicated that the use of free/total PSA ratio in patients with PSA levels of 4–10 ng/mL should enhance the specificity of PSA screening and decrease the number of unnecessary biopsies [35]. However, a free/total ratio is not available with this method. We will test more samples in the near future to further examine the suitability of such kits for mass screening.

Conclusions

The results of this study showed that this PSA rapid quantitative test with a GICA strip based on a Chromogenic Rapid Test Reader yielded good results and was appropriate for the quantitative determination of PSA concentration. We do not believe that a PSA rapid quantitative test and clinical chemistry tests are mutually exclusive methods. Clearly laboratory-based methods have a better analytical performance [36]. Thus, if time is not critical and the appropriate equipment is available, laboratory-based methods may still be preferable. However, for many clinical situations and for many point-of-care measurements, PSA rapid quantitative testing may be the preferred method, particularly when the results can be sent directly to a hospital data management system as is possible with the PSA Chromogenic Reader.

Abbreviations
PSA: Prostate specific antigen; CMIA: Chemiluminescent microparticle immunoassay; ARM: Advanced RISC machine; GICA: Gold immunochromatographic assay.

Competing interests
The authors declare that they have no competing interests.

Authors' contributions
Conceived and designed the experiments: Wu CC, Wang CP, Lin HY, Lee YJ, and Hu JJ. Performed the experiments: Lu LF, Yu TH, Houng JY, and Hung WC. Analyzed the data: Chung FM and Houng JY. Contributed reagents/materials/analysis tools: Wu CC, Lin HY, and Hu JJ. Wrote the paper: Wu CC,

Chung FM, Lee YJ, and Hu JJ. All authors have read and approved the final version of the manuscript.

Acknowledgements

The authors would like to thank E-Da Hospital and National Cheng-Kung University Hospital of the Republic of China, Taiwan, for financially supporting this research under Contract NCKUEDA 10413 and EDAHP104058.

Author details

[1]Institute of Biomedical Engineering, National Cheng Kung University, Tainan 70101, Taiwan. [2]Department of Urology, E-Da Hospital, I-Shou University, Kaohsiung 82445, Taiwan. [3]Division of Cardiac Surgery, Department of Surgery, E-Da Hospital, I-Shou University, Kaohsiung 82445, Taiwan. [4]Department of Medical Nutrition, Institute of Biotechnology and Chemical Engineering and I-Shou University, Kaohsiung 82445, Taiwan. [5]Lee's Endocrinology Clinic, Pingtung 90000, Taiwan. [6]Division of Cardiology, Department of Internal Medicine, E-Da Hospital, I-Shou University, Kaohsiung 82445, Taiwan. [7]School of Medicine for International Students, I-Shou University, Kaohsiung 82445, Taiwan.

References

1. Dok An C, Yoshiki T, Lee G, Okada Y. Evaluation of a rapid qualitative prostate specific antigen assay, the One Step PSA(TM) test. Cancer Lett. 2001;162(2):135–9.
2. Hochmeister MN, Budowle B, Rudin O, Gehrig C, Borer U, Thali M, et al. Evaluation of prostate-specific antigen (PSA) membrane test assays for the forensic identification of seminal fluid. J Forensic Sci. 1999;44(5):1057–60.
3. Jung K, Zachow J, Lein M, Brux B, Sinha P, Lenk S, et al. Rapid detection of elevated prostate-specific antigen levels in blood: performance of various membrane strip tests compared. Urology. 1999;53(1):155–60.
4. Lein M, Jung K, Schnorr D, Henke W, Brux B, Loening SA. Rapid screening of PSA: evaluation of an immunochemical membrane strip test. Clin Chem. 1995;41(10):1545–7.
5. Lein M, Jung K, Schnorr D, Henke W, Loening SA. Strip test for the quick detection of increased concentrations of prostate-specific antigen in blood. Eur J Clin Chem Clin Biochem. 1996;34(6):511–4.
6. Madersbacher S, Mian C, Maier U, Simak R. Validation of a 10-min dipstick test for serum prostate-specific antigen. Eur Urol. 1996;30(4):446–50.
7. Graves HC. Issues on standardization of immunoassays for prostate- specific antigen: a review. Clin Invest Med. 1993;16(6):415–24.
8. Berg W, Linder C, Eschholz G, Link S, Schubert J. Possibility of improving the acceptance rate of early detection testing for prostate cancer with a one-step test for prostate-specific antigen in whole blood. Urol Int. 1999;63(2):102–6.
9. Müller-Bardorff M, Freitag H, Scheffold T, Remppis A, Kübler W, Katus HA. Development and characterization of a rapid assay for bedside determinations of cardiac troponin T. Circulation. 1995;92(10):2869–75.
10. Jiang H, Min D, Ke D. A Rapid Quantitative Determination Method of AFP Concentration with Gold Immunochromatographic Strip. Journal of Computers. 2012;7(12):2868–75.
11. Li Y, Zeng N, Min D. A novel image methodology for interpretation of gold immunochromatographic strip. Journal of Computers. 2011;6(3):540–7.
12. Catalona WJ, Richie JP, Ahmann FR, Hudson MA, Scardino PT, Flanigan RC, et al. Comparison of digital rectal examination and serum prostate specific antigen in the early detection of prostate cancer: results of a multicenter clinical trial of 6,630 men. J Urol. 1994;151(5):1283–90.
13. Littrup PJ, Kane RA, Mettlin CJ, Murphy GP, Lee F, Toi A, et al. Cost-effective prostate cancer detection. Reduction of low-yield biopsies. Investigators of the american cancer society national prostate cancer detection project. Cancer. 1994;74(12):3146–58.
14. Potter SR, Horniger W, Tinzl M, Bartsch G, Partin AW. Age, prostate- specific antigen, and digital rectal examination as determinants of the probability of having prostate cancer. Urology. 2001;57(6):1100–4.
15. Richie JP, Catalona WJ, Ahmann FR, Hudson MA, Scardino PT, Flanigan RC, et al. Effect of patient age on early detection of prostate cancer with serum prostate-specific antigen and digital rectal examination. Urology. 1993;42(4):365–74.

16. Merrill RM, Stephenson RA. Trends in mortality rates inpatients with prostate cancer during the era of prostate specific antigen screening. J Urol. 2000;163(2):503–10.
17. Bartsch G, Horninger W, Klocker H, Reissigl A, Oberaigner W, Schönitzer D, et al. Prostate cancer mortality after the introduction of prostate-specific antigen mass screening in the Federal State of Tyrol, Austria. Urology. 2001;58(3):417–24.
18. Meyer F, Moore L, Bairati I, Fradet Y. Downward trend in prostate cancer mortality in Quebec and Canada. J Urol. 1999;161(4):1189–91.
19. Tarone RE, Chu KC, Brawley OW. Implications of stage-specific survival rates in assessing recent declines in prostate cancer mortality rates. Epidemiology. 2000;11(2):167–70.
20. Do T, Dave G, Parker R, Kagan AR. Serum PSA evaluations during salvage radiotherapy for post-prostatectomy biochemical failures as prognosticators for treatment outcomes. Int J Radiat Oncol Biol Phys. 2001;50(5):1220–5.
21. McLeod DG. The effective management of biochemical recurrence in patients with prostate cancer. Rev Urol. 2005;7 Suppl 5:S29–36.
22. Berg W, Linder C, Eschholz G, Schubert J. Pilot study of the practical relevance of a one-step test for prostate-specific antigen in capillary blood to improve the acceptance rate in the early detection program of prostate carcinoma. Int Urol Nephrol. 2001;32(3):381–8.
23. Miano R, Mele GO, Germani S, Bove P, Sansalone S, Pugliese PF, et al. Evaluation of a new, rapid, qualitative, one-step PSA Test for prostate cancer screening: the PSA RapidScreen test. Prostate Cancer Prostatic Dis. 2005;8(3):219–23.
24. Fernández-Sánchez C, McNeil CJ, Rawson K, Nilsson O, Leung HY, Gnanapragasam V. One-step immunostrip test for the simultaneous detection of free and total prostate specific antigen in serum. J Immunol Methods. 2005;307(1–2):1–12.
25. Oberpenning F, Hetzel S, Weining C, Brandt B, De Angelis G, Heinecke A, et al. Semi-quantitative immunochromatographic test for prostate specific antigen in whole blood: tossing the coin to predict prostate cancer? Eur Urol. 2003;43(5):478–84.
26. Semjonow A, De Angelis G, Oberpenning F, Schmid HP, Brandt B, Hertle L. The clinical impact of different assays for prostate specific antigen. BJU Int. 2000;86(5):590–7.
27. Semjonow A, Brandt B, Oberpenning F, Roth S, Hertle L. Discordance of assay methods creates pitfalls for the interpretation of prostate-specific antigen values. Prostate Suppl. 1996;7:3–16.
28. Graves HCB. Standardization of immunoassays for prostate-specific antigen. A problem of prostate-specific antigen complexation or a problem of assay design? Cancer. 1993;72(11):3141–4.
29. Vessella RL, Lange PH. Issues in the assessment of PSA immunoassays. Urol Clin North Am. 1993;20(4):607–19.
30. Zhou AM, Tewari PC, Bluestein BI, Caldwell GW, Larsen FL. Multiple forms of prostate-specific antigen in serum: differences in immunorecognition by monoclonal and polyclonal assays. Clin Chem. 1993;39(12):2483–91.
31. Rittenhouse HG, Finlay JA, Mikolajczyk SD, Partin AW. Human Kallikrein 2 (hK2) and prostate-specific antigen (PSA): two closely related, but distinct, kallikreins in the prostate. Crit Rev Clin Lab Sci. 1998;35(4):275–368.
32. McCormack RT, Rittenhouse HG, Finlay JA, Sokoloff RL, Wang TJ, Wolfert RL, et al. Molecular forms of prostate-specific antigen and the human kallikrein gene family: a new era. Urology. 1995;45(5):729–44.
33. Wener MH, Daum PR, Close B, Brawer MK. Method-tomethod and lot-to-lot variation in assays for prostate-specific antigen. Am J Clin Pathol. 1994;101:387–8.
34. Roehl KA, Antenor JA, Catalona WJ. Robustness of free prostate specific antigen measurements to reduce unnecessary biopsies in the 2.6-4.0 ng/ml range. J Urol. 2002;168(3):922–5.
35. Erol B, Gulpinar MT, Bozdogan G, Ozkanli S, Onem K, Mungan G, et al. The cutoff level of free/total prostate specific antigen (f/t PSA) ratios in the diagnosis of prostate cancer: a validation study on a Turkish patient population in different age categories. Kaohsiung J Med Sci. 2014;30(11):545–50.
36. Vickers AJ, Cronin AM, Björk T, Manjer J, Nilsson PM, Dahlin A, et al. Prostate specific antigen concentration at age 60 and death or metastasis from prostate cancer: case–control study. BMJ. 2010;341:c4521.

19

Prognostic factors and risk stratification in patients with castration-resistant prostate cancer receiving docetaxel-based chemotherapy

Shimpei Yamashita*, Yasuo Kohjimoto, Takashi Iguchi, Hiroyuki Koike, Hiroki Kusumoto, Akinori Iba, Kazuro Kikkawa, Yoshiki Kodama, Nagahide Matsumura and Isao Hara

Abstract

Background: While novel drugs have been developed, docetaxel remains one of the standard initial systemic therapies for castration-resistant prostate cancer (CRPC) patients. Despite the excellent anti-tumor effect of docetaxel, its severe adverse effects sometimes distress patients. Therefore, it would be very helpful to predict the efficacy of docetaxel before treatment. The aims of this study were to evaluate the potential value of patient characteristics in predicting overall survival (OS) and to develop a risk classification for CRPC patients treated with docetaxel-based chemotherapy.

Methods: This study included 79 patients with CRPC treated with docetaxel. The variables, including patient characteristics at diagnosis and at the start of chemotherapy, were retrospectively collected. Prognostic factors predicting OS were analyzed using the Cox proportional hazard model. Risk stratification for overall survival was determined based on the results of multivariate analysis.

Results: PSA response ≥50 % was observed in 55 (69.6 %) of all patients, and the median OS was 22.5 months. The multivariate analysis showed that age, serum PSA level at the start of chemotherapy, and Hb were independent prognostic factors for OS. In addition, ECOG performance status (PS) and the CRP-to-albumin ratio were not significant but were considered possible predictors for OS. Risk stratification according to the number of these risk factors could effectively stratify CRPC patients treated with docetaxel in terms of OS.

Conclusions: Age, serum PSA level at the start of chemotherapy, and Hb were identified as independent prognostic factors of OS. ECOG PS and the CRP-to-albumin ratio were not significant, but were considered possible predictors for OS in Japanese CRPC patients treated with docetaxel. Risk stratification based on these factors could be helpful for estimating overall survival.

Keywords: Castration-resistant prostate cancer, Docetaxel, Prognostic factor

Background

Prostate cancer is currently the most common malignancy in men from Western countries, and its occurrence has recently been increasing in Japan.

Because most prostate cancers grow in an androgen-dependent manner, androgen-deprivation therapy has been the initial treatment for recurrent or metastatic

* Correspondence: keito608@wakayama-med.ac.jp
Department of Urology, Wakayama Medical University, 811-1 Kimiidera, Wakayama 641-0012, Japan

prostate cancer [1, 2]. However, under prolonged androgen deprivation, prostate cancer finally becomes refractory to hormonal manipulation and is then defined as castration-resistant prostate cancer (CRPC) [3, 4].

Recently, possible therapeutic strategies for CRPC have been increasing [5–8]. Novel therapies including enzalutamide, abiraterone acetate, cabazitaxel, sipuleucel-T, and radium 223 have been approved for therapy of CRPC patients. Enzalutamide and abiraterone acetate have shown their efficacy in not only the post-docetaxel setting but also the pre-docetaxel setting [9, 10]. In patients with no visceral metastasis, enzalutamide and abiraterone are recommended as well as docetaxel in the NCCN guideline. Moreover, in patients with visceral metastasis, these novel agents have been approved by FDA in the pre-chemotherapy setting. However, it was in 2014 that these agents were approved in Japan. In addition, the efficacy of novel therapies is still limited, and the prognoses of CRPC patients still remain poor.

To date, docetaxel, a natural taxane from *Taxus baccata*, has been established as effective and has been widely used in CRPC treatment [11, 12]. While novel drugs have been developed, docetaxel remains one of the standard initial systemic therapies for CRPC patients. In the EAU guideline 2014, docetaxel is still recommended as the first-line chemotherapeutic agent, especially in patients with evidence of progressive disease. Docetaxel is also recommended as the first-line drug in the NCCN guideline 2015. Despite of the excellent antitumor effect of docetaxel, its severe adverse effects, including myelosuppression, sometimes distress patients. Therefore, it would be helpful to predict the efficacy of docetaxel before treatment. Since novel agents such as enzalutamide and abiraterone acetate are now available, appropriate selection of CRPC patients using prognostic factors is crucial when choosing first-line therapy.

A predictive factor is a measurement that is associated with response or lack of response to a particular therapy. In contrast, a prognostic factor is a measurement that is associated with patient's prognoses with or without treatment. Several prognostic factors in CRPC patients have been reported, and some nomograms or risk classifications have been developed. However, the magnitude of the benefit provided by each factor has varied among studies.

We previously reported that visceral metastases, including lung, liver and lymph nodes and excluding bone, and pretreatment anemia (hemoglobin < 11.3 g/dL) were two independent factors predicting overall survival in patients who received docetaxel chemotherapy for prostate cancer [13]. In a previous study, we collected the data from not only our hospital but also our related hospitals. Thus, the cohort in that study was rather heterogeneous regarding the indications, chemotherapy regimens, and amount of missing data. In the present study, patients only from our institute were targeted, and more variables, such as the neutrophil-to-lymphocyte ratio (NLR) and the C-reactive protein (CRP)-to-albumin ratio, were evaluated as predictors of overall survival.

The aims of this study were to evaluate the potential value of patient characteristics in predicting overall survival (OS) and to develop a risk classification for CRPC patients treated with docetaxel-based chemotherapy.

Methods
Patients and treatment
Patients with CRPC treated with docetaxel chemotherapy at the Wakayama Medical University Hospital (Wakayama, Japan) from June 2005 to May 2014 were included in this study. The eligibility criteria included histopathologically diagnosed adenocarcinoma of the prostate and confirmed failure of prior androgen deprivation therapy. If PSA increased after confirmation of the existence of anti-androgen withdrawal syndrome and alternative antiandrogen therapy, we judged that prior androgen deprivation therapy was a failure. No patient was administered abiraterone or enzalutamide or sipuleucel-T. In general, patients received 70 mg/m^2 of docetaxel intravenously every 3 or 4 weeks. The recommended dose of docetaxel in the NCCN guidelines is 75 mg/m^2, however the 70 mg/m^2 dose is commonly used in Japan. This is because severe myelosuppression is more likely to develop in Japanese than Europeans and Americans. If necessary, dose reduction and interval extension were allowed, based on the patient's overall condition. Prednisone 5 mg was routinely administered twice daily simultaneously with hormonal therapy for medical or surgical castration. Treatment with docetaxel was continued until disease progression, unacceptable adverse events, or the patient's refusal. Disease progression was defined as increases in the number of evaluable lesions observed or in size of existing lesions by RECIST 1.1 on imaging tests and/or biological progression characterized by an elevated serum PSA level of 25 % and an absolute increase of ≥2 ng/mL than the nadir. As a general rule, PSA increase required at least two times.

This study was approved by the institutional review board of Wakayama Medical University (approval number 1672). Written informed consent to participate in this study was not obtained from patients since this study was a retrospective observational study for ordinary medical practice. Instead, information about this clinical study was disclosed at the web page of our hospital and posted at visitor consultation rooms in our hospital. If patients refused the use of their clinical data, we should have excluded their data from our study. However, no patient refused to provide his data for our study.

Assessment
The variables, including patients' characteristics at diagnosis (serum PSA level, Gleason score, and metastatic sites) and characteristics at the start of chemotherapy (age, ECOG performance status (PS), significant clinical pain, precedent treatment, serum PSA level, duration from initiation of androgen deprivation therapy, complete blood count, biochemical profile, combined drugs) were collected retrospectively. The NLR was calculated from

the circulating neutrophil and lymphocyte counts. The CRP-to-albumin ratio was calculated from the CRP value and the albumin value using the formula: CRP value/albumin value) × 100.

The goal of the of the study was to determine the effect of patient characteristics on OS, calculated as the interval between the first day of docetaxel administration and the date of death or the last follow-up visit for censored (living) patients.

Statistical analysis

All statistical analyses were performed using SPSS software. OS was determined according to the Kaplan-Meier method. Univariate and multivariate analyses of OS were performed to compare the prognostic factors in a Cox proportional hazards analysis. Continuous data were divided into 2 groups according to their median values. $P < 0.05$ was considered significant.

Results

During the study period, 79 CRPC patients received docetaxel-based chemotherapy at our institution. The patients' characteristics at diagnosis and at the start of chemotherapy are shown in Table 1. The median age was 72 years (range: 52–86 years). ECOG PS was <1 in 52 (65.8 %) patients and ≥1 in 27 (34.2 %) patients. Most patients had one or more metastases when they were diagnosed with prostate cancer. Overall, 9 (11.4 %) and 17 (21.5 %) patients underwent radical prostatectomy and radiation therapy, respectively. The median androgen deprivation therapy administration period was 31.4 months (range: 2.8–152.6 months). The median serum PSA level at chemotherapy initiation was 43.2 ng/mL (range: 2.7–3133.7 ng/mL). 54 patients (68.4 %) simultaneously received estramustine. Oral estramustine (560 mg) was administered on days 1 to 5 and days 8 to 12. However, adverse events associated with estramustine, such as thromboembolic events, did not develop.

The median number of chemotherapy cycles was 6 (range: 1–43). 20 patients (25.3 %) required dose reduction due to treatment intolerance or side effects. A total of 71 patients (89.9 %) discontinued docetaxel treatment because of disease progression ($N = 39$, 54.9 %), adverse events ($N = 24$, 33.8 %), patient's refusal ($N = 3$, 4.2 %), and other reasons ($N = 5$, 7.0 %), respectively. The remaining 8 patients (10.1 %) were still undergoing docetaxel treatment during the course of the study. The median number of chemotherapy cycles in patients who discontinued treatment because of adverse events was 2.5 (range: 1–14).

Waterfall plots of the PSA response are shown in Fig. 1. PSA responses ≥0 %, ≥30 %, and ≥50 % were observed in 69 (87.3 %), 64 (81.0 %), and 55 (69.6 %) of the total patients, respectively.

Table 1 Patient characteristics

	$n = 79$
Median age (range), years	72 (52–86)
ECOG performance status, n (%)	
0	52 (65.8)
1	15 (19.0)
> = 2	12 (15.2)
Significant pain, n (%)	32 (40.5)
Median PSA at prostate cancer dianosis (range), ng/mL	125.2 (6.8–18778.0)
Gleason score, n (%)	
> =8	43 (54.4)
< =7	36 (45.6)
Metastatic site, n (%)	
bone	41 (51.9)
Lymph nodes	35 (44.3)
Lung	2 (2.5)
Liver	2 (2.5)
Prior treatment, n (%)	
Prostatectomy	9 (11.4)
Radiotherapy	17 (21.5)
Combined androgen blockade	79 (100)
Combination treatment, n (%)	
Bisphosphonate	23 (29.1)
Estramustine	54 (68.4)
Median PSA at docetaxel initiation (range), ng/mL	43.2 (2.7–3133.7)
Median androgen deprivation therapy administration period (range), months	31.4 (2.8–152.6)
Median serum markers at the start of docetaxel therapy (range)	
Hemoglobin, g/dL	11.9 (6.6–14.9)
NLR	2.9 (0.8–18.6)
Cre, mg/dL	0.8 (0.5–2.1)
ALP, IU/L	277 (1.9–4151.0)
LDH, IU/L	231 (123–594)
CRP-to-Albumin Ratio	7.3 (0.5–225.3)

Abbreviations: ECOG eastern cooperative oncology group, *PSA* prostate-specific antigen, *NLR* neutrophil-to-lymphocyte ratio, *Cre* creatinine, *ALP* alkaline phosphatase, *LDH* lactate dehydrogenase

During the observation period (median 15.1 months, range: 1.8–53.4 months), 36 of all 79 patients (53.2 %) died of prostate cancer, and 6 (7.6 %) died of another cause. The median OS was 22.5 months, and the 1-year OS rate was 78.8 %.

Univariate and multivariate Cox proportional hazards regression models were used to investigate pre-treatment predictors of OS (Table 2). Among several predictors, age ≥ 72 years, ECOG PS ≥ 1, serum PSA level at the start of chemotherapy ≥ 40 ng/mL, duration from initiation of

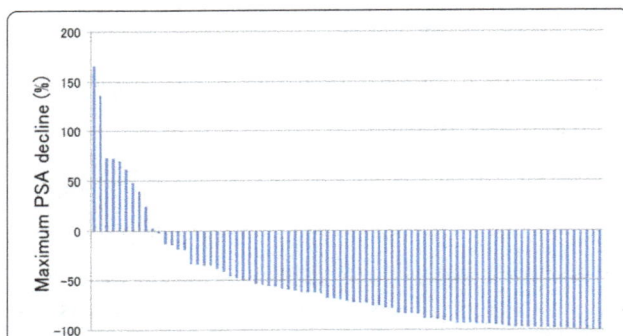

Fig. 1 Waterfall plot of PSA response. PSA responses of ≥0 %, ≥30 %, and ≥50 % are seen in 69 (87.3 %), 64 (81.0 %), and 55 (69.6 %) patients, respectively

androgen deprivation therapy ≥ 30 months, Hb ≥ 12.0 g/dL, ALP ≥ 300 IU/L, and LDH ≥ 230 IU/L were identified as significant predictors for OS on univariate analysis. Furthermore, significant clinical pain, NLR ≥ 3, CRP-to-albumin ratio ≥ 7, and combination use of

estramustine were not significant, but were considered possible predictors for OS. Of these factors, age ≥ 72 years and serum PSA level at the start of chemotherapy ≥ 40 ng/mL were independent unfavorable predictors of OS and Hb ≥ 12.0 g/dL was an independent favorable predictor of OS on multivariate analysis. ECOG PS ≥ 1 and CRP-to-albumin ratio ≥ 7 were not significant, but they were considered possible unfavorable predictors for OS.

To develop a risk classification model to help in the appropriate selection of docetaxel chemotherapy in patients with CRPC, five pre-treatment factors, including advanced age (age ≥ 72 years), poor PS (ECOG PS ≥ 1), high serum PSA level at the start of chemotherapy (PSA ≥ 40 ng/mL), anemia (Hb < 12 g/dL), and high CRP-to-albumin ratio (CRP-to albumin ratio ≥ 7) were used, and the cohort was classified into three groups according to the presence of these five risk factors. Patients with 0–1, 2–3, and 4–5 risk factors were classified as low ($N = 21$), intermediate ($N = 37$), and high ($N = 21$) risk groups, respectively. This model effectively stratified patients in

Table 2 Univariate and multivariate analyses of associations between various pre-treatment parameters and overall survival

Variable	Univariate analysis			Multivariate analysis		
	HR	95 % CI	P value	HR	95 % CI	P value
Age > = 72 years	2.38	1.23–4.60	0.01	4.07	1.68–9.90	<0.01
ECOG PS > =1	2.92	1.59–5.51	<0.01	2.18	1.00–4.77	0.05
Significant pain	1.72	0.94–3.15	0.08	1.37	0.63–2.96	0.43
PSA at prostate cancer diagnosis > = 125 ng/mL	1.06	0.58–1.95	0.85			
Gleason score > = 8	0.7	0.38–5.78	0.26			
Metastatic site						
Bone	1.49	0.80–2.77	0.21			
Lymph node	1.05	0.57–1.93	0.89			
Prior treatment						
Prostatectomy	0.81	0.32–2.07	0.66			
Radiotherapy	1.14	0.57–2.27	0.72			
Combination therapy						
Bisphosphonate	1.02	0.52–1.99	0.96			
Estramustine	2.52	0.99–6.47	0.05	1.35	0.49–3.68	0.56
PSA at docetaxel initiation	3.45	1.76–6.77	<0.01	2.36	1.02–5.45	<0.05
Androgen deprivation therapy administration period > = 30 months	0.46	0.25–0.85	0.01	0.76	0.37–1.54	0.44
Serum markers at the start of docetaxel therapy						
Hemoglobin > = 12 g/dL	0.24	0.12–0.48	<0.01	0.24	0.10–0.59	<0.01
NLR > = 3	1.71	0.93–3.15	0.09	1.33	0.62–2.85	0.46
Cre > = 0.8 mg/dL	0.68	0.37–1.26	0.22			
ALP > =300 IU/L	3.27	1.70–6.30	<0.01	0.87	0.34–2.22	0.76
LDH > =230 IU/L	1.88	1.02–3.49	<0.05	1.24	0.62–2.46	0.55
CRP-to-Albumin Ratio > =7	1.7	0.92–3.12	0.09	2.34	0.91–6.05	0.08

Abbreviations: ECOG Eastern Cooperative Oncology Group, *PSA* prostate-specific antigen, *NLR* Neutrophil-to-Lymphocyte Ratio, *Cre* creatinine, *ALP* alkaline phosphatase, *LDH* lactate dehydrogenase

terms of OS according to risk group ($p < 0.001$), as shown in Fig. 2.

Discussion

Two randomized trials demonstrated significant survival improvements in CRPC patients treated with docetaxel-based chemotherapy [11, 12], and it is widely used, including in Japan. Recently, several novel agents, including enzaltamide and abiraterone acetate, were shown to prolong overall survival in CRPC patients and have appeared on the market [5, 8]. However, docetaxel still remains a standard option, especially in CRPC patients with evidence of progressive disease. Accordingly, this provides clinicians with a wide choice between docetaxel and novel agents [14]. Therefore, it is crucial to identify prognostic factors and develop a risk stratification for CRPC patients treated with docetaxel.

Many prognostic models in patients with CRPC have been developed using pre and post chemotherapeutic factors. Although post chemotherapeutic factors, including PSA decline, tumor response, and pain response, are often used to evaluate patient's prognosis [15, 16], it might be more beneficial for CRPC patients to predict the response and outcome before the initiation of chemotherapy. Armstrong et al. reported that four independent risk factors, including visceral metastases, bone scan progression, significant pain, and anemia (hemoglobin level < 13 g/dL), predicted OS well, and they developed a risk stratification model for CRPC patients treated with docetaxel [16]. This Armstrong risk classification (ARC) is highly reliable because it was developed from 656 CRPC patients treated with docetaxel and was also internally validated in 333 CRPC patients who were administered mitoxantrone from among the 1006 CRPC patients in the TAX 327 study [11]. However, few reports have externally validated the ARC in CRPC patients who were treated with docetaxel. Nakano et al. reported that the ARC could predict the prognosis in docetaxel-treated CRPC patients [17]. On the other hand, Shiota et al. reported that the ARC failed to stratify the cohort satisfactorily [18]. They showed that ALP

value, visceral metastasis, and duration from initiation of hormone treatment were independent prognostic factors on multivariate analysis. Indeed, the reported prognostic factors for CRPC patients have differed widely among studies. The prognostic factors for CRPC patients reported in previous studies are shown in Table 3. Other than the above, Bamias et al. reported that baseline PSA >100, pain, weight loss, and simultaneous extraosseous and bone disease were associated with worse prognosis in CRPC patients [19]. Matsuyama et al. reported that a decrease of ≥ 50 % in the PSA, serum markers at the start of docetaxel therapy (PSA, ALP, and CRP), and the number of docetaxel courses were independent predictors of OS, and ALP, hemoglobin, and age at the start of docetaxel therapy were useful for deciding the duration of docetaxel therapy in CRPC patients [20].

The pre-chemotherapeutic prognostic factors are divided broadly into two categories. The first category reflects cancer progression. PSA value, PSADT, bone scan progression, and significant pain are included in this category. The second category represents the patient's general condition. Age, ECOG PS, and CRP are included in the second category. The magnitude of the benefit provided by each factor has varied among studies.

In this retrospective study, prognostic factors were identified using only prechemotherapeutic factors in a single-institute Japanese cohort. The serum PSA level at the start of chemotherapy and anemia have been reported to be prognostic factors for CRPC patients in previous studies [16, 21, 22], and these factors were shown to be independent prognostic factors for CRPC patients treated with docetaxel in the present study. In addition, this study showed that age was also an independent prognostic factor and suggested that ECOG PS and the CRP-to-albumin ratio could be prognostic factors for CRPC patients. Accumulating evidence has indicated that cancer and inflammation are linked [23], and inflammation-based prognostic scores, including the NLR, Glasgow Prognostic Score (GPS), and Prognostic Nutritional Index (PNI), have been reported to have prognostic value in patients with various types of cancer

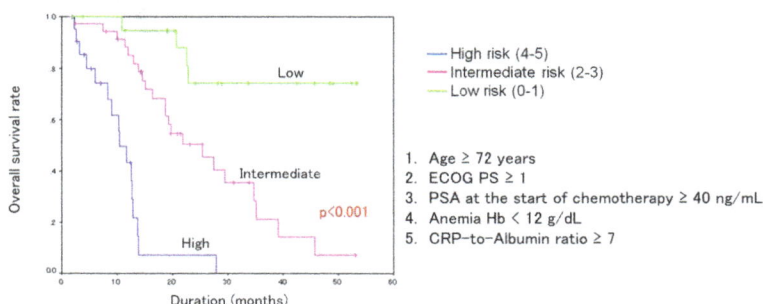

Legend:
- High risk (4-5)
- Intermediate risk (2-3)
- Low risk (0-1)

1. Age ≥ 72 years
2. ECOG PS ≥ 1
3. PSA at the start of chemotherapy ≥ 40 ng/mL
4. Anemia Hb < 12 g/dL
5. CRP-to-Albumin ratio ≥ 7

Fig. 2 Kaplan-Meier curves for overall survival (OS) according to risk group classification

Table 3 The prognostic factors for CRPC patients reported in previous studies

	Patient characteristics							Prognostic factor											
	Number of patients	PSA at DTX median	Age median	% bone meta	% visceral meta	% PSA >50% reduction	OS median	Age	PS	Hb (Anemia)	CRP	PSA	PSA DT	PSA >50% reduction	Pain	Bone scan progression	ALP	Visceral meta	Duration from initial ADT
Armstrong et al.	656	110	69	91	23	45–48	17.8–19.2	x	x	o		x	x		o	o	o	o	x
Nakano et al.	78	19.7	70	54	5	23		x	x	x		x	o		o※1	o※1		o※1	x
Shiota et al.	97	81.3	70	83.5	15.5	44.3	20.8	x	x	x		x	x		x	x	o	o	o
Bamias et al.	94	84	71	87		54	16.2	x	x	x		o			o		o		x
Matsuyama et al.	279	35.2	71	60.5	7.9	57.5	26	x	x	x	o	o		o			o	x	
Ito et al.	80						14.5	x	x	o	o	x			x		x	x	
Nuhn et al.	238	91.2–112.9	68.3	90.3	16.5		14.4–18.3	x	x	o	o	o			x		x	x	
Present study	79	43.2	72	51.9	5	69.6	22.5	o	x	o	o※2	o			x		x	x	x

Abbreviations: PSA prostate-specific antigen, *DTX* docetaxel, *OS* overall survival, *PS* performance status, *Hb* haemoglibin, *CRP* C-reactive protein, *PSA DT* prostate-specific antigen doubling time, *ALP* alkaline phosphatase, *ADT* androgen deprivation therapy

o: Significant

x: Not significant

※1: The Armstrong risk classification was independent prognostic factor

※2: CRP-to-Albumin Ratio was independent prognostic factor

Prognostic factors and risk stratification in patients with castration-resistant prostate cancer receiving...

149

in the last few years [24–28]. It has been reported that CRP and the NLR are useful clinical markers of the systemic inflammatory response in predicting OS in patients with CRPC treated with docetaxel [21, 22]. However, Kinoshita et al. reported that the CRP-to-albumin ratio might be an independent prognostic marker in patients with hepatocellular carcinoma and may have comparable prognostic ability to other established inflammation-based prognostic scores [29]. The present study suggested that this novel inflammation-based prognostic score could be a valuable prognostic marker in CRPC patients.

Our risk stratification could effectively stratify CRPC patients treated with docetaxel in terms of OS. Most of the prognostic factors included in the ARC, such as visceral metastases, bone scan progression, and significant pain, reflect the metastases of cancer. On the other hand, the prognostic factors included in the present risk stratification reflect the patient's general condition. This difference was likely caused by the differences in the baseline characteristics of target patients. In the TAX 327 study, the median serum PSA level at chemotherapy initiation of the patients was over 100 ng/mL [11]. Bone metastases were observed in more than 90 % of patients, and visceral metastases were seen in about 20 %. However, in the present study, the median serum PSA level at chemotherapy initiation was 43.2 ng/mL, and the frequency of bone metastases or visceral metastases was less. Therefore, in the present study, a PSA response of $\geq$ 50 % from baseline was observed in about 70 % patients, and this PSA response rate was better than in previous clinical trials performed in Western countries, including the TAX327 trial [11, 12]. Moreover, the median OS duration in this cohort was 22.5 months, while the median OS duration in the TAX327 cohort was <20 months. The difference of disease burden between our cohort and the TAX327 cohort caused these differences of PSA response and OS. Considering these facts, it appears that factors representing disease progression might be associated with OS in patients with progressive disease, while factors reflecting the patient's general condition might be correlated with OS in patients with less progressive disease – namely, prostate cancer with low serum PSA level at chemotherapy initiation or without bone metastases and visceral metastases. Lower disease burden in our cohort might be one of the reasons that significant pain, included in ARC, was not a significant factor in this study.

With the advent of novel agents, the demand for docetaxel in CRPC patients might slightly decrease. However, the results of the CHAARTED trial indicate the new effect of docetaxel for prostate cancer, and the importance of docetaxel will never be lost. Our study focused on the prognostic factors in CRPC patients receiving docetaxel-based chemotherapy, but the study about the prognostic factors in hormone sensitive prostate cancer (HSPC) patients receiving docetaxel-based chemotherapy will be needed.

This study had some limitations. First, the sample size was small, and the observation period might not have been long enough to determine the actual OS. Second, this study was a retrospective study using data from a single institution. Thirdly, many patients in our cohort received estramustine. It is less likely to combine estramustine to docetaxel based chemotherapy in Europe and United States. In fact, EAU and NCCN guidelines do not recommend to combine estramustine with docetaxel based chemotherapy. However, serious adverse events of estrogen, such as embolism, are reported to be rather rare in Japanese patients [30]. Finally, most patients required docetaxel dose reductions because of adverse events. Additional larger confirmatory studies are warranted to validate our results.

Conclusions

Age, serum PSA level at the start of chemotherapy, and Hb were identified as independent prognostic factors of OS, and ECOG PS and the CRP-to-albumin ratio were not significant but were considered as possible predictors for OS in Japanese CRPC patients treated with docetaxel. Risk stratification based on these factors could be helpful for estimating OS.

Abbreviations
ALP: alkaline phosphatase; ARC: Armstrong risk classification; CRP: C-reactive protein; CRPC: castration-resistant prostate cancer; EAU: European Association of Urology; ECOG: Eastern Cooperative Oncology Group; GPS: Glasgow Prognostic Score; Hb: hemoglobin; LDH: lactate dehydrogenase; NCCN: National Comprehensive Cancer Network; NLR: neutrophil-to-lymphocyte ratio; OS: overall survival; PNI: Prognostic Nutritional Index; PS: performance status; PSA: prostate specific antigen; PSADT: PSA doubling time.

Competing interests
The authors declare that they have no competing interests.

Authors' contributions
Study conception and design: SY and YK Acquisition of data: TI, HK, HK, AI, KK and YK Analysis and interpretation of data: SY and NM Drafting of manuscript: SY Critical revision: IH. All authors read and approved the final manuscript.

Acknowledgements
None.

References
1. Sharifi N, Gulley JL, Dahut WL. An update on androgen deprivation therapy for prostate cancer. Endocrine-Related Cancer. 2010;17(4):R305–15.
2. Miyamoto H, Messing EM, Chang C. Androgen deprivation therapy for prostate cancer: current status and future prospects. Prostate. 2004;61(4):332–53.
3. Shiota M, Yokomizo A, Naito S. Pro-survival and anti-apoptotic properties of androgen receptor signaling by oxidative stress promote treatment resistance in prostate cancer. Endocrine-related Cancer. 2012;19(6):R243–53.

4. Sadar MD. Small molecule inhibitors targeting the "achilles' heel" of androgen receptor activity. Cancer Res. 2011;71(4):1208–13.

5. Scher HI, Fizazi K, Saad F, Taplin ME, Sternberg CN, Miller K, et al. Increased survival with enzalutamide in prostate cancer after chemotherapy. New England J Med. 2012;367(13):1187–97.

6. Kantoff PW, Higano CS, Shore ND, Berger ER, Small EJ, Penson DF, Redfern CH, Ferrari AC, Dreicer R, Sims RB et al. Sipuleucel-T immunotherapy for castration-resistant prostate cancer. N Engl J Med. 2010;363(5):411–22.

7. de Bono JS, Oudard S, Ozguroglu M, Hansen S, Machiels JP, Kocak I, Gravis G, Bodrogi I, Mackenzie MJ, Shen L et al. Prednisone plus cabazitaxel or mitoxantrone for metastatic castration-resistant prostate cancer progressing after docetaxel treatment: a randomised open-label trial. Lancet. 2010; 376(9747):1147–54.

8. de Bono JS, Logothetis CJ, Molina A, Fizazi K, North S, Chu L, Chi KN, Jones RJ, Goodman OB, Jr., Saad F, et al. Abiraterone and increased survival in metastatic prostate cancer. N Engl J Med. 2011;364(21):1995–2005.

9. Beer TM, Armstrong AJ, Rathkopf DE, Loriot Y, Sternberg CN, Higano CS, et al. Enzalutamide in metastatic prostate cancer before chemotherapy. N Engl J Med. 2014;371(5):424–33.

10. Ryan CJ, Smith MR, de Bono JS, Molina A, Logothetis CJ, de Souza P, et al. Abiraterone in metastatic prostate cancer without previous chemotherapy. N Engl J Med. 2013;368(2):138–48.

11. Tannock IF, de Wit R, Berry WR, Horti J, Pluzanska A, Chi KN, et al. Docetaxel plus prednisone or mitoxantrone plus prednisone for advanced prostate cancer. N Engl J Med. 2004;351(15):1502–12.

12. Petrylak DP, Tangen CM, Hussain MH, Lara Jr PN, Jones JA, Taplin ME, et al. Docetaxel and estramustine compared with mitoxantrone and prednisone for advanced refractory prostate cancer. N Engl J Med. 2004;351(15):1513–20.

13. Kuramoto T, Inagaki T, Fujii R, Sasaki Y, Nishizawa S, Nanpo Y, et al. Docetaxel in combination with estramustine and prednisolone for castration-resistant prostate cancer. Int J Clin Oncol. 2013;18(5):890–7.

14. Shiota M, Yokomizo A, Fujimoto N, Kuruma H, Naito S. Castration-resistant prostate cancer: novel therapeutics pre- or post- taxane administration. Curr Cancer Drug Targets. 2013;13(4):444–59.

15. Armstrong AJ, Garrett-Mayer E, de Wit R, Tannock I, Eisenberger M. Prediction of survival following first-line chemotherapy in men with castration-resistant metastatic prostate cancer. Clin Cancer Res Off J Am Assoc Cancer Res. 2010;16(1):203–11.

16. Armstrong AJ, Tannock IF, De Wit R, George DJ, Eisenberger M, Halabi S. The development of risk groups in men with metastatic castration-resistant prostate cancer based on risk factors for PSA decline and survival. Eur J Cancer (Oxford, England 1990). 2010;46(3):517–25.

17. Nakano K, Komatsu K, Kubo T, Natsui S, Nukui A, Kurokawa S, et al. External validation of risk classification in patients with docetaxel-treated castration-resistant prostate cancer. BMC Urol. 2014;14:31.

18. Shiota M, Yokomizo A, Adachi T, Koga H, Yamaguchi A, Imada K, et al. The oncological outcomes and risk stratification in docetaxel chemotherapy for castration-resistant prostate cancer. Jpn J Clin Oncol. 2014;44(9):860–7.

19. Bamias A, Bozas G, Antoniou N, Poulias I, Katsifotis H, Skolarikos A, et al. Prognostic and predictive factors in patients with androgen-independent prostate cancer treated with docetaxel and estramustine: a single institution experience. Eur Urol. 2008;53(2):323–31.

20. Matsuyama H, Shimabukuro T, Hara I, Kohjimoto Y, Suzuki K, Koike H, et al. Combination of hemoglobin, alkaline phosphatase, and age predicts optimal docetaxel regimen for patients with castration-resistant prostate cancer. Int J Clin Oncol. 2014;19(5):946–54.

21. Nuhn P, Vaghasia AM, Goyal J, Zhou XC, Carducci MA, Eisenberger MA, et al. Association of pretreatment neutrophil-to-lymphocyte ratio (NLR) and overall survival (OS) in patients with metastatic castration-resistant prostate cancer (mCRPC) treated with first-line docetaxel. BJU Int. 2014;114(6b):E11–7.

22. Ito M, Saito K, Yasuda Y, Sukegawa G, Kubo Y, Numao N, et al. Prognostic impact of C-reactive protein for determining overall survival of patients with castration-resistant prostate cancer treated with docetaxel. Urology. 2011;78(5):1131–5.

23. Roxburgh CS, McMillan DC. Role of systemic inflammatory response in predicting survival in patients with primary operable cancer. Future Oncol (London, England). 2010;6(1):149–63.

24. Ishizuka M, Kubota K, Kita J, Shimoda M, Kato M, Sawada T. Impact of an inflammation-based prognostic system on patients undergoing surgery for hepatocellular carcinoma: a retrospective study of 398 Japanese patients. Am J Surg. 2012;203(1):101–6.

25. Gomez D, Farid S, Malik HZ, Young AL, Toogood GJ, Lodge JP, et al. Preoperative neutrophil-to-lymphocyte ratio as a prognostic predictor after curative resection for hepatocellular carcinoma. World J Surg. 2008;32(8):1757–62.

26. Pinato DJ, North BV, Sharma R. A novel, externally validated inflammation-based prognostic algorithm in hepatocellular carcinoma: the prognostic nutritional index (PNI). Br J Cancer. 2012;106(8):1439–45.

27. McMillan DC. The systemic inflammation-based Glasgow Prognostic Score: a decade of experience in patients with cancer. Cancer Treat Rev. 2013;39(5):534–40.

28. Kinoshita A, Onoda H, Imai N, Iwaku A, Oishi M, Tanaka K, et al. The Glasgow Prognostic Score, an inflammation based prognostic score, predicts survival in patients with hepatocellular carcinoma. BMC Cancer. 2013;13:52.

29. Kinoshita A, Onoda H, Imai N, Iwaku A, Oishi M, Tanaka K, Fushiya N, Koike K, Nishino H, Matsushima M: The C-Reactive Protein/Albumin Ratio, a Novel Inflammation-Based Prognostic Score, Predicts Outcomes in Patients with Hepatocellular Carcinoma. Ann Surgical Oncol. 2015;22(3):803-10.

30. Izumi K, Kadono Y, Shima T, Konaka H, Mizokami A, Koh E, et al. Ethinylestradiol improves prostate-specific antigen levels in pretreated castration-resistant prostate cancer patients. Anticancer Res. 2010;30(12):5201–5.

Quality of life and functional outcome after infravesical desobstruction and HIFU treatment for localized prostate cancer

G. Hatiboglu[*], I. V. Popeneciu, M. Deppert, J. Nyarangi-Dix, B. Hadaschik, M. Hohenfellner, D. Teber[†] and S. Pahernik[†]

Abstract

Background: To evaluate quality of life, functional and oncological outcome after infravesical desobstruction and HIFU treatment for localized prostate cancer.

Methods: One hundred thirty-one patients, treated with TURP and HIFU in a single institution were followed up for oncological and functional outcome. Oncological outcome was quantified by biochemical recurrence free survival using the Stuttgart and Phoenix criteria. Quality of life was assessed by usage of standardized QLQ-C30 and QLQ-PR25 questionnaires. In addition, functional questionnaires such as IPSS and IIEF-5 were used. Complications were assessed by the Clavien-Dindo classification.

Results: One hundred thirty-one patients with a mean age of 72.8 years (SD: 6.0) underwent HIFU for prostate cancer (29.0% low risk, 58.8% intermediate risk, 12.2% high risk). PSA nadir was 0.6 ng/ml (SD: 1.2) after a mean of 4.6 months (SD: 5.7). Biochemical recurrence free survival defined by Stuttgart criteria was 73.7%, 84.4% and 62.5% for low-, intermediate- and high-risk patients after 22.2 months. Complications were grouped according to Clavien-Dindo and occurred in 10.7% (grade II) and 11.5% (grade IIIa) of cases. 35.1% of patients needed further treatment for bladder neck stricture. Regarding incontinence, 14.3%, 2.9% and 0% of patients had de novo urinary incontinence grade I°, II° and III° and 3.8% urge incontinence due to HIFU treatment. Patients were asked for the ability to have intercourse: 15.8%, 58. 6% and 66.7% of patients after non-, onesided and bothsided nervesparing procedure were able to obtain sufficient erection for intercourse, respectively. Regarding quality of life, mean global health score according to QLQ-C30 was 69. 4%.

Conclusion: HIFU treatment for localized prostate cancer shows acceptable oncological safety. Quality of life after HIFU is better than in the general population and ranges within those of standard treatment options compared to literature. HIFU seems a safe valuable treatment alternative for patients not suitable for standard treatment.

Keywords: HIFU, Quality of life, Outcome

Background

High intensified focused ultrasound (HIFU) is a minimal invasive, thermoablative treatment option for patients with localized prostate cancer. Its aim is equivalent oncological safety with reduced toxicity, compared to standard treatment options [1]. HIFU can be performed in general or spinal anesthesia via transrectal approach.

* Correspondence: gencay.hatiboglu@med.uni-heidelberg.de
†Equal contributors
Department of Urology, University of Heidelberg, Im Neuenheimer Feld 110, 69120 Heidelberg, Germany

Focused, high energetic ultrasound waves cause thermal alteration and cavitation, causing coagulative necrosis and thereby destroying malignant tissue [2, 3].

Since the initial presentation in 1995 [4], several studies have evaluated oncological and functional outcome after HIFU. Recent publications report of 76%, 63% and 57% biochemical free survival after 8 years for low-, intermediate- and high-risk patients [5]. The 10-year prostate cancer specific survival rate and metastasis-free survival rate were 97% and 94%, respectively [5]. Regarding morbidity of HIFU treatment, severe incontinence rates of 3.1% and erectile function preservation of up to 42.3% are described [5]. Patients rejecting standard treatment and preferring HIFU do this with the expectation for less complications and less invasiveness compared to standard treatment. Especially incontinence, erectile dysfunction after radical prostatectomy as well as gastrointestinal and genitourinary side effects after radiotherapy are feared by many patients and can impair their quality of life [6]. Recent studies have evaluated quality of life for prostate cancer patients after local therapy, showing good results with moderate alteration in erectile and lower urinary tract function with minimal decrease in quality of life [7, 8]. The authors utilized standardized questionnaires for this evaluation like the European Organisation for Research and Treatment of cancer (EORTC) quality of life questionnaire QLQ-C30 and the prostate specific module QLQ-PR25. The QLQ-C30 questionnaire evaluates overall health related quality of life as well as several functional domains and general cancer related symptoms. The QLQ-PR25 assesses urinary symptoms, sexual activity and function, as well as bowel symptoms. Both questionnaires have been evaluated and validated extensively [9, 10]. Regarding quality of life for prostate cancer patients, both questionnaires are routinely used.

To our knowledge, data about quality of life after HIFU therapy using standardized questionnaires are rare and have not been evaluated in a standardized fashion so far. The aim of the study was to investigate prospectively quality of life after HIFU ablation of the prostate for the local treatment of prostate cancer.

Methods

One hundred thirty-one patients undergoing infravesical desobstruction and HIFU treatment for localized prostate cancer between 02/2008 and 12/2012 were followed up in a prospectively conducted database. The study protocol was approved by the ethics committee of the University of Heidelberg (S-182/2012). All patients gave written informed consent.

All patients were treated with the Ablatherm HIFU device (Ablatherm integrated imaging device; EDAP-TMS, Vaulx-en-Velin, France). Before HIFU treatment an infravesical desobstruction was routinely done one day prior to HIFU treatment, normally by transurethral resection of the prostate (TURP) or by greenlight laservaporisation of the prostate [11]. The mode of infravesical desobstruction was at patients' preference (TUR-P was recommended, some patients explicitly wished to undergo greenlight laservaporisation). HIFU treatment was performed as inpatient procedure in combined spinal and epidural anesthesia. Nervesparing procedure was only done in patients explicitly demanding for this. All these patients were intensively informed about

higher risk for recurrent prostate cancer but wished to undergo nervesparing anyway and with awareness of all risks (this was also documented in informed consent). In these cases, mainly one sided nervesparing was done - if prostate biopsy showed cancer infiltration on only one side the nervesparing was done on the contralateral side. However, some patients explicitly wished both sided nervesparing, taking into account the risk for tumor recurrence. For all patients, the following parameters were assessed and entered in a prospective conducted database: patient age, body mass index, prostate volume, PSA value at diagnosis, Gleason Score, clinical stage, risk classification (according to D'Amico et al. [12, 13]), PSA nadir and time to PSA nadir, biochemical recurrence according to Stuttgart criteria [14] and Phoenix criteria [15]. In addition, treatment related data were evaluated and included: type of preoperative infravesical desobstruction, duration and number of applied lesions during HIFU treatment, nervesparing (non-,unilateral-,bilateral nervesparing), hospital stay, indwelling time for transurethral and suprapubic catheter, uroflowmetry and residual volume (pre-HIFU and 2 weeks post-HIFU). In addition, complication were evaluated according to Clavien-Dindo [16]. Patients were asked to fill out the international prostate symptom score (IPSS) and international index for erectile function (IIEF-5) questionnaire before and 3 months after HIFU treatment. Continence was evaluated and graduated during follow-up, the usage and number of used pads was evaluated. Patients were also asked for sexual activity after HIFU treatment including the usage of adjuvant medication for erection.

Assessment of quality of life

All patients were asked to complete the European Organisation for Research and Treatment of cancer (EORTC) quality of life questionnaire QLQ-C30 (Version 3.0) and the prostate specific module QLQ-PR25 retrospectively in 12/2012. Both questionnaires are internationally validated and used in cancer patients. They were used in German translation. The QLQ-C30 questionnaire consists of 30 questions, the QLQ-PR25 of 25 questions. The QLQ-C30 measures global health related quality of life, five functional domains (physical, role, emotional, cognitive and role function) and nine symptom scales (fatigue, nausea and vomiting, pain, dyspnoe, insomnia, appetite loss, constipation, diarrhea, financial difficulties). The QLQ-PR25 questionnaire, consisting of 25 questions, assesses urinary symptoms, bowel symptoms, treatment-related symptoms and sexual symptoms and functioning. In both instruments, all answers ranged from 1 (not at all) to 4 (very much), despite 2 questions in the QLQ-C30 considering global health related quality of life ranging from 1 (very poor) to 7 (excellent).

Both questionnaires have been interpreted according to the EORTC guidelines. The scores have been converted to linear scales ranging from 0 to 100. Higher values in functional scales and health related quality of life represent better results. Lower values in symptom scales represent less symptoms.

Statistical analysis

Above mentioned variables were evaluated by descriptive statistics. Median, mean, standard deviation and range were calculated for every variable using Microsoft Excel and IBM SPSS statistics version 20.

Results

One hundred thirty-one patients with a mean age of 72.8 ± 6.0 years have been included to this analysis. PSA values at prostate cancer diagnosis were 9.6 ± 14.9 ng/ml. Gleason score was 6 in 57 patients (43.5%), 7 in 66 patients (50.4%) and ≥ 8 in 8 patients (6.1%). 29.0% of patients had a low risk, 58.8% an intermediate risk and 12.2% a high risk prostate cancer (Table 1). When presenting for HIFU treatment, 28 patients (21.4%) have been on neoadjuvant hormonal therapy, that has been stopped directly after HIFU treatment. Bothsided nervesparing was performed in 21.1%, 9.6% and 6.7%, onesided nervesparing in 28.9%, 26.0% and 6.7% of low-, intermediate- and high-risk patients, respectively. After HIFU the mean PSA nadir was 0.6 ± 1.2 ng/ml (median: 0.1 ng/ml; range 0.01-6.50 ng/ml) and reached after 4.7 months (SD: 5.7) (Table 2). Mean follow up was 22.2 months (SD: 16.1). 28 patients (21.4%) developed a biochemical recurrence, defined as PSA Nadir + 1.2 ng/ml (according to Stuttgart criteria [14]) after a mean

Table 1 Demographics

	n (%)	mean (SD)
Age (years)	131	72.8 (6.0)
Clinical stage		
cT1	83 (63.8%)	
≥ cT2	47 (36.2%)	
Gleason Score		
≤ 6	57 (43.5%)	
7	66 (50.4%)	
≥ 8	8 (6.1%)	
inital PSA (ng/ml)	130	9.6 (14.9)
Risk stratification (D'Amico)		
Low - risk	38 (29.0%)	
Intermediate - risk	77 (58.8%)	
High - risk	16 (12.2%)	
Prostate volume (ml)	130	43.7 (25.6)
Prostate volume after resection	123	26.0 (12.5)

Table 2 Perioperative parameter

	n (%)	mean (SD)
Treated HIFU volume (ml)	126	27.7 (9.9)
Duration of HIFU treatment (minutes)	127	104.3 (28.8)
Applied lesions	127	433.8 (136.2)
Nervesparing		
No nervesparing	79 (60.3%)	
One-sided nervesparing	31 (23.7%)	
Both-sided nervesparing	16 (12.2%)	
Data missing	5 (3.8%)	
Transurethral catheter indwelling time	125	4.0 (2.5)
Suprapubic catheter indwelling time	78	14.5 (15.0)

time of 15.5 ± 11.6 months. Among them, 10 patients (26.3%), 12 patients (15.6%) and 6 patients (37.5%) of low-, intermediate-and high-risk profile, respectively. Therefore, biochemical recurrence free survival was 73.7%, 84.4% and 62.5% for low-, intermediate- and high-risk patients at latest follow-up. In addition, 3 patients had histological confirmed recurrence that was confirmed in prostate biopsy in patients undergoing biopsy after 6 months at own wish or after bladder neck resection due to infravesical obstruction.

Of these 31 patients with recurrent prostate cancer, 18 patients (58.1%) underwent active therapy. Twelve of these patients were lost to follow-up. Five patients underwent salvage radiotherapy, two 2 patients salvage-HIFU therapy, one patient prostatectomy and one patient brachytherapy and pelvic lymphadenectomy. The other 9 patients (29.0%) did not wish salvage therapy and received antiandrogen treatment. During follow-up, 7 patients (5.3%) deceased – 1 patient because of systemic progression of the prostate cancer, the other 6 patients due to cardiovascular events (Table 3).

When defining biochemical recurrence according to Phoenix criteria, 20 patients (15.5%) showed biochemical recurrence with a mean time to recurrence of 17.4 ± 12.5 months. Biochemical recurrence free survival was therefore 81.6%, 89.6% and 68.8% for low-, intermediate-and high-risk patients at latest follow-up, respectively.

Regarding treatment data, 109 patients (83.2%) underwent TUR-P, 18 patients greenlight-laser vaporization (13.7%) and 1 patient (0.8%) combination of both in advance to HIFU treatment. Resection was done the day prior to HIFU. Mean prostate size was thereby reduced from 43.7 ml (±25.6) to 26.0 ml (±12.5). Three patients (2.3%) had no prior infravesical desobstruction. During HIFU treatment, a one-sided nervesparing was done in 31 patients (23.7%), a both sided nervesparing in 16 patients (12.2%). Perioperative side effects up to 30 days after HIFU treatment were assessed and grouped according to Clavien-Dindo classification and occurred in

Table 3 Oncological outcome

	n (%)	Mean (SD)
PSA – nadir (ng/ml)	101	0.6 (1.2) median: 0.1 (range: 0.01–6.50)
Time to nadir (months)	99	4.7 (5.7)
Recurrencies	31 (23.7%)	
Biochemical recurrence (BCR) Suttgart criteria	28 (21.4%)	
low - risk - PCa	10 (7.6%)	
intermediate - risk – PCa	12 (9.2%)	
high - risk – PCa	6 (4.6%)	
Time to BCR (in months) (Stuttgart criteria)	28	15.5 (11.6)
Time to BCR (in months) (Phoenix criteria)		17.4 (12.5)
low - risk - PCa	10	14.1 (8.2)
intermediate - risk - PCa	12	19.8 (13.8)
high - risk – Pca	6	11.3 (5.4)
Recurrence without BCR	3 (2.3%)	

25 patients (19.1%), 4 patients had 2 complications. Main complications were infravesical obstruction and urinary tract infections. With respect to infravesical obstruction, grade II and grade IIIa complications occurred in 14 (10.7%) and 15 (11.5%) cases, respectively. Regarding late complications beyond 30 days, 47 patients (35.9%) needed further treatment. 46 patients (35.1%) needed catheterization or suprapubic catheter insertion and transurethral resection because of bladder neck obstruction. One patients needed DJ insertion because progression of prostate cancer.

IPSS score before and after HIFU treatment was 10.9 ± 7.1 and 9.2 ± 6.2, respectively. Uroflowmetrie before and after HIFU treatment showed max. flow of 14.0 ml/s (SD 8.2) and 14.1 ml/s (SD 8.7) with post voiding residual volume of 45.5 ml (SD 69.4) and 54.0 ml (SD 93.6), respectively. Regarding incontinence, 14.3%, 2.9% and 0% of patients had de novo urinary incontinence grade I°, II° and III° and 3.8% urge incontinence due to HIFU treatment. Before HIFU treatment 97.1% of patients did not need a pad. After HIFU treatment, 9.5%, 6.7% and 1.9% of patients needed 1pad, 2pads or >2pads, respectively, meaning 81.9% did not need a pad at all at latest follow-up.

IIEF-5 scores showed 17.2 ± 7.3 and 9.7 ± 8.0 before and after HIFU treatment in all patients, respectively. When grouped according to nervesparing procedure, mean IIEF-5 score before and after HIFU was 15.1 ± 8.1 vs. 7.5 ± 7.4 for the non-nervesparing group, 19.7 ± 4.8 vs. 12.5 ± 8.3 for the one-sided nervesparing group and 20.7 ± 5.3 and 12.1 ± 7.5 for the both sided nervesparing

group, respectively. Regarding the ability to have sexual intercourse, 15.8%, 58.6% and 66.7% of patients after non-, onesided and bothsided nervesparing procedure were able to obtain sufficient erection for intercourse, respectively. 33.3% of these patients used PDE5 inhibitors, 3 patients mechanical devices to obtain erection. Functional outcomes after HIFU therapy are displayed in Table 4.

Quality of life was evaluated using the QLQ-C30 questionnaire and showed a global health status of 69.4% (SD: 20.6). Functional scales revealed physical functioning of 86.2% (SD 17.7) after HIFU treatment. Regarding symptom scales, fatigue and insomnia were the most frequent symptoms with 25.9% (SD: 24.8) and 31.4% (SD: 31.4) of cases in a cohort of men aged 72.8 ± 6.0 years. For further evaluation of prostate specific symptoms the QLQ-PR25 questionnaire was used and showed sexual activity and functioning of 56.9% (SD: 28.1) and 49.6% (SD: 20.5), respectively. Evaluation of symptom scales showed urinary symptoms in 28.3% (SD: 18.4) and

Table 4 Functional outcome after HIFU treatment (mean(SD))

	Pre - HIFU	Post - HIFU
Continence and micturation symptoms		
IPSS – Score	10.9 (7.1)	9.2 (6.2)
Micturation volume (ml)	207.7 (116.5)	189.2 (92.4)
Post voiding Residual volume(ml)	45.5 (69.4)	54.0 (93.6)
Qmax (ml/sec)	14.0 (8.2)	14.1 (8.7)
Continence		
Continent	93 (88.6%)	71 (67.6%)
Incontince grade I°	5 (4.8%)	20 (19.0%)
Incontince grade II°	0 (0.0%)	3 (2.9%)
Incontince grade III°	1 (1.0%)	1 (1.0%)
Urge incontinence	6 (5.7%)	10 (9.5%)
Pad usage		
No pads	102 (97.1%)	86 (81.9%)
1 pad	1 (1.0%)	10 (9.5%)
2 pads	1 (1.0%)	7 (6.7%)
> 2 pads	1 (1.0%)	2 (1.9%)
Sexual function		
Sexual intercourse after HIFU		
Yes		36 (35.6%)
No		65 (64.4%)
Due to HIFU treatment		46 (45.5%)
Other reason		55 (54.5%)
IIEF – 5		
IIEF - 5 – score	17.2 (7.3)	9.7 (8.0)
IIEF - 5 - non – nervesparing	15.1 (8.1)	7.5 (7.4)
IIEF - 5 - onesided - nervesparing	19.7 (4.8)	12.5 (8.3)
IIEF - 5 - bothsided – nervesparing	20.7 (5.3)	12.1 (7.5)

urinary bother in 38.6% (SD: 35.6) of patients after HIFU. Bowel symptoms did appear in 6.7% (SD: 11.2) of patients. The overall quality of life did not change before and after HIFU (evaluated by the IPSS questionnaire). All results are displayed in Table 5.

Discussion

The present study was performed to evaluate quality of life after HIFU treatment for prostate cancer. To our knowledge, this is the first study investigating this topic. Quality of life was assessed by standardized questionnaires. In addition, functional outcome and oncological results were evaluated with respect to limited followup.

Regarding oncological results, recent reports from Crouzet et al. showed 7 years biochemical free survival

Table 5 Quality of life – post-HIFU outcome of QLQ-C30, QLQ-PR25 and IPSS-QoL questionnaires (n = 105). Data are shown as mean with standard deviation

QLQ - C30	
Global health status/QoL (QL2)	69.4 (20.6)
Functional scales	
Physical functioning (PF2)	86.2 (17.7)
Role functioning (RF2)	79.0 (29.9)
Emotional functioning (EF)	74.8 (23.5)
Cognitive functioning (CF)	83.3 (20.5)
Social functioning (SF)	74.8 (25.0)
Symptom scales/items	
Fatigue (FA)	25.9 (24.8)
Nausea and vomiting (NV)	1.5 (6.7)
Pain (PA)	17.1 (27.8)
Dyspnoea (DY)	18.1 (26.6)
Insomnia (SL)	31.4 (31.4)
Appetite loss (AP)	4.8 (16.9)
Constipation (CO)	16.2 (27.0)
Diarrhoea (DI)	7.3 (19.6)
Financial difficulties (FI)	10.5 (23.3)
QLQ - PR25	
Functional scales	
Sexual activity(PRSAC)(n = 104)	56.9 (28.1)
Sexual functioning (PRSFU)(n = 71)	49.6 (20.5)
Symptom scales/items	
Urinary symptoms (PRURI)	28.3 (18.4)
Urinary bother (PRAID)	38.6 (35.6)
Bowel symptoms (PRBOW)	6.7 (11.2)
ADT – treatments symptoms (PRHTR)	16.4 (16.4)
Quality - of - life; IPSS	
Prä - HIFU	2.1 (1.4)
Post - HIFU	2.0 (1.3)

(Phoenix Criteria) in 75%, 63% and 62% for low-, intermediate- and high-risk prostate cancer patients [5]. Using the recently supposed stricter Stuttgart criteria (meaning PSA nadir +1.2 ng/ml [14]), Pfeiffer et al. described 5 years biochemical free survival as 85%, 65% and 55% for low-, intermediate- and high-risk prostate cancer [17]. The present series mainly consisted of intermediate risk patients (58.8%) because high risk patients were consulted for standard treatment and low risk patients for active surveillance. In this cohort, biochemical recurrence free survival was 76.3%, 84.4% and 64.7% (using Stuttgart criteria) and 81.6%, 89.6% and 68.8% (using Phoenix criteria) for low-, intermediate- and high-risk patients with a mean follow up of 22.2 months. However, 3 patients of our cohort also had histological proven recurrence without biochemical recurrence. Previous studies by Ganzer et al. showed, that negative biopsy rates correlate with postoperative PSA nadir. Ganzer et al. described negative biopsy rates of 91.6% for patients with PSA nadir ≤ 0.2 ng/ml. Thus, 8.4% of patients had remaining prostate cancer tissue in control biopsies after 3–6 months [14] with a PSA value < 0.2 ng/ml.

In our cohort, side effects were limited in severity. Main complications were urinary tract infections and infravesical obstruction. While infections were mainly managed successfully by antibiotic treatment, 25% of patients needed further surgical treatment in form of transurethral resection of bladder neck strictures. These complications and rates were also described in other publications as the most frequent re-interventions [18–20]. More severe complications like fistulas did not occur in our cohort. Regarding postoperative micturition and continence, IPSS and uroflowmetry data did not change after HIFU treatment. Previous studies could show, that combining TURP and HIFU is mandatory to reduce postoperative voiding dysfunction [21]. However, even previous TURP cannot reduce infravesical obstruction completely. During followup, 35.1% of patients needed further treatment for infravesical obstruction after HIFU treatment. Previous studies confirm, that bladder neck obstruction or urethral strictures are the most common side effects of HIFU treatment [5, 18]. Crouzet et al. described up to 16% bladder neck obstruction in their group, when TUR-P and HIFU were combined in one session. To reduce these side effects, an interval of up to 6 weeks between TUR-P and HIFU has been proposed [11] with reduction of infravesical obstruction to 11%, as described by Crouzet et al. [5]. Compared to our cohort, median pre-HIFU prostate volume was smaller in the cohort described by Crouzet et al. (22–24.5 ml) compared to our cohort (38.5 ml), which could explain the higher bladder neck obstruction rates in the present study due to a selection bias.

Evaluation of erectile function in our group revealed, that postoperative erectile function depends on nervesparing procedure. Most studies do not report of nervesparing as this means sparing a few millimeters of prostatic tissue and therefore increasing the risk for biochemical recurrence [22]. As expected, the PSA nadir ranges were higher (up to 6.5 ng/ml), most likely because of nervesparing procedure, that has been done in 35.9% of patients. Warmuth et al. [18] reviewed 20 studies with a total of 3018 patients undergoing whole gland ablation and reported of erectile dysfunction rates ranging from 20–39%. Crouzet et al. [5] recently reported their results of 1002 patients and described preservation of erectile function in 42.3% patients (<70 years: 55.6%; >70 years: 25.6%). None of these trials took nervesparing procedure into account. In our cohort, erectile function could be preserved in only 15% in patients undergoing whole gland ablation. These patients tended to be of advanced age (mean age in non-nervesparing group was 74.4 years), that is known to be associated with impaired baseline potency status [23] and therefore these patients normally do not wish nervesparing procedure. In contrast, both sided nervesparing HIFU could preserve erectile function in up to 66% of our patients (median age in this group was 69.7 years).

Patients undergoing HIFU ablation instead of standard treatment commonly expect less side effects and better preservation of quality of life. As quality of life represents a multidimensional construct that includes physical, social, psychological and functional domains, its assessment needs complex and standardized questionnaires. Shoji et al. examined the changes in quality of life for patients at a mean age 68 years undergoing HIFU by using the japanese versions of the FACT-G and FACT-P questionnaires (functional assessment of cancer therapy – general and prostate cancer module) [24]. The authors reported, that general quality of life improves after HIFU therapy while the values for FACT-P questionnaire did not change. However, patients undergoing HIFU may be biased as they actively rejected standard therapy for a new, minimal invasive therapy option. We evaluated quality of life after HIFU therapy using the standardized QLQ-C30 and QLQ-PR25 questionnaire. Mean global health score after HIFU treatment was 69.4% for all patients, 66.4% for patients ≤70 years and 70.9% for patients >70 years. Schwarz et al. evaluated QLQ-C30 data for the general german population [25] and described global health scores of 65.6% and 61.5% for patients ≤70 and >70 years, respectively. When compared to the general german population, patients after HIFU treatment show better quality of life with respect to global health scores. Drummond et al. evaluated quality of life after standard therapy in more than 6000 patients within the PiCTure study (prostate cancer treatment, your experience) [8]. They described global health scores ranging from 73.4% for radical prostatectomy and 69.4% for external beam radiation therapy. With respect to the younger patient collective in the PiCTure study, global health score after HIFU treatment in our collective ranged within the scores after standard treatment options described by Drummond et al. Comparing the results of QLQ-PR25 items revealed more urinary symptoms (28.3% for HIFU vs. 19.8% for standard treatment [8]) and more urinary bother (38.6% for HIFU vs. 15.6% for standard treatment [8]) and less sexual activity (56.9% for HIFU vs. 67.8% for standard treatment [8]).

Limitations of the study include short followup. Results predicting oncological safety need longer followup periods, that should be considered in further studies. Another limitation is the missing, preoperative assessment for quality of life to compare changes for this parameter.

Conclusion

In conclusion, HIFU treatment for localized prostate cancer shows acceptable oncological safety in limited follow up. However, local recurrence is not always indicated by biochemical recurrence. Compared to literature, the quality of life after HIFU showed better results compared to general population of equivalent age. Patients' satisfaction ranges within those of standard treatment options. Further studies are needed to compare changes in quality of life before and after HIFU therapy. In addition, nearly 25% of patients needed further treatment for bladder neck obstruction. HIFU seems a safe valuable treatment alternative for patients not suitable for standard treatment.

Abbreviations

EORTC: European Organisation for Research and Treatment of cancer; HIFU: High intensified focused ultrasound; IIEF-5: International index for erectile function; IPSS: International prostate symptom score; QLQ: Quality of life questionnaire; TURP: Transurethral resection of the prostate

Authors' contribution

GH, IVP and MD carried out data acquisition and data analysis. GH participated in design of the study and drafted the manuscript. JND, DT and BH helped in designing the study and revised the manuscript critically. SP, DT and MH made substantial contribution to conception and design, analysis of data, critically revising the manuscript and final approval. DT and SP contributed equally. All authors read and approved the final manuscript.

Competing interests

The authors declare that they have no competing interests.

Ethics approval and consent to participate

The study protocol was approved by the ethics committee of the University of Heidelberg (S-182/2012). All patients gave written informed consent. Nervesparing was only done in patients, explicitly demanding for this with full awareness of higher risk of tumor recurrence. This was also documented in the informed consent.

Quality of life and functional outcome after infravesical desobstruction and HIFU treatment for localized...

157

References

1. Heidenreich A, Bellmunt J, Bolla M, Joniau S, Mason M, Matveev V, et al. EAU guidelines on prostate cancer. Part 1: screening, diagnosis, and treatment of clinically localised disease. Eur Urol. 2011;59(1):61–71. doi:10. 1016/j.eururo.2010.10.039.

2. Chaussy CG, Thuroff S. Transrectal high-intensity focused ultrasound for local treatment of prostate cancer: current role. Arch Esp Urol. 2011;64(6):493–506.

3. Madersbacher S, Marberger M. High-energy shockwaves and extracorporeal high-intensity focused ultrasound. J Endourol. 2003;17(8):667–72. doi:10. 1089/089277903322518680.

4. Madersbacher S, Pedevilla M, Vingers L, Susani M, Marberger M. Effect of high-intensity focused ultrasound on human prostate cancer in vivo. Cancer Res. 1995;55(15):3346–51.

5. Crouzet S, Chapelon JY, Rouviere O, Mege-Lechevallier F, Colombel M, Tonoli-Catez H, et al. Whole-gland ablation of localized prostate cancer with high-intensity focused ultrasound: oncologic outcomes and morbidity in 1002 patients. Eur Urol. 2014;65(5):907–14. doi:10.1016/j.eururo.2013.04.039.

6. Osoba D. Health-related quality of life and cancer clinical trials. Ther Adv Med Oncol. 2011;3(2):57–71. doi:10.1177/1758834010395342.

7. Miller DC, Sanda MG, Dunn RL, Montie JE, Pimentel H, Sandler HM, et al. Long-term outcomes among localized prostate cancer survivors: health-related quality-of-life changes after radical prostatectomy, external radiation, and brachytherapy. J Clin Oncol. 2005;23(12):2772–80. doi:10.1200/JCO.2005.07.116.

8. Drummond FJ, Kinnear H, O'Leary E, Donnelly, Gavin A, Sharp L. Long-term health-related quality of life of prostate cancer survivors varies by primary treatment. Results from the PiCTure (Prostate Cancer Treatment, your experience) study. J Cancer Surviv. 2015. doi:10.1007/s11764-014-0419-6.

9. Groenvold M, Klee MC, Sprangers MA, Aaronson NK. Validation of the EORTC QLQ-C30 quality of life questionnaire through combined qualitative and quantitative assessment of patient-observer agreement. J Clin Epidemiol. 1997;50(4):441–50.

10. Niezgoda HE, Pater JL. A validation study of the domains of the core EORTC quality of life questionnaire. Qual Life Res. 1993;2(5):319–25.

11. Chaussy C, Thuroff S. The status of high-intensity focused ultrasound in the treatment of localized prostate cancer and the impact of a combined resection. Curr Urol Rep. 2003;4(3):248–52.

12. D'Amico AV, Moul J, Carroll PR, Sun L, Lubeck D, Chen MH. Cancer-specific mortality after surgery or radiation for patients with clinically localized prostate cancer managed during the prostate-specific antigen era. J Clin Oncol. 2003;21(11):2163–72. doi:10.1200/JCO.2003.01.075.

13. D'Amico AV, Whittington R, Malkowicz SB, Schultz D, Blank K, Broderick GA, et al. Biochemical outcome after radical prostatectomy, external beam radiation therapy, or interstitial radiation therapy for clinically localized prostate cancer. JAMA. 1998;280(11):969–74.

14. Ganzer R, Robertson CN, Ward JF, Brown SC, Conti GN, Murat FJ, et al. Correlation of prostate-specific antigen nadir and biochemical failure after high-intensity focused ultrasound of localized prostate cancer based on the Stuttgart failure criteria - analysis from the @-Registry. BJU Int. 2011;108(8 Pt 2):E196–201. doi:10.1111/j.1464-410X.2011.10091.x.

15. Roach 3rd M, Hanks G, Thames Jr H, Schellhammer P, Shipley WU, Sokol GH, et al. Defining biochemical failure following radiotherapy with or without hormonal therapy in men with clinically localized prostate cancer: recommendations of the RTOG-ASTRO Phoenix Consensus Conference. Int J Radiat Oncol Biol Phys. 2006;65(4):965–74. doi:10.1016/j.ijrobp.2006.04.029.

16. Dindo D, Demartines N, Clavien PA. Classification of surgical complications: a new proposal with evaluation in a cohort of 6336 patients and results of a survey. Ann Surg. 2004;240(2):205–13.

17. Pfeiffer D, Berger J, Gross AJ. Single application of high-intensity focused ultrasound as a first-line therapy for clinically localized prostate cancer: 5-year outcomes. BJU Int. 2012;110(11):1702–7. doi:10.1111/j.1464-410X.2012.11375.x.

18. Warmuth M, Johansson T, Mad P. Systematic review of the efficacy and safety of high-intensity focussed ultrasound for the primary and salvage treatment of prostate cancer. Eur Urol. 2010;58(6):803–15. doi:10.1016/j.eururo.2010.09.009.

19. Blana A, Rogenhofer S, Ganzer R, Lunz JC, Schostak M, Wieland WF, et al. Eight years' experience with high-intensity focused ultrasonography for treatment of localized prostate cancer. Urology. 2008;72(6):1329–33. doi:10.1016/j.urology.2008.06.062. discussion 33–4.

20. Ganzer R, Fritsche HM, Brandtner A, Brundl J, Koch D, Wieland WF, et al. Fourteen-year oncological and functional outcomes of high-intensity focused ultrasound in localized prostate cancer. BJU Int. 2013;112(3):322–9. doi:10.1111/j.1464-410X.2012.11715.x.

21. Chaussy CG, Thuroff SF. Robotic high-intensity focused ultrasound for prostate cancer: what have we learned in 15 years of clinical use? Curr Urol Rep. 2011;12(3):180–7. doi:10.1007/s11934-011-0184-2.

22. Chaussy C, Thuroff S. Results and side effects of high-intensity focused ultrasound in localized prostate cancer. J Endourol. 2001;15(4):437–40. doi:10.1089/089277901300189501. discussion 47–8.

23. Burke RM, Evans JD. Avanafil for treatment of erectile dysfunction: review of its potential. Vasc Health Risk Manag. 2012;8:517–23. doi:10.2147/VHRM.S26712.

24. Shoji S, Nakano M, Nagata Y, Usui Y, Terachi T, Uchida T. Quality of life following high-intensity focused ultrasound for the treatment of localized prostate cancer: a prospective study. Int J Urol. 2010;17(8):715–9. doi:10.1111/j.1442-2042.2010.02568.x.

25. Schwarz R, Hinz A. Reference data for the quality of life questionnaire EORTC QLQ-C30 in the general German population. Eur J Cancer. 2001; 37(11):1345–51.

Epididymal anomalies in boys with undescended testis or hydrocele: Significance of testicular location

Sun-Ouck Kim[*], Seong Woong Na, Ho Song Yu and Dongdeuk Kwon

Abstract

Background: Epididymal anomalies and patent processus vaginalis are frequently found in boys with cryptorchidism or hydrocele. We conducted this study to evaluate the association between epididymal anomalies and testicular location or patent processus vaginalis in boys with undescended testis or hydrocele.

Methods: Children undergoing surgery with undescended testis (group A, 136 boys and 162 testes) or communicating hydrocele (group B, 93 boys and 96 testes) were included. Testicular locations and epididymal anomalies were investigated prospectively. An anomalous epididymis was defined as anomalies of epididymal fusion that consisted of loss of continuity between the testis, the epididymis, and the long looping epididymis. The epididymis was considered normal when a normal, firm attachment between the testis, the caput, and the cauda epididymis was present.

Results: The mean ages of groups A and B were 24.6 ± 19.7 (range, 8–52 months) and 31.4 ± 20.6 months (range, 10–59 months). The incidence of epididymal anomalies was significantly higher in group A than that in group B (65.4 % vs. 13.5 %, $P < 0.001$). The incidence of epididymal anomalies in boys with undescended testis was significantly different according to testis location. Epididymal anomalies were observed in 100 %, 91.4 %, and 39.3 % of cases when the testis was located in the abdomen, inguinal canal, and distal to the external inguinal ring, respectively ($P < 0.001$).

Conclusion: We conclude that epididymal anomalies were more frequent in boys with undescended testis than in boys with hydrocele, and that these anomalies were more frequent when undescended testis was at a higher level. These results suggest that testicular location is associated with epididymal anomalies rather than patent processus vaginalis.

Keywords: Undescended testis, Epididymis, Hydrocele

Background

Epididymal and vasal anomalies are associated with undescended testis. These anomalies occur in association with undescended testis at varying degrees of 32–79 % according to various epididymal anomaly diagnostic criteria [1–7]. These anomalies can be found either during orchiopexy or hydrocelectomy/hernia repair. The patency of processus vaginalis is also strongly related with epididymal anomalies [8].

The surgeon must be aware of associated epididymal anomalies when operating to correct undescended testes or hydrocele and not to dissect an elongated epididymis, a cranially located testis with a descended long or dissociated epididymis, or a cranially located testis [5]. Although epididymal anomalies in children with undescended testis or hydrocele are detected frequently during the surgery, only limited and sporadic reports are available on this subject.

Some reports have suggested that epididymal anomalies associated with more cranially located testis are more severe than those associated with more caudally located testis among boys with undescended testis [4]. However,

---
* Correspondence: seinsena@hanmail.net
From the Department of Urology, Chonnam National University Medical School, Gwangju, South Korea

no study has evaluated epididymal anomalies based on the location of undescended testis, which represents the exact incidence rate. We prospectively evaluated the relationship between epididymal anomalies in boys with undescended testis or hydrocele. The aim of this study was to clarify whether patent processus vaginalis or undescended testis is a more important factor in epididymal anomalies. We specially focused on the severity of epididymal anomalies according to testicular location in boys with undescended testis to better understand the relationship between epididymal morphology and testicular descent.

Methods

Patients and study design

We included children undergoing an inguinal exploration for undescended testis or a communicating hydrocele in the urologic department of our hospital between January 2011 and July 2013. A communicating hydrocele was defined by the size change history and a sac extending to the groin on ultrasound sonography. We performed a cross-sectional study to determine the incidence of epididymal anomalies in these children. Boys with any of the following were excluded from the study: associated disorders, such as hypospadias, exstrophy, imperforated anus, sex development disorders, ectopic testes, or vanishing testis. The spermatic cord was isolated after incising the cremasteric fascia, and the hernia sac was high-ligated when present. Orchiopexy was performed by placing the testis into the subdartos pouch. Hydrocelectomy was performed using a typical inguinal approach, and the testis was delivered to the groin so the epididymal anomaly could be examined. Written informed consent for data collection and participation in the study was obtained from a parent or guardian. This study received approval from the local ethics committee (CNUH institutional review board). The study procedures complied with the guidelines provided by the Declaration of Helsinki.

Definition of epididymal anomalies

Testicular locations and epididymal anomalies were investigated carefully. According to morphological classification by Barthold and Redman [9], an anomalous epididymis was defined as an anomaly of epididymal fusion consisting of loss of continuity between the testis and the epididymis or long looping epididymis. The epididymis was considered normal when a normal firm attachment between the testis and the caput and cauda epididymis was present.

Statistical analyses

SPSS ver. 17 for Windows software (SPSS Inc., Chicago, IL, USA) was used for statistical analyses. Data were analyzed with the chi-square test. P-values < 0.05 were deemed significant.

Results

A total of 229 boys (258 testes) with undescended testis (group A: 136 boys and 162 testes) or with hydrocele (group B: 93 boys and 96 testes) were included in this study. The mean ages in groups A and B were 24.6 ± 19.7 (range, 8–52 months) and 31.4 ± 20.6 months (range, 10–59 months), respectively. In total, 110 patients (left: 52, right: 58) in group A had unilateral lesions and 26 patients had bilateral lesions. A total of 90 boys in group B had unilateral lesions (left: 55, right: 35) and three had bilateral lesions. The patient demographic data are shown in Table 1.

The incidence of epididymal anomalies was significantly higher in group A than that in B (65.4 % [106/162] vs. 13.5 % [13/96], $P < 0.001$) (Table 2). The incidence of epididymal anomalies in group A was 100 % (20/20) when the affected testis was found in the abdomen, 91.4 % (53/58) when it was found in the inguinal canal and 39.3 % (33/84) when it was found in the distal to external inguinal ring. This result indicates that higher testicular locations were associated with higher frequencies of epididymal anomalies ($P < 0.001$) (Table 3).

Discussion

We evaluated the associations between epididymal anomalies and testicular location or patent processus vaginalis in boys with undescended testis or hydrocele, specially focusing on severity of the epididymal anomalies according to testicular location in boys with undescended testis. The incidence of epididymal anomalies was significantly higher in boys with undescended testis (65.4 %) than in boys with hydrocele (13.5 %).

The estimated overall incidence of epididymal anomalies in boys with undescended testis and hydrocele was 46.1 %, suggesting that testicular location contribute more to epididymal anomalies than patent processus vaginalis. Epididymal anomalies were found more frequently in boys with a higher testicular location. All boys

Table 1 Patient characteristics

	Group A	Group B
Mean age (months)	24.6 ± 19.7	31.4 ± 20.6
No. of boys (n)	136	93
No. of testis (n)	162	96
Bilaterality (n)		
Lt.	52	55
Rt.	58	35
Bilateral	26	3

No. = number, Lt = left, Rt = right, Group A: undescended testis, Group B: hydrocele

Table 2 Type of epididymis in cases of undescended testis and hydrocele

Type of epididymis	No. of boys (%)	
	Group A	Group B
Normal epididymis	56 (34.6)	83 (86.5)
Normal firm attachment	32 (19.8)	45 (46.9)
Widening of the mesentery	24 (14.8)	38 (39.6)
Abnormal epididymis[a]	106 (65.4)	13 (13.5)
Complete separation of the caput	27 (16.7)	0 (0)
Complete separation of the cauda	32 (19.8)	7 (7.3)
Complete separation of the caput and cauda	20 (12.3)	6 (6.3)
Long looping type	27 (16.7)	0 (0)

No. = number, Group A: undescended testis, Group B: hydrocele. [a]Fisher's exact test, $P = 0.001$

with undescended testis located in intra-abdominal area had epididymal anomalies, 91.4 % when the undescended testis was in the inguinal canal, and 39.3 % when it was distal to external inguinal ring.

Controversies exist regarding the role of the epididymis in testicular descent, as epididymal anomalies have been found in 36–79 % of boys with undescended testis. Most studies that have reported anatomical abnormalities of epididymis in boys with undescended testis have been sporadic and used different methods, and no recent data were found [1–7]. Mollaeian et al. reported that epididymal and vas anomalies occur with an overall frequency of 36 % in boys with undescended testis [7]. Gill et al. reported that epididymal anomalies were detected in 43 % of boys with undescended and vanishing testis [4]. In the present study 65.4 % of boys with undescended testis had epididymal anomalies. The reason for the discrepancy may be due to different evaluation tools used in the studies. We used the most recently reported and most widely used epididymal anomaly classification [9].

Factors that have been suggested as important for normal testicular descent include normal gubernaculum, epididymis, and intra-abdominal pressure, and innervation by the genitofemoral nerve of the gubernaculums [10, 11]. However, some boys with normally descended testis have epididymal and vassal anomalies [12]. Elder evaluated the incidence of epididymal anomalies based

Table 3 Epididymal anomalies according to location of undescended testis

Location of testis	Epididymal anomalies No. of testis (%)	P-value
Intra-abdominal	20/20 (100)	
Inguinal canal	53/58 (91.4)	<0.001*
Distal to external inguinal ring	33/84 (39.3)	
Total	106/162 (65.4)	

No number; *Fisher's exact test

on patency of the processus vaginalis in patients with hernia, hydrocele, and undescended testis and suggested that most epididymal abnormalities probably do not contribute to the testicular descent process [6]. That author insisted that an abnormal epididymis with undescended testis maybe an associated finding and not a cause, as he reported that 64 % of cases showed an epididymal anomaly when the processus vaginalis was completely patent, whereas 11 % were abnormal when the processus vaginalis was incompletely patent [6]. We found a rather low incidence of boys with patent processus vaginalis compared to that in Elder's study. We found that 13.3 % of boys with a communicating hydrocele and completely patent processus vaginalis and normally descended testis had epididymal anomalies. This discrepancy may be due to different inclusion criteria for the studies. We compared the incidence of epididymal anomalies between boys with normal descended testis with patent processus vaginalis/hydrocele and boys with undescended testis.

Knowledge of normal testicular anatomy is necessary to understand epididymal anomalies. The normal epididymis curves along the testis but the epididymal body may be slightly detached from the testis body. The epididymal head remains in close proximity with the cranial pole of the testis, while the cauda epididymis disappears within the gubernaculum [13]. The testis and caput epididymis arise from the genital ridge, whereas the body of the epididymis and vassal structure arise from the mesonephric tubules and Wolffian duct. Then, union of the rete testis and mesonephric tubules begins at 12 weeks of gestation. During involution of the mesonephric duct, the testis receives blood from the internal spermatic artery, and the vessel structures derive blood supply from the internal iliac artery. Ductal or epididymal atresia or segmental anomalies may occur die to a vascular accident related to this difference in vascular supply [14].

Epididymal anomalies are associated with maldescent of the testis and may account for impaired future fertility [3, 4]. A clinically important point to consider is possible infertility due to epididymal or vassal malformation of the sperm transporting mechanism. Infertility problems in patients with undescended testis may partly result from obstruction associated with an abnormal epididymis [3, 4]. Koff and Scaletscky reported that an elongated epididymis may present problems for sperm maturation and transportation, and may be associated with severe impairment in future fertility, despite early surgical correction of undescended testis [5].

In the present study, epididymal anomalies were detected in all boys when the affected testis was found in the intra-abdominal area, whereas 91.4 % showed an abnormal condition when the testis was in the inguinal canal and 39.3 % when it was found distal to the external inguinal ring. More severe epididymal anomalies and vassal anomalies are encountered in boys with testis located in the intra-abdominal or high inguinal position in a small case series [1, 4]. Our results suggest that higher testicular locations were associated with more frequent epididymal anomalies, as shown previously. It appears that future fertility issue should be considered when epididymal anomalies are detected at orchiopexy, particularly when the affected testis is located in a high cranial position.

Conclusions

We conclude that epididymal anomalies were more frequent in boys with undescended testis than in boys with hydrocele, and that these anomalies were more frequent when the undescended testis was at a higher level. This result suggests that testicular location, rather than patent processus vaginalis, is associated with epididymal anomalies.

Competing interests
The authors declare no competing interests.

Authors' information
Sun-Ouck Kim, Seong Woong Na, Ho Song Yu, and Dongdeuk Kwon
Department of Urology, Chonnam National University Medical School, Gwangju, Korea.

Authors' contributions
SOK help conceive and design the study and drafted the manuscript. SWN collected the data and performed the statistical analyses. HSY assisted with conception and design of the study. DDK conceived and supervised the study and helped draft the manuscript. All authors have read and approved the final version of the manuscript.

References

1. Marshall FF, Shermeta DW. Epididymal abnormalities associated with undescended testis. J Urol. 1979;121(3):341–3.
2. Mininberg DT, Schlossberg S. The role of the epididymis in testicular descent. J Urol. 1983;129(6):1207–8.
3. Heath AL, Man DW, Eckstein HB. Epididymal abnormalities associated with maldescent of the testis. J Ped Surg. 1984;19(1):47–9.
4. Gill B, Kogan S, Starr S, Reda E, Levitt S. Significance of epididymal and ductal anomalies associated with testicular maldescent. J Urol. 1989;142(2 Pt 2):556–8.
5. Koff WJ, Scaletscky R. Malformations of the epididymis in undescended testis. J Urol. 1990;143(2):340–3.
6. Elder JS. Epididymal anomalies associated with hydrocele/hernia and cryptorchidism: implications regarding testicular descent. J Urol. 1992;148(2 Pt 2):624–6.
7. Mollaeian M, Mehrabi V, Elahi B. Significance of epididymal and ductal anomalies associated with undescended testis: study in 652 cases. Urology. 1994;43(6):857–60.
8. Han CH, Kang SH. Epididymal anomalies associated with patent processus vaginalis in hydrocele and cryptorchidism. J Korean Med Sci. 2002;17(5):660–2.
9. Barthold JS, Redman JF. Association of epididymal anomalies with patent processus vaginalis in hernia, hydrocele and cryptorchidism. J Urol. 1996;156(6):2054–6.
10. Elder JS, Isaacs JT, Walsh PC. Androgenic sensitivity of the gubernaculums testis: evidence for hormonal/mechanical interaction in testicular descent. J Urol. 1982;127(1):170–6.
11. Hutson JM, Beasley SW. Embryological controversies in testicular descent. Semin Urol. 1988;6(2):68–73.
12. Parker RM, Robison JR. Anatomy and diagnosis of torsion of the testicle. J Urol. 1971;106(2):243–7.
13. Scorer CG, Farrington GH. Congenital deformities of the testis and epididymis. London: Butterworths & Co; 1971. p. 136–46.
14. Dickinson SJ. Structural abnormalities in the undescended testis. J Pediatr Surg. 1973;8(4):523–7.

22

A rare presentation of metastatic prostate cancer, initially a suspect for urothelial cell carcinoma of the ureter

Ho Seok Chung[1], Myung Soo Kim[1], Yang Hyun Cho[1], Eu Chang Hwang[1*] ⓘ, Seung Il Jung[1], Taek Won Kang[1], Dong Deuk Kwon[1], Suk Hee Heo[2] and Chan Choi[3]

Abstract

Background: The most common metastatic sites of prostate cancer are the lymph nodes and bone. Ureteral metastasis from prostate cancer is very unusual and only a few cases have been reported.

Case presentation: We describe a 76-year-old male with ureteral metastasis of prostate cancer along with a review of the literature. Initially, based on the diagnostic evaluation, urothelial cell carcinoma of the left distal ureter was suspected. Nephroureterectomy with bladder cuff excision was performed. The final pathologic diagnosis was prostate cancer metastatic to the ureter.

Conclusion: Although rare and the mechanistic link between prostate cancer and distant ureteral metastasis has not been clarified on a clinical basis, this would be included in the differential diagnosis of ureteral lesions in patients with a history of prostate cancer. It is important to recognize this unusual manifestation so that timely appropriate treatment can be initiated.

Keywords: Neoplasm metastasis, Prostate cancer, Ureter

Background

Prostate cancer, one of the most common malignancies in aging men, commonly spreads to lymph nodes and bone [1]. Ureteral metastasis from other primary cancers is very rare, and prostate cancer metastatic to the ureter is extremely rare, as only 45 cases have been reported worldwide in the last century [2, 3]. Herein, we describe a patient with hydronephrosis secondary to a ureteral tumor caused by metastasis from prostate cancer.

Case presentation

A 76-year-old male visited the emergency room in June 2014 because of left flank pain. His past medical history was significant for advanced prostate cancer treated with androgen deprivation therapy (ADT). According to medical records, he first presented at our outpatient department with urinary obstructive symptoms and was

diagnosed with prostate cancer (clinical stage T3bN0M0), with an initial serum prostate specific antigen (PSA) level of 80.69 ng/ml 2 years earlier. At that time, we recommended ADT plus radiation for the treatment of the prostate cancer. However, the patient only received ADT. After 9 months of complete androgen blockade therapy, the PSA had decreased to 0.39 ng/ml, but the patient was lost to follow-up and treatment.

When he again presented at the emergency room in June 2014, the PSA level was 6.75 ng/ml. Abdominal computed tomography (CT) revealed a left distal ureteral enhancing mass about 2.1 cm in length causing hydronephrosis, and no lymphadenopathy (Fig. 1). We initially performed left percutaneous nephrostomy for symptomatic hydronephrosis. Retrograde pyelography showed smooth, marginated filling defects in the left distal ureter (Fig. 2). Cytology showed no pathological results.

Because of suspected urothelial cell carcinoma of the left distal ureter, nephroureterectomy with bladder cuff excision was performed. Pathological examination revealed a lesion consisting of hyperchromatic cells around

---
* Correspondence: urohwang@gmail.com
[1]Department of Urology, Chonnam National University Medical School, 42 Jebongro, Donggu, Gwangju 501-757, Republic of Korea
Full list of author information is available at the end of the article

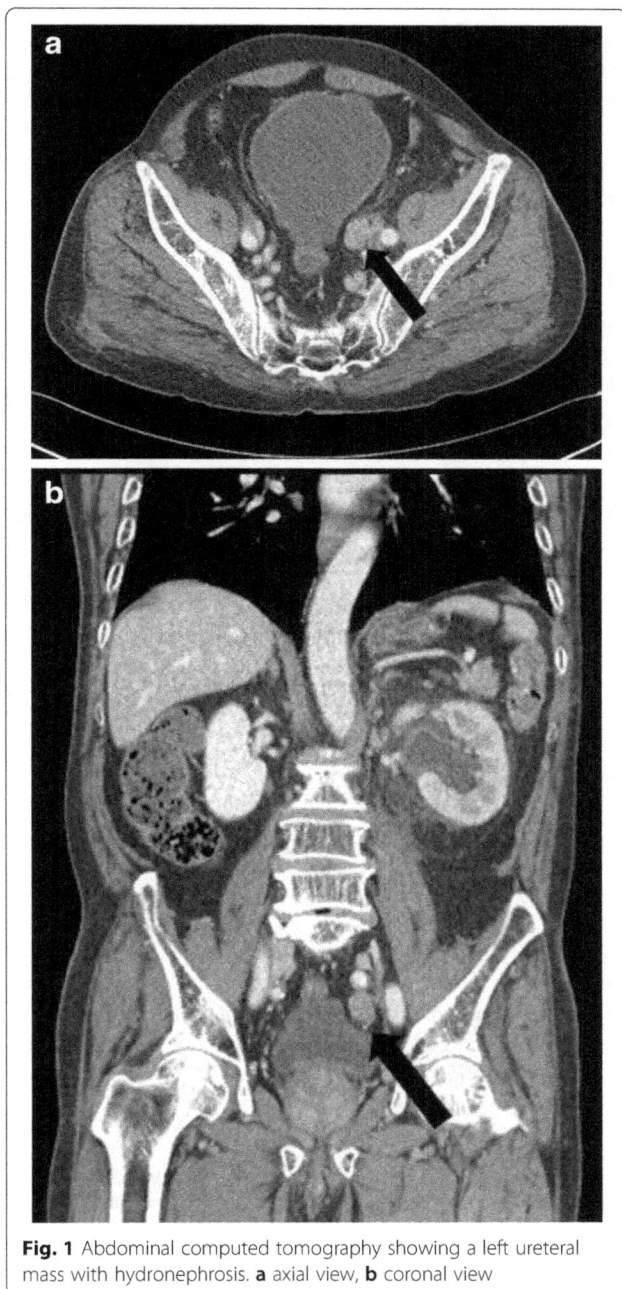

Fig. 1 Abdominal computed tomography showing a left ureteral mass with hydronephrosis. **a** axial view, **b** coronal view

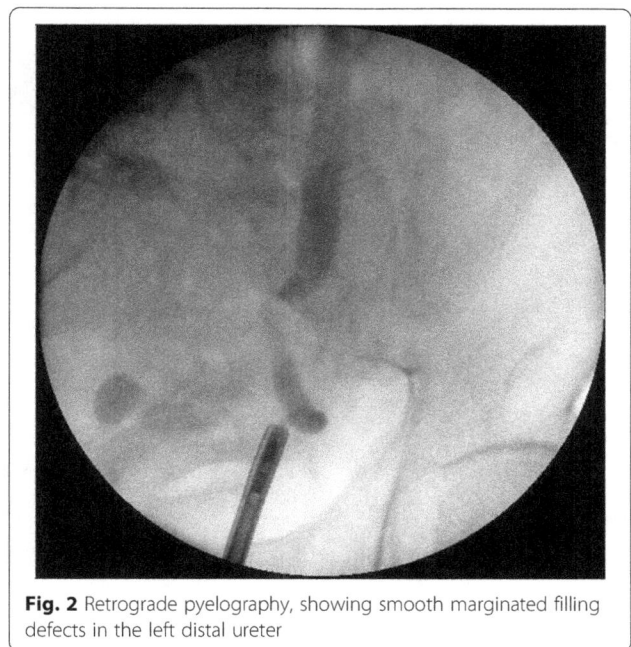

Fig. 2 Retrograde pyelography, showing smooth marginated filling defects in the left distal ureter

the ureter (Fig. 3a). Immunohistochemical staining was strongly positive for prostate cancer markers, including p504S, PSA, and ERG, and negative for p63 (Fig. 3b-e). These findings confirmed a diagnosis of prostate carcinoma metastatic to the left ureter, with no evidence of urothelial cell carcinoma. The tumor invaded the adventitia and muscularis of the ureter, but the distal ureteral surgical margin was not involved by tumor cells.

After the operation, the patient was treated with complete androgen blockade therapy. However, at the 3-month follow-up, the PSA level increased to 8.73 ng/ml.

At the 1-year follow up, further progression with multiple bone metastases, metastatic lymphadenopathy, and right ureteral metastasis led to docetaxel chemotherapy following enzalutamide therapy, but terminating in death after the year.

Discussion

There is increasing discussion about the risk of development of a second primary cancer in prostate cancer patients [4]. Braisch et al. reported an increased risk of a subsequent primary cancer in the renal pelvis and ureter [5]. Ureteral lesions can also occur by metastasis from primary cancer. The most common malignancies that metastasize to the ureter are breast cancer, gastric cancer, and colorectal cancer [6]. However, ureteral metastasis from any type of primary cancer is unusual, because the ureters have segmental lymphatic circulation without continuation in the ureteral wall. Moreover, ureteral metastasis from prostate cancer is extremely rare, because there is no direct periureteral sheath drainage from the prostate [7]. The ureters can be affected by prostate cancer causing hydronephrosis through direct invasion of the tumor around the intravesical ureter. Prostate cancer may metastasize to the ureter through dissemination of malignant cells to the retroperitoneal lymph nodes near the ureter, via the periureteral lymphatic pathway [8].

A total of 38 cases of ureteral metastases from prostate cancer were described by Haddad in 1999 [2]. Since then, few cases have been reported [3, 6]. In these cases, the most common symptom was flank pain caused by ureteral obstruction, as in our case. In addition, most ureteral metastases were treated by nephroureterectomy

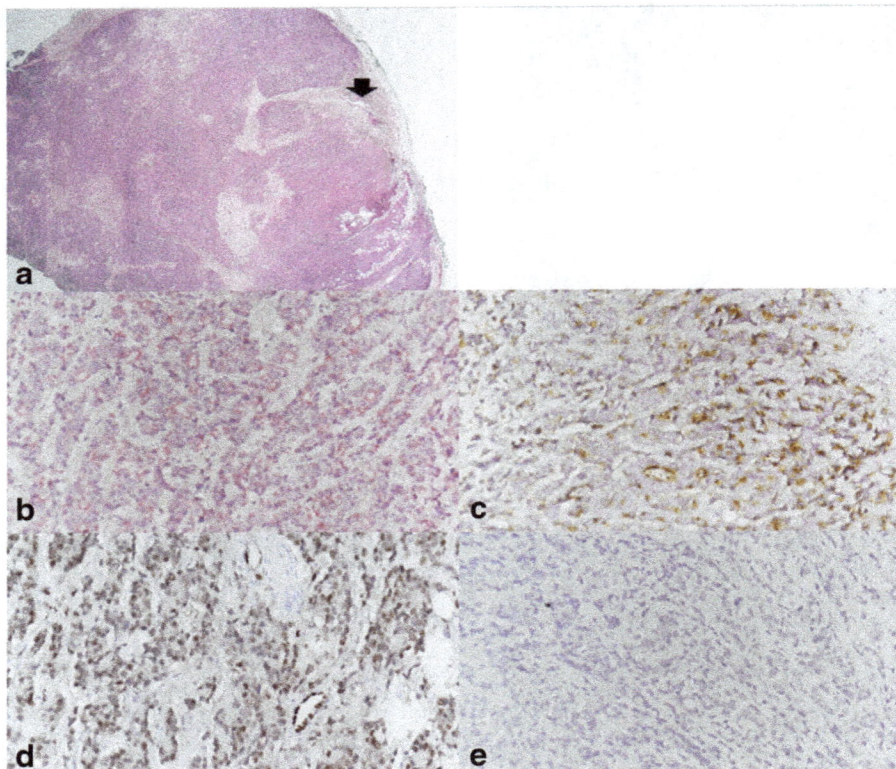

Fig. 3 Pathological features of the involved ureter. **a** Solid sheet of hyperchromatic cells are noted around the ureter. Arrow indicates ureter. (hematoxylin-eosin staining, ×10) (**b, c, d, e**) The tumor cells were positive for p504S, prostate specific antigen (PSA), and ERG, and negative for p63 (immunohistochemical stain, ×200)

because of presumed upper urothelial carcinoma [3]. However, before surgery, diagnostic ureteroscopy and biopsy would be reasonable options for the differential diagnosis [9]. Because nephroureterectomy might have been avoided, and the ureteral mass could be regressed under antiandrogen treatment. For severe flank pain with hydronephrosis, immediate percutaneous nephrostomy or double J stent might be a good choice. Gross hematuria is rarely observed, possibly because most ureteral metastasis occurs beneath the mucosa and by invasion from surrounding tissues [6]. Most case series reported that primary prostate cancer metastatic to ureter had a Gleason score (GS) ≥ 7 [3]. In our case, transrectal ultrasound (TRUS)-guided biopsy revealed prostate cancer with GS 9 (4 + 5). It is possible that prostate cancer with a high GS is associated with the risk of ureteral metastasis [3].

Conclusion

Although rare, the urologist should consider metastatic disease in the differential diagnosis of ureteral lesions in a patient with a history of prostate cancer with a high GS. If ureteral metastasis is confirmed by ureteroscopic biopsy before definitive treatment such as nephroureterectomy,

segmental ureterectomy and ureteroureterostomy could be applied in this condition for preservation of ipsilateral kidney. In addition, conservative treatment using nephrostomy or double J stenting may be helpful to relieve urinary obstructive symptoms.

Abbreviation

ADT: Androgen deprivation therapy; CT: Computed tomography; GS: Gleason score; PSA: Prostate specific antigen; TRUS: Transrectal ultrasound

Acknowledgments

None.

Funding

None.

Authors' contributions

HSC and ECH made contributions to conception and design, of acquisition of data. MSK, SIJ, TWK, and DDK have been involved in revising it critically. YHC, SHH, and CC analyzed and interpreted the patient data. All authors read and approved the final manuscript.

Competing interests

The authors declare that they have no competing interests.

Author details
[1]Department of Urology, Chonnam National University Medical School, 42 Jebongro, Donggu, Gwangju 501-757, Republic of Korea. [2]Department of Radiology, Chonnam National University Medical School, Gwangju, Republic of Korea. [3]Department of Pathology, Chonnam National University Medical School, Gwangju, Republic of Korea.

References
1. Gandaglia G, Abdollah F, Schiffmann J, Trudeau V, Shariat SF, Kim SP, Perrotte P, Montorsi F, Briganti A, Trinh QD, Karakiewicz PI, Sun M. Distribution of metastatic sites in patients with prostate cancer: a population-based analysis. Prostate. 2014;74:210–6.
2. Haddad FS. Metastases to the ureter. Review of the world literature, and three new case reports. J Med Liban. 1999;47:265–71.
3. Huang TB, Yan Y, Liu H, Che JP, Wang GC, Liu M, Zheng JH, Yao XD. Metastatic prostate adenocarcinoma posing as urothelial carcinoma of the right ureter: a case report and literature review. Case Rep Urol. 2014;2014:230852.
4. Van Hemelrijck M, Feller A, Garmo H, Valeri F, Korol D, Dehler S, Rohrmann S. Incidence of second malignancies for prostate cancer. PLoS One. 2014;9: e102596.
5. Braisch U, Meyer M, Radespiel-Tröger M. Risk of subsequent primary cancer among prostate cancer patients in Bavaria, Germany. Eur J Cancer Prev. 2012;21:552–9.
6. Zhang D, Li H, Gan W. Hydronephrosis associated with ureteral metastasis of prostate cancer: a rare case report. Mol Clin Oncol. 2016;4:597–8.
7. Hulse CA, O'Neill TK. Adenocarcinoma of the prostate metastatic to the ureter with an associated ureteral stone. J Urol. 1989;142:1312–3.
8. Zhang T, Wang Q, Min J, Yu D, Xie D, Wang Y, Ding D, Chen L, Zou C, Zhang Z, Wang D. Metastasis to the proximal ureter from prostatic adenocarcinoma: a rare metastatic pattern. Can Urol Assoc J. 2014;8:E859–61.
9. Schneider S, Popp D, Denzinger S, Otto W. A rare location of metastasis from prostate cancer: hydronephrosis associated with ureteral metastasis. Adv Urol. 2012;2012:656023.

23

Bone management in Japanese patients with prostate cancer: hormonal therapy leads to an increase in the FRAX score

Takashi Kawahara[1,2†], Shusei Fusayasu[1†], Koji Izumi[1], Yumiko Yokomizo[1], Hiroki Ito[1], Yusuke Ito[1], Kayo Kurita[1], Kazuhiro Furuya[1], Hisashi Hasumi[1], Narihiko Hayashi[1], Yasuhide Myoshi[2], Hiroshi Miyamoto[3], Masahiro Yao[1] and Hiroji Uemura[1,2*]

Abstract

Background: Osteoporosis is a common consequence of androgen deprivation therapy (ADT) for prostate cancer. Up to 20 % of men on ADT have suffered from fractures within 5 years. The WHO Fracture Risk Assessment Tool (FRAX) has been utilized to predict the 10-year probability of major osteoporotic and hip fracture. However, to date, no large studies assessing the utility of the FRAX score in prostate cancer patients with or without ADT have been performed. We herein evaluated the impact of ADT on the FRAX score in prostate cancer patients.

Methods: The assessment of the FRAX score was performed in a total of 1220 prostate cancer patients, including patients who underwent brachytherapy ($n = 547$), radical prostatectomy ($n = 200$), external beam radiation therapy ($n = 264$) and hormonal therapy alone ($n = 187$) at Yokohama City University Hospital (Yokohama, Japan). We evaluated the effect of ADT on the FRAX score.

Results: Using the FRAX model, the median and mean 10-year probability of a major osteoporotic fracture according to the clinical risk factors alone was 7.9 % (8.8 ± 4.3 %), while the 10-year probability of hip fracture risk was 2.7 % (3.5 ± 3.1 %). In the ADT group, the duration of ADT was correlated with both major osteoporotic risk and hip fracture risk ($R^2 = 0.141$, $p < 0.001$ and $R^2 = 0.166$, $p < 0.001$, respectively). A comparison between the ADT ($n = 187$) and non-ADT ($n = 399$) groups demonstrated that the major fracture risk was > 20 % higher and the hip fracture risk was > 3 % higher in the ADT group than in the non-ADT group (ADT: 10 (5.3 %) and 118 (63.1 %), non-ADT 13 (3.3 %) and 189 (47.4 %), $p < 0.001$ and $p < 0.001$, respectively).

Conclusions: These results suggested that the longer duration of ADT led to an increased FRAX score, and the FRAX score may be a predictor of bone management treatment, particularly in prostate cancer patients.

Keywords: Androgen deprivation therapy, FRAX, Prostate cancer, Bone fracture

Background

Following the widespread implementation of PSA screening, the incidence of prostate cancer has been increasing in Japan [1, 2]. By the end of 2015, 98,400 men will have been newly diagnosed and 12,200 men will

have died of prostate cancer. Many patients diagnosed with prostate cancer are elderly and must be treated with hormonal therapy [3]. Men with prostate cancer are often at risk for other age-related adverse events, such as hip fractures. The risk of hip fractures can increase in men with prostate cancer because the bone density often decreases due to androgen deprivation therapy (ADT), occult bone metastases, or a combination thereof [4–8]. The mechanism is believed to be due to a decrease in sexual hormone levels, which induces receptor activator of nuclear factor-kappa-B ligand (RANKL) expression from osteoblasts. Consequently,

* Correspondence: hu0428@yokohama-cu.ac.jp
†Equal contributors
[1]Department of Urology, Yokohama City University, Graduate School of Medicine, Yokohama, Japan
[2]Department of Urology and Renal Transplantation, Yokohama City University Medical Center, 4-57 Urafune-cho, Minami-ku, Yokohama, Kanagawa 232-0024, Japan
Full list of author information is available at the end of the article

osteoclasts are involved in bone resorption [9]. The skeleton is the third most common site of metastatic cancers, and one-third to one-half of all cancers metastasize to the bone. In prostate cancer, bone metastasis is the most common site for tumor development [10]. Osteoporosis or low bone mineral density (BMD) is a highly prevalent health problem in the elderly as well as in prostate cancer patients treated with ADT. The FRAX score is a fracture risk assessment tool developed by the World Health Organization (WHO) to predict the fracture risk of patients according to clinical risk factors alone or in combination with BMD at the femoral neck [11]. It is a computer-based algorithm which provides the 10-year probability of hip and major osteoporotic fractures (e.g., clinical spine, forearm, hip, or shoulder fracture) according to age, sex, body mass index, and clinical risk factors [12, 13]. There have been no proven methods for predicting pathologic fractures in patients with skeletal metastasis thus far [14].

The fracture risk varies depending on the geographic location and ethnicity, and the FRAX algorithm has been calibrated to account for this [11]. Algorithms are available for diverse ethnic groups, including Asians, based largely on data from Japan and China [13]. Despite its importance, there have been few studies which investigated the fracture risk among Asians with prostate cancer living in Japan [13]. The present study evaluates the risk of developing hip fractures in Japanese men treated at one institute for prostate cancer [4] by examining whether or not ADT could influence the FRAX score.

Methods

Patients

A total of 1220 patients were enrolled in this study. All patients were pathologically diagnosed with prostate cancer and followed-up at Yokohama City University Hospital (Yokohama, Japan) and the FRAX score was calculated once during prostate cancer therapy. Written informed consent was obtained from all patients and this study protocol was approved by the Institutional Review Board at Yokohama City University Hospital.

The study cohort comprised 547 (44.8 %) patients who received brachytherapy, 200 (16.4 %) who received radical prostatectomy, 267 (21.9 %) who received external beam radiation therapy (EBRT), 187 (15.3 %) who received ADT monotherapy, and 19 (1.6 %) who received active surveillance. Excluding the ADT monotherapy group, 615 (50.4 %) patients received ADT in combination with surgical or radiation therapy. (Table 1) In the present study, EBRT was performed as a high-dose intensity-modulated radiation therapy. Some of the patients in the hormonal therapy group had bone metastasis at the time of diagnosis. To exclude bias, men with castration-resistant prostate cancer were not included in the present study. Data from

Table 1 Patients' background

Variables	number (%)
Total	1220 (100.0 %)
Brachy Therapy	547 (44.8 %)
with neo-adjuvant HTx	336 (27.5 %)
without HTx	211 (17.3 %)
Total Prostatectomy	200 (16.4 %)
with adjuvant HTx	50 (4.1 %)
without HTx	150 (12.3 %)
EBRT	267 (21.9 %)
with HTx	229 (18.8 %)
without HTx	38 (3.1 %)
Hormonal Tx only	187 (15.3 %)
Active surveillance	19 (1.6 %)

each subject were entered into the FRAX algorithm and 10-year fracture probabilities were calculated using the clinical risk factors (CRFs) alone. Due to the differences between the FRAX score alone or in combination with BMD, we excluded the FRAX score using the BMD measurement. BMD was measured using dual-energy X-ray absorptiometry of the femoral neck.

The FRAX tool (available at http://www.shef.ac.uk/FRAX/tool.jsp?lang=en) was used to compute the probability of a major osteoporotic event and hip fracture. The date of birth, weight (kg), height (cm), and a yes or no response for various CRFs were entered into the FRAX questionnaire, and the fracture probability was calculated for each subject. Childhood fractures reported by the subjects were not considered to be fragility fractures.

Statistical analysis

All continuous variables were expressed as the means ± SD. The numerical data were compared using Student's t-test. The correlation between 148 variables was determined using Spearman's correlation coefficient. A p-value 149 of 0.05 or less was considered to be statistically significant.

Results

A total of 1220 men were recruited to participate in this study. Their demographic characteristics are presented in Table 2. There were no differences in terms of age, body weight, body height, previous fractures, parent fractured hip, current smoking, use of glucocorticoids, rheumatoid arthritis, secondary osteoporosis, and alcohol consumption of 3 or more units per day, which are risk factors for fracture that are included in the FRAX score (Table 2).

Using the FRAX model, the median and mean 10-year probability of a major osteoporotic fracture according to the CRFs alone was 7.9 % (8.8 ± 4.3 %), while the 10-year probability of hip fracture risk was 2.7 % (3.5 ± 3.1 %).

Table 2 Results in each therapy with prostate cancer patients

Number (%) or median (Mean ± SD)

Variables	Total (1220)	Brachy Tx (547)	Prostatectomy (200)	EBRT (267)	Hormonal monotherapy (187)
Age	74 (73.3 ± 7.1)	73 (72.1 ± 6.4)	72.5 (72.1 ± 7.1)	75 (74.6 ± 6.5)	77 (76.3 ± 8.2)
Weight (kg)	64 (64.3 ± 8.9)	64 (64.6 ± 8.7)	63.6 (63.7 ± 8.3)	65 (65.1 ± 9.2)	63 (63.3 ± 9.9)
Height (cm)	165 (165.5 ± 6.0)	165 (165.7 ± 6.1)	165 (165.4 ± 5.8)	166 (165.7 ± 5.9)	165 (164.6 ± 6.0)
Previous fracture	255 (20.9 %)	111 (20.2 %)	40 (20.0 %)	63 (23.6 %)	35 (18.7 %)
Parent Fractured Hip	90 (7.4 %)	38 (6.9 %)	19 (8.5 %)	18 (6.7 %)	12 (6.4 %)
Current Smoking	138 (11.3 %)	71 (13.0 %)	26 (13.0 %)	22 (8.2 %)	16 (8.6 %)
Glucocorticoid	38 (3.1 %)	3 (0.5 %)	4 (2.0 %)	8 (3.0 %)	19 (10.2 %)
Rheumatoid arthritis	13 (1.1 %)	3 (0.5 %)	3 (1.5 %)	3 (1.1 %)	4 (2.1 %)
Secondary osteoporosis	108 (8.9 %)	45 (8.2 %)	20 (10.0 %)	26 (9.7 %)	18 (9.6 %)
Alcohol 3 or more units per day	380 (31.1 %)	174 (31.8 %)	72 (36.0 %)	95 (35.6 %)	38 (20.3 %)

Forty-nine patients (4.0 %) had a major osteoporotic fracture risk of more than 20 % and 643 patients (52.7 %) had a hip fracture risk of more than 3 %. A comparison between the ADT monotherapy ($n = 187$) and non-ADT ($n = 399$) groups showed that the major osteoporotic fracture risk > 20 % and hip fracture risk > 3 % was significantly higher in the ADT group than in the non-ADT group (ADT: 10 (5.3 %) and 118 (63.1 %), non-ADT 13 (3.3 %) and 189 (47.4 %), $p < 0.001$ and $p < 0.001$, respectively).

The major osteoporotic risk of patients who received periodical ADT in combination with brachytherapy tended to be higher than that of the patients who did not receive ADT ($p = 0.12$). On the other hand, the hip fracture risk of the patients who received ADT in combination with brachytherapy was significantly higher than that of the patients who did not receive ADT ($p = 0.04$) (Fig. 1).

Regarding the therapies for prostate cancer, the major osteoporotic risk was 7.9 % (8.8 ± 4.3 %) in the

brachytherapy group, 8.2 % (9.3 ± 5.2 %) in the radical prostatectomy group, 9.2 % (19.2 ± 5.0) in the EBRT group, and 9.1 % (10.4 ± 5.4 %) in the ADT group. The EBRT and ADT monotherapy groups showed significantly higher major osteoporotic risk than the brachytherapy group ($p < 0.001$ and $p < 0.001$, respectively). The hip fracture risk was 2.7 % (3.5 ± 3.1 %) in the brachytherapy group, 2.9 % (3.7 ± 3.3 %) in the radical prostatectomy group, 3.6 % (4.5 ± 4.0 %) in the EBRT group, and 4.0 % (5.2 ± 4.6 %) in the ADT group. The EBRT and ADT groups showed significantly higher hip fracture risk than both the brachytherapy and prostatectomy groups ($p < 0.001$, $p < 0.001$ and $p = 0.02$, $p < 0.001$, respectively) (Fig. 2).

The major osteoporotic risk > 20 % and hip fracture risk > 3 % were 2.7 and 46.6 % in the brachytherapy group, 3.5 and 48.5 % in the radical prostatectomy group, 5.6 and 60.7 % in the EBRT group, and 5.9 and 70.1 % in the ADT group.

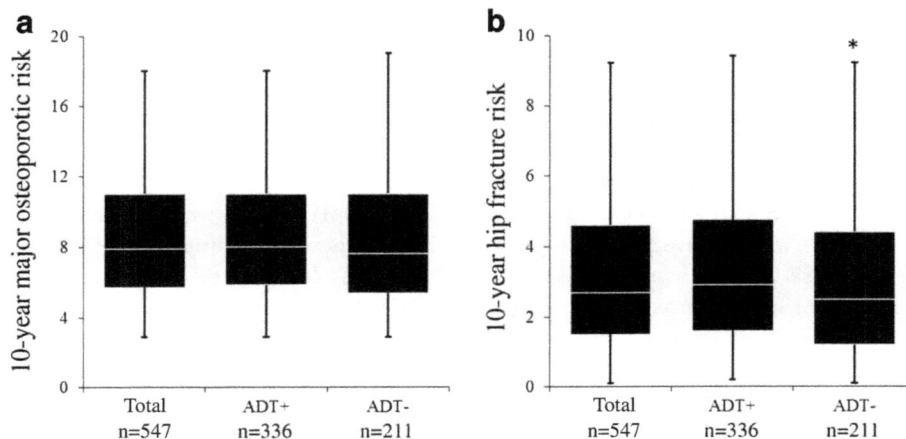

Fig. 1 The FRAX score with or without ADT in the patients who received brachytherapy. The FRAX score between prostate cancer patients who received brachytherapy with ADT and those without ADT was compared. **a** According to the 10-year major osteoporotic risk, the ADT group showed a tendency toward a higher FRAX score ($p = 0.12$). **b** According to the 10-year hip fracture risk, the ADT group showed a significantly higher FRAX score than the non-ADT group ($p = 0.04$)

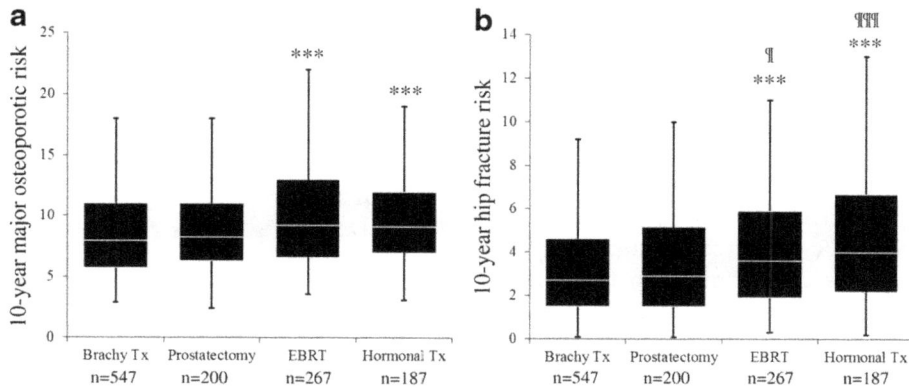

Fig. 2 The FRAX score among various prostate cancer therapies. **a**: The 10-year major osteoporotic risk. The EBRT and ADT monotherapy groups showed significantly higher FRAX scores than the brachytherapy group ($p < 0.001$, $p < 0.001$, respectively). **b**: The 10-year hip fracture risk. The EBRT and ADT monotherapy groups showed higher FRAX scores than both the brachytherapy group ($p < 0.001$, $p < 0.001$, respectively) and the prostatectomy group ($p < 0.05$, $p < 0.001$, respectively)

When analyzed in the ADT monotherapy group, the duration of ADT correlated with both the major osteoporotic risk and hip fracture risk ($R^2 = 0.141$, $p < 0.001$ and $R^2 = 0.166$, $p < 0.001$, respectively) (Fig. 3).

Discussion

This study revealed that ADT increased the FRAX score and that the duration of ADT correlated with the FRAX score. In particular for prostate cancer patients treated with hormonal therapy, fractures are a major complication which can influence both the activities of daily life and life expectancy. Although the median 10-year probability of major osteoporotic and hip fracture risks were not higher than expected, 7.9 and 2.7 %, respectively, ADT elevated those probabilities as expected. It is plausible that patients who received ADT were comparatively older than those who received brachytherapy or RRP. We found that the

FRAX score correlated with the duration of ADT. In most of the patients in the brachytherapy-treated group, ADT was performed within one year. Consequently, there were no large differences occurred within the brachytherapy group regardless of whether the patients received ADT or not. ADT, a common treatment option for patients with prostate cancer that reduces circulating testosterone levels, has a detrimental effect on BMD, leading to a substantial increase in the fracture risk [8, 15, 16]. Men undergoing ADT are four times more likely to develop significant bone deficiency [8, 15]. ADT is known to cause a decrease in BMD, and therefore patients who receive ADT should be assumed to have secondary osteoporosis when calculating the fracture risk using the FRAX score [2, 11]. It has been well established that fractures are associated with significant morbidity and mortality. This study showed that the increase in FRAX score by ADT correlated with the duration

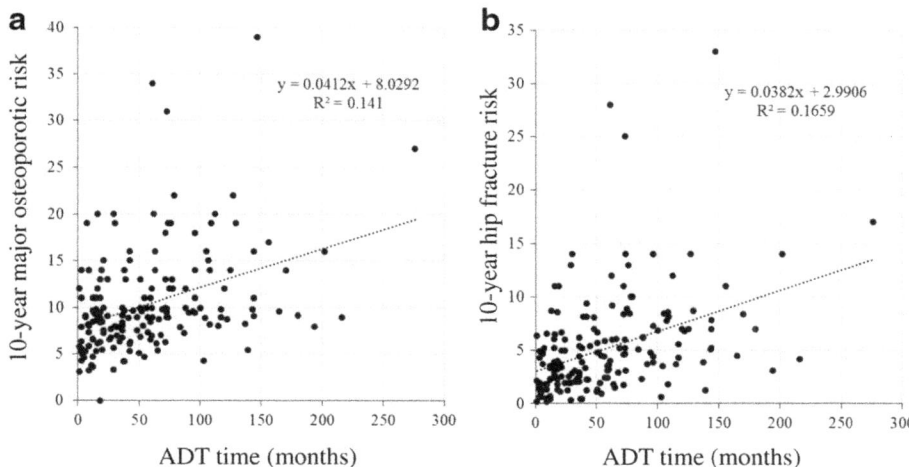

Fig. 3 The FRAX score correlated with the duration of ADT. **a**: The 10-year major osteoporotic risk was positively correlated with the duration of ADT ($R^2 = 0.141$, $p < 0.0001$). **b**: The 10-year hip fracture risk was positively correlated with the duration of ADT ($R^2 = 0.1659$, $p < 0.0001$)

of ADT. During ADT, it might be recommended that patients, especially those who have received ADT for longer periods of time, perform regular muscle-strengthening exercises or increase their vitamin D intake [17].

Although ADT use was positively correlated with the FRAX score ($R^2 = 0.141$), the correlation was not so high. We speculate that the relatively weak correlation resulted from the use of the FRAX score for assessment rather than the DEXA score. We are presently conducting another study to reveal the correlation between the ADT time and the risk of fracture using the DEXA score and some bone related biomarkers. Although there were some indications for intervention to prevent fracture, we set the cut-off point as 20 % in patients with major osteoporosis and 3 % in patients with hip fracture because a 10-year probability of major osteoporotic risk >20 % and hip fracture >3 % is considered to represent a clinically-relevant degree of risk [11] according to the American National Osteoporosis Foundation Clinician's Guide to Prevention and Treatment of Osteoporosis. Our study also found that the ADT group showed a significantly higher fracture risk, which requires fracture prevention.

There are two limitations associated with the present study. First, we assessed the FRAX score and did not determine the patients' real fracture incidences over the 10-year follow-up period. The FRAX was developed by the WHO to predict the fracture risk; however, this score has some ethnicity-related differences, although there are algorithms available for various ethnic groups. In addition, this score is typically used during the clinical courses. Therefore, assessing the fracture risk using the FRAX score is valuable. Second, we did not include the BMD score in this study. BMD is a useful tool to predict fractures and initiate the intervention for bone management [12, 13]. The National Osteoporosis Foundation and other groups have recommended guidelines for BMD testing according to clinical factors. Additionally, the FRAX score may be used with or without BMD. In the present study we did not use BMD testing in our assessment of the FRAX score. In several cases, we also performed dual-energy X-ray absorptiometry (DEXA) to calculate the BMD and found that the FRAX score was reduced when we used BMD (data not shown). In the present study FRAX was therefore used as a screening tool to determine whether or not BMD testing should be performed. The 10-year probability of a major osteoporotic fracture increases when the femur neck T-scores are added to the CRFs in the FRAX algorithm, and this population has a high fracture probability even in the absence of CRFs [18, 19]. However, in clinical use, not all patients undergo DEXA due to the medical costs. Accordingly, we recommend the use of the FRAX score for prostate cancer patients, especially those treated with ADT, as a screening tool in addition to bone management therapy. The FRAX algorithm without the BMD values was superior to BMD alone in identifying the patients at a higher risk of fractures. Therefore, patients with high FRAX scores should receive DEXA in order to avoid additional bone management therapy.

Conclusion

The duration of ADT can influence the FRAX score and the ADT group showed a significantly higher FRAX score and an increased need for additional bone management treatment. This large study is needed to show that ADT influenced the FRAX scores.

Abbreviations

ADT, Androgen deprivation therapy; FRAX, fracture risk assessment tool; BMD, bone mineral density; DEXA, dual-energy X-ray absorptiometry; CRF, clinical risk factors; RRP, radical retropubic prostatectomy

Acknowledgement

We thank S Honjo, T Iijima and S Uchiyama for statistical survey. This study was supported by a MEXT/JSPS KAKENHI Grant.

Authors' contributions

TK and HU contributed to drafting the manuscript, HU and SF were involved in the design of the study. KI, YY, HI, YI, KK, KF, HH, NH, YM, and HM were study investigators, MY was responsible for clinical trial management. TK was responsible for the statistical analysis. All authors read and approved the final manuscript.

Competing interests

The authors declare that they have no competing interests.

Author details

[1]Department of Urology, Yokohama City University, Graduate School of Medicine, Yokohama, Japan. [2]Department of Urology and Renal Transplantation, Yokohama City University Medical Center, 4-57 Urafune-cho, Minami-ku, Yokohama, Kanagawa 232-0024, Japan. [3]Departments of Pathology and Urology, Johns Hopkins University School of Medicine, Baltimore, USA.

References

1. Polascik TJ, Oesterling JE, Partin AW. Prostate specific antigen: a decade of discovery—what we have learned and where we are going. J Urol. 1999; 162(2):293–306.
2. Kawahara T, Ishiguro H, Hoshino K, Teranishi J, Miyoshi Y, Kubota Y, Uemura H. Analysis of NSAID-activated gene 1 expression in prostate cancer. Urol Int. 2010;84(2):198–202.
3. Rosenberg L, Lawlor GO, Zenlea T, Goldsmith JD, Gifford A, Falchuk KR, Wolf JL, Cheifetz AS, Robson SC, Moss AC. Predictors of endoscopic inflammation in patients with ulcerative colitis in clinical remission. Inflamm Bowel Dis. 2013;19(4):779–84.
4. Valery R, Mendenhall NP, Nichols Jr RC, Henderson R, Morris CG, Su Z, Mendenhall WM, Williams CR, Li Z, Hoppe BS. Hip fractures and pain following proton therapy for management of prostate cancer. Acta Oncol. 2013;52(3):486–91.
5. Wadhwa VK, Weston R, Mistry R, Parr NJ. Long-term changes in bone mineral density and predicted fracture risk in patients receiving androgen-deprivation therapy for prostate cancer, with stratification of treatment based on presenting values. BJU Int. 2009;104(6):800–5.

6.   Hatano T, Oishi Y, Furuta A, Iwamuro S, Tashiro K. Incidence of bone
     fracture in patients receiving luteinizing hormone-releasing hormone
     agonists for prostate cancer. BJU Int. 2000;86(4):449–52.
7.   Melton 3rd LJ, Lieber MM, Atkinson EJ, Achenbach SJ, Zincke H, Therneau
     TM, Khosla S. Fracture risk in men with prostate cancer: a population-based
     study. J Bone Mineral Res Off J Am Soc Bone Mineral Res. 2011;26(8):1808–15.
8.   Shahinian VB, Kuo YF, Freeman JL, Goodwin JS. Risk of fracture after
     androgen deprivation for prostate cancer. N Engl J Med. 2005;352(2):154–64.
9.   Schulman C, Irani J, Aapro M. Improving the management of patients with
     prostate cancer receiving long-term androgen deprivation therapy. BJU Int.
     2012;109 Suppl 6:13–21.
10. Michaeli DA, Inoue K, Hayes WC, Hipp JA. Density predicts the activity-
     dependent failure load of proximal femora with defects. Skelet Radiol. 1999;
     28(2):90–5.
11. Kanis JA, Oden A, Johansson H, Borgstrom F, Strom O, McCloskey E. FRAX
     and its applications to clinical practice. Bone. 2009;44(5):734–43.
12. Johansson H, Kanis JA, Oden A, Johnell O, McCloskey E. BMD, clinical risk
     factors and their combination for hip fracture prevention. Osteoporosis Int J
     Established Result Cooperation Between Eur Foundation Osteoporosis
     National Osteoporosis Foundation USA. 2009;20(10):1675–82.
13. Kuruvilla K, Kenny AM, Raisz LG, Kerstetter JE, Feinn RS, Rajan TV. Importance
     of bone mineral density measurements in evaluating fragility bone fracture
     risk in Asian Indian men. Osteoporosis Int J Estab Result Cooperation
     Between Eur Foundation Osteoporosis National Osteoporosis Foundation
     USA. 2011;22(1):217–21.
14. Hipp JA, Springfield DS, Hayes WC. Predicting pathologic fracture risk in the
     management of metastatic bone defects. Clin Orthop Relat Res. 1995;312:
     120–35.
15. James 3rd H, Aleksic I, Bienz MN, Pieczonka C, Iannotta P, Albala D, Mariados
     N, Mouraviev V, Saad F. Comparison of fracture risk assessment tool score to
     bone mineral density for estimating fracture risk in patients with advanced
     prostate cancer on androgen deprivation therapy. Urology. 2014;84(1):164–8.
16. Saad F, Abrahamsson PA, Miller K. Preserving bone health in patients with
     hormone-sensitive prostate cancer: the role of bisphosphonates. BJU Int.
     2009;104(11):1573–9.
17. Cosman F, de Beur SJ, LeBoff MS, Lewiecki EM, Tanner B, Randall S, Lindsay R,
     National Osteoporosis F. Clinician's Guide to Prevention and Treatment of
     Osteoporosis. Osteoporos Int. 2014;25(10):2359–81.
18. Lewiecki EM, Watts NB, McClung MR, Petak SM, Bachrach LK, Shepherd JA,
     Downs RW, Jr., International Society for Clinical D: Official positions of the
     international society for clinical densitometry. J Clin Endocrinol Metab. 2004;
     89(8):3651–5.
19. Force USPST. Screening for osteoporosis in postmenopausal women:
     recommendations and rationale. Ann Intern Med. 2002;137(6):526–5.

24

Frequent mismatch-repair defects link prostate cancer to Lynch syndrome

Mev Dominguez-Valentin[1], Patrick Joost[1], Christina Therkildsen[2], Mats Jonsson[1], Eva Rambech[1] and Mef Nilbert[1,2]*

Abstract

Background: A possible role for prostate cancer in Lynch syndrome has been debated based on observations of mismatch-repair defective tumors and reports of an increased risk of prostate cancer in mutation carriers. Potential inclusion of prostate cancer in the Lynch syndrome tumor spectrum is relevant for family classification, risk estimates and surveillance recommendations in mutation carriers.

Methods: We used the population-based Danish HNPCC-register to identify all prostate cancers that developed in mutation carriers and in their first-degree relatives from 288 Lynch syndrome families. The tumors were evaluated for clinicopathologic features and mismatch-repair status, and the cumulative risk of prostate cancer was determined.

Results: In total, 28 prostate cancers developed in 16 mutation carriers and in 12 first-degree relatives at a median age of 63 years. The majority of the tumors were high-grade tumors with Gleason scores 8–10. Prostate cancer was associated with mutations in *MSH2, MLH1* and *MSH6* with loss of the respective mismatch repair protein in 69 % of the tumors, though a MSI-high phenotype was restricted to 13 % of the tumors. The cumulative risk of prostate cancer at age 70 was 3.7 % (95 % CI: 2.3–4.9).

Conclusion: We provide evidence to link prostate cancer to Lynch syndrome through demonstration of MMR defective tumors and an increased risk of the disease, which suggests that prostate cancer should be considered in the diagnostic work-up of Lynch syndrome.

Keywords: Mismatch repair deficiency, Microsatellite instability, *MLH1, MSH2, MSH6*

Background

Lynch syndrome is a multi-tumor syndrome with the highest risks for colorectal cancer and endometrial cancer though a number of other tumor types, e.g. cancer of the urinary tract, the small bowel and the ventricle, ovarian cancer, brain tumors and skin tumors develop at increased incidence [1, 2]. Other tumor types assumed to represent sporadic tumors in families with hereditary cancer, e.g. breast cancer, pancreatic cancer and sarcoma may indeed develop as part of the syndrome. This is suggested based on identification of mismatch repair (MMR) defective tumors of these subtypes and demonstration of an increased risk of these tumor types in mutation carriers [3–10].

Prostate cancer is the most common tumor type in men in the Western world with an estimated lifetime risk of 18 % and a median age at diagnosis of 67 years [1]. Worldwide, prostate cancer is the sixth common tumor with more than 250,000 deaths annually [11]. In Denmark, prostate cancer constitutes 23 % of all male cancers with an estimated risk of 10 % for disease development before age 75 [12]. The role of prostate cancer in Lynch syndrome is unresolved though molecular investigations and epidemiologic studies have suggested a potential link to the syndrome [1, 8, 13]. The MMR system has been suggested to influence prostate carcinogenesis e.g. through an increased risk of prostate cancer linked to single nucleotide polymorphisms in *MLH1* and *MSH3*, and a role for complex structural rearrangements in *MSH2* and *MSH6* as a mechanism underlying the hypermutation in aggressive prostate cancer [14–20]. We assessed the role of prostate cancer in the Danish Lynch syndrome cohort with characterization of MMR status and risk estimates.

* Correspondence: mef.nilbert@med.lu.se
[1]Institute of Clinical Sciences, Division of Oncology and Pathology, Lund University, SE-22381 Lund, Sweden
[2]HNPCC-Register, Clinical Research Centre, Copenhagen University Hospital, Hvidovre, Denmark

Methods

Patients and tumor samples

The Danish Hereditary Non-Polyposis Colorectal Cancer (HNPCC) Register is a national Danish register containing all families identified with proven or suspected hereditary cancer. Through research collaborations, data from the register is freely available. We obtained data on all adeno-carcinomas of the prostate that had developed in carriers of a disease-predisposing MMR gene mutation in *MLH1, MSH2, MSH6* or *PMS2* and in their first-degree relatives. Clinical data were obtained from pathology reports and clinical files. All patients provided an informed consent for inclusion into the Danish HNPCC register during genetic counseling sessions. Ethical approval for the study was granted from the Ethical Committee at The Capital Region of Copenhagen, Denmark (H-D-2007–0032). All tumor specimens available were collected for analysis of MMR status. The tumors were pathologically reviewed regarding their Gleason scores and the presence of tumor-infiltrating lymphocytes (TIL) (cut-off ≥4 per high-power field) [8, 21] by a pathologist (PJ), who was blinded to MMR status.

Immunohistochemistry and analysis of microsatellite instability

All tumors were immunohistochemically stained for the MMR proteins MLH1, PMS2, MSH2 and MSH6. Briefly, 4-μm sections were placed on SuperFrost® Plus microscope slides. Antigen retrieval was performed in a pressure boiler in Target Retrieval Solution, pH 9 (Dako, Glostrup, Denmark) and stained in an automated immunostainer (Autostainer Plus, Dako, Glostrup, Denmark) using Dako EnVision™FLEX+ Detection System, Peroxidase/DAB, Rabbit/Mouse (Dako, Glostrup, Denmark), according to the manufacturers' instructions. The antibodies used were MLH1, clone ES05 (Dako, Glostrup, Denmark, dilution 1:100), PMS2, clone A16-4 (BD Pharmingen, San Diego, CA, dilution 1:300), MSH2, clone FE11 (Calbiochem, Merck KgaA, Darmstadt, Germany, dilution 1:100), and MSH6, clone EPR3945 (Epitomics, Burlingame, dilution 1:100). Tumor MMR protein expression was assessed as retained (normal), lost, or reduced (i.e. tumor cell staining intensity was reduced compared with that of the normal internal control).

For analysis of microsatellite instability (MSI), non-necrotic tumor areas were macro-dissected from the paraffin-embedded tumor blocks. DNA extraction was performed from three 5-mm sections using the Qiagen FFPE Kit (Qiagen Valencia, CA) according to the manufacturer's instructions. DNA concentration was determined using a Qubit Fluorometric Quantitation (Invitrogen) and the products run on a 3130XL Genetic Analyzer (Applied Biosystems, Foster City, CA). The analysis was performed using the MSI Analysis System, Version 1.2 (Promega, Madison, WI) and included the 5 mononucleotide markers BAT-25 BAT-26, NR-21, NR-24, and MONO-27 (Promega, MSI Analysis System, Version 1.2, Madison, WI). The results were evaluated using GeneMapper Software Version 4.0 (Applied Biosystems, Foster City, CA) and defined as MSI high when ≥2 markers were unstable, MSI low when one marker was unstable and MSS when none of the markers were unstable.

Statistical analysis

Genotypic and phenotypic data from all mutation carriers and their first-degree relatives were transferred into R i386 3.1.0 (R: A Language and Environment for Statistical Computing, 2011, R Foundation for Statistical Computing, Vienna, Austria). *EPCAM* mutations (identified in one family) were pooled together with *MSH2* mutations, while 7 *PMS2* mutation families (none of which contained any prostate cancers) were excluded from the analyses. Mutation carriers were weighted by 1 and first-degree relatives by 0.5 motivated by a 50 % risk of carrying the inherited mutation. The event times used were age at diagnosis, age at death or current age (censored at May 14, 2014). Cumulative incidences were calculated with death as a competing risk (cmprsk: Subdistribution Analysis of Competing Risks, 2011, Bob Gray, R package version 2.2-2). Confidence intervals were calculated at age 70 using a non-parametric bootstrap. Permutation tests with 10,000 replicates were used to calculate p-values with significance set at $p < 0.05$.

Results

In total, 288 Lynch syndrome families with disease-predisposing germline mutations in *MLH1, MSH2, MSH6* or *PMS2* were identified in the Danish HNPCC register. In this cohort of 1609 males (677 mutation carriers and 932 first-degree relatives), prostate cancer developed in 16 mutation carriers and in 12 first-degree relatives. The median age at diagnosis of prostate cancer was 61 (range 52–78) years for the mutation carriers and 63 (range 53–81) years for the first-degree relatives. All tumors were adenocarcinomas with Gleason scores between 6 and 10. The tumors were linked to disease-predisposing mutations in *MSH2* ($n = 14$), *MLH1* ($n = 8$) and *MSH6* ($n = 6$) (Table 1). Among the 28 men diagnosed with prostate cancer, 16 had a previous cancer diagnosis, which included colon cancer in 15 cases. Four prostate cancers had developed among the 593 male non-mutation carriers (0.67 %) compared to 2.22 % of the mutation carriers and 1.39 % of the first-degree relatives.

Tumor tissue could be retrieved for MMR analysis from 16 tumors (derived from 10 mutation carriers and 6 first-degree relatives), with loss of expression for the respective MMR proteins in 11/16 tumors (including 7/

Table 1 Prostate cancers analyzed for mismatch-repair function

ID no.	Status	Age at diagnosis	Gleason score	TILs ≥4/HPF	MMR gene mutation	Immunohistochemical staining				MSI
						MLH1	PMS2	MSH2	MSH6	
P32	Carrier	56	9 (4 + 5)	NA	MSH2 c.(?_-68)_366 + ?del			NA		
P7	Carrier	53	8 (4 + 4)	y	MSH2 c.560G > T	+	+	−	−	MSI-L
P14	FDR	63	9 (5 + 4)	y	MSH2 c.646-?_1276 + ?del	+	+	−	−	MSI-L
P8	Carrier	69	9 (4 + 5)	y	MSH2 c.892C > T	+	+	−	−	MSI-L
P33	FDR	77	NA	NA	MSH2 c. 942 + 3A > T			NA		
P34	FDR	62	NA	NA	MSH2 c. 942 + 3A > T			NA		
P5	Carrier	69	8 (3 + 5)	NA	MSH2 c. 942 + 3A > T			NA		
P31	FDR	56	10 (5 + 5)	NA	MSH2 c. 942 + 3A > T			NA		
P10	Carrier	76	7 (4 + 3)	y	MSH2 c.1786_788delAAT	+	+	−	−	MSI-L
P20	FDR	81	10 (5 + 5)	y	MSH2 c.1786_788delAAT	+	+	−	−	MSI-H
P9	Carrier	52	8 (4 + 4)	y	MSH2 c.1906G > C	+	+	−	−	MSS
P30	Carrier	60	NA	NA	MSH2 c.2038C > T			NA		
P12	Carrier	57	6 (3 + 3)	y	MSH2 c.2347delC	+	+	−	−	MSI-H
P35	Carrier	67	NA	NA	MLH1 c. 350C > T			NA		
P11	Carrie	63	7 (4 + 3)	n	MLH1 c.588 + 5G > A	+	+	+	+	MSS
P22	FDR	56	7 (3 + 4)	y	MLH1 c.1537_1547delInsC	−	−	+	+	MSS
P2	Carrier	60	8 (4 + 4)	n	MLH1 c.1667 + 2delTAAATCAinsATTT	+	+	+	+	MSS
P13	FDR	63	9 (4 + 5)	y	MLH1 c.1667 + 2delTAAATCAinsATTT	−	−	+	+	MSI-L
P18	FDR	63	7 (3 + 4)	y	MLH1 c.1667 + 2delTAAATCAinsATTT	+	+	+	+	MSS
P6	FDR	80	7 (3 + 4)	n	MLH1 c.1732-2A > T	+	+	+	+	MSS
P1	Carrier	72	NA	NA	MLH1 c.1732-2A > T			NA		
P16	Carrier	74	10 (5 + 5)	n	MLH1 c.1852_54delAAG	+	+	+	+	MSS
P37	Carrier	58	NA	NA	MSH6 C.1444C > T			NA		
P3	Carrier	58	8 (4 + 4)	y	MSH6 c.1483C > T	+	+	−	−	MSI-L
P15	Carrier	78	6 (3 + 3)	y	MSH6 c.3647-1G > A	+	+	+	−	MSS
P38	FDR	81	NA	NA	MSH6 c. 3609_3612delTGCA			NA		
P36	FDR	53	NA	NA	MSH6 c.3992 + 1 T > C			NA		
P17	FDR	57	7 (3 + 4)	NA	MSH6 c.3992 + 1 T > C			NA		

Abbreviations: FDR first-degree relatives, *HPF* high-power field, *MMR* mismatch repair, *MSI* microsatellite instability high/low, *MSS* microsatellite stability, *n* no, *TIL* tumour-infiltrating lymphocytes, *y* yes, *NA* Not available

10 tumors from mutation carriers (Table 1). Notably, MMR protein loss was detected in all *MSH2* and *MSH6* associated tumors prostate cancers. MSI analysis applied standard diagnostic markers and revealed a MSI-high phenotype in 2 tumors, a MSI-low phenotype in 6 tumors and a MSS phenotype in 8 tumors (Table 1, Fig. 1). Notably, all *MLH1*-associated tumors has a microsatellite stable phenotype. Pathologic review revealed TIL in 12/16 tumors, including all MMR defective tumors. Gleason scores tended to be high in MMR defective prostate cancer with Gleason scores of 8–10 in 7/11 MMR defective prostate cancers (Table 1).

Risk analysis could be performed based on 1488/1609 males from whom complete data were available. The cumulative risk for prostate cancers at age 70 was 3.7 % (95 % CI: 2.32–4.92) in mutation carriers and first-degree relatives compared to 593 for non-mutation carriers in these families (Fig. 2a). No significant differences could be demonstrated in relation to disease-predisposing gene; *MLH1* 4.4 % (95 % CI: 1.44; 7.04), *MSH2* 3.9 % (95 % CI: 1.96–5.70) and *MSH6* 2.5 % (95 % CI: 0.56–4.12) (Fig. 2b).

Discussion

In the Danish Lynch syndrome cohort, 28 prostate cancers were identified. These tumors were diagnosed at a median age of 63 years, which is in line with reports of prostate cancers diagnosed at median 59–65 years in Lynch syndrome [9, 22–26]. MMR protein loss in line with the underlying MMR gene mutation was identified in

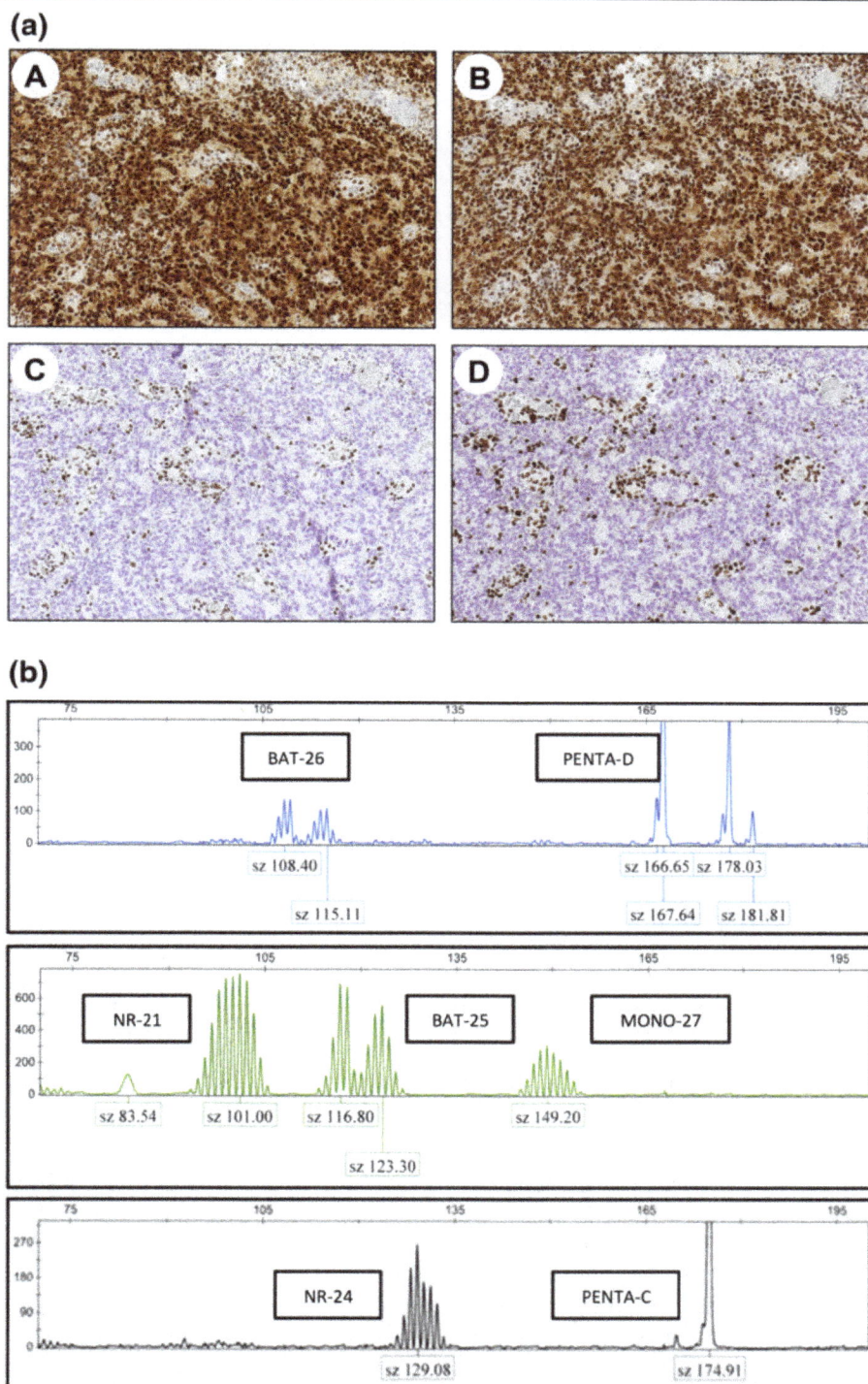

Fig. 1 a A prostate cancer from an individual with a *MSH2* mutation showing normal expression for MLH1 and PMS2 (**A** and **B**) and loss of expression for MSH2 and MSH6 (**C** and **D**); **b** microsatellite instability for the markers BAT-26, NR-21, BAT-25, NR-24 and MONO-27 in the same prostate cancer

11/16 prostate cancers, including all *MSH2* and *MSH6* mutant tumors and supports observations of a high degree, 69–100 %, of MMR deficiency in prostate cancers in Lynch syndrome [8, 24, 27]. *MSH2* mutations were found in 14/28 prostate cancers and this MMR gene has been linked to an expanded spectrum of extracolonic tumors

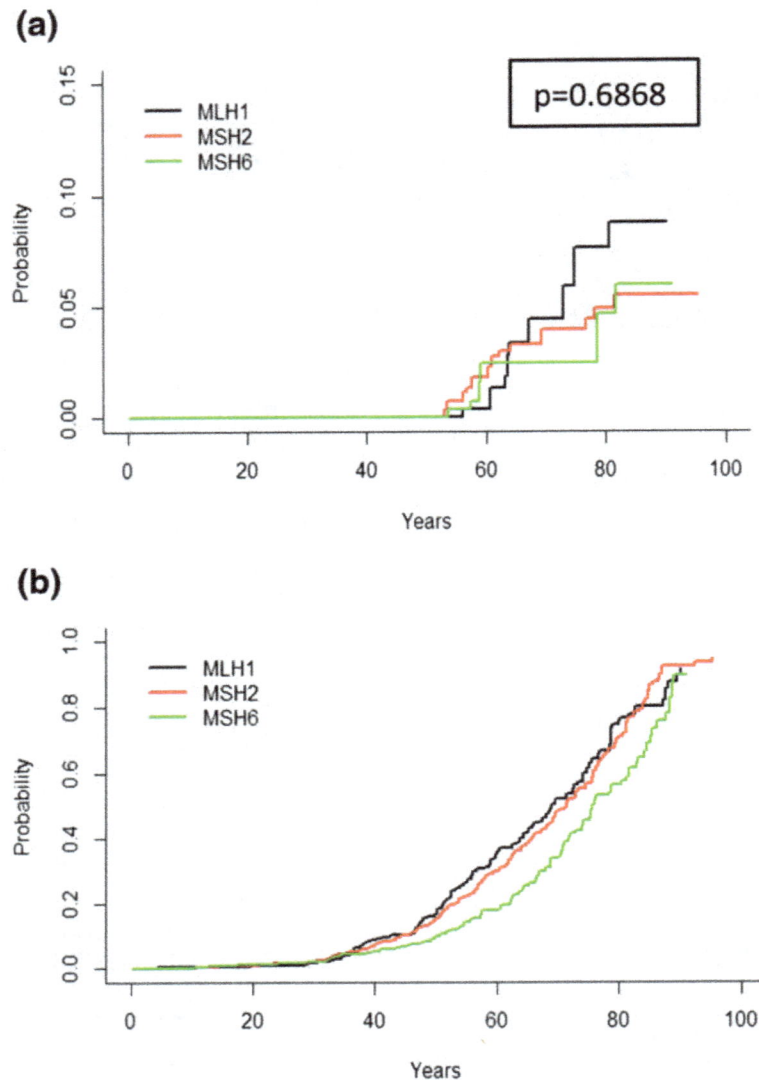

Fig. 2 Non-parametric risk estimates showing **a** age-specific cumulative risks for prostate cancer; **b** mortality rates in *MLH1*, *MSH2* and *MSH6* families

with an increased risk for e.g. urothelial cancer, brain tumors and skin tumors [6, 8–10, 22–24, 28, 29]. A MSI-high phenotypes was identified only in 2 prostate cancers using a standard MSI markers panel with an additional number of tumors showing a MSI-low phenotype. This observation supports an earlier report of MSI defects in 4–10 % of Lynch syndrome associated prostate cancers [30]. MSI phenotypes were predominantly observed in *MSH2* and *MSH6* associated tumors and could potentially reflect alternate mechanisms by which MSI is acquired in prostate cancer or an association with tumor differentiation [19] [31]. These observations support a role for MMR defects in prostate carcinogenesis and link germline MMR defects to the development of prostate cancer.

MMR-defective tumors show histopathologic characteristics that include poor differentiation and lymphocytic reactions with an increased number of TIL [8]. Blinded analysis of TIL showed a striking correlation with MMR defects with TIL in all MMR defective prostate cancer and in only 1/5 MSS and MMR proficient prostate cancers. TIL has been suggested to represent an adverse prognostic factor in prostate cancer [32–34]. Of the 11 MMR defective prostate cancers in our study, 7 had a Gleason score of ≥8 suggesting aggressive tumors. Hereditary prostate cancers, also associated with *BRCA2* mutations, have been suggested to have an accelerated tumor development an aggressive phenotype. Knowledge about prostate cancer in Lynch syndrome is scarce, but early age at onset, frequent TIL and an aggressive phenotype warrants further investigation related to a possible role for surveillance and potential therapeutic implications from e.g. immunotherapy with PD-1 inhibitors [35].

The cumulative risk of prostate cancer at age 70 was 3.7 % in mutation carriers. No significant differences were discerned in relation to disease-predisposing gene, but this analysis is based on very limited numbers. Under the assumption that MMR-defective prostate cancer signifies Lynch syndrome, mutation carriers can be estimated to be at a 2- to 3-fold increased risk of prostate cancer compared to the general population [1, 13]. Growing data suggest that MMR defects in prostate cancer may signify chromoplexy, whereby a single hit infers genetic complexity of relevance for prostate cancer initiation, progression and therapeutics [18, 19].

Conclusions

The Danish Lynch syndrome cohort contains 28 prostate cancers that developed at a median age of 63 years, showed high Gleason scores and frequent TILs. The tumors were predominantly linked to *MSH2* mutations. Frequent MMR defects consistent with the underlying germline defects suggest that prostate cancer is included in Lynch syndrome tumor spectrum and should be considered during genetic counseling.

Availability of data and materials

All available data from the cases included are summarized in Table 1. Additional data on these individuals and their families (e.g. detailed mutation data and family data) are freely available from the Danish HNPCC-register though contact with the principal investigator, Mef.Nilbert@regionh.dk.

Abbreviations

CI: confidence interval; HNPCC: hereditary nonpolyposis colorectal cancer; MMR: mismatch repair; MSI: microsatellite instability; MSS: microsatellite stable; TIL: tumor-infiltrating lymphocytes..

Competing interests

The authors declare that they have no competing interests.

Authors' contributions

All authors have read and approved of the final version of the manuscript. MDV: Protocol/project development, experimental analysis, data collection and analysis, manuscript writing/editing. PJ: Protocol/project development, data analysis, manuscript writing/editing. CT: Data collection or management, data analysis, manuscript writing/editing. MJ: Experimental support, manuscript writing/editing. ER: Experimental support, manuscript writing/editing. MN: Protocol/project development, data management, manuscript editing.

Acknowledgments

Financial support was granted from the Swedish Cancer Society, the Danish Cancer Society, the Nilsson Cancer Fund and the Kamprad Cancer Fund and the ALF Funds at the Lund University Medical Faculty.

References

1. Raymond VM, Mukherjee B, Wang F, Huang SC, Stoffel EM, Kastrinos F, Syngal S, Cooney KA, Gruber SB. Elevated risk of prostate cancer among men with Lynch syndrome. J Clin Oncol. 2013;31(14):1713–8.
2. Win AK, Lindor NM, Winship I, Tucker KM, Buchanan DD, Young JP, Rosty C, Leggett B, Giles GG, Goldblatt J, et al. Risks of colorectal and other cancers after endometrial cancer for women with Lynch syndrome. J Natl Cancer Inst. 2013;105(4):274–9.
3. Antoniou A, Pharoah PD, Narod S, Risch HA, Eyfjord JE, Hopper JL, Loman N, Olsson H, Johannsson O, Borg A, et al. Average risks of breast and ovarian cancer associated with BRCA1 or BRCA2 mutations detected in case Series unselected for family history: a combined analysis of 22 studies. Am J Hum Genet. 2003;72(5):1117–30.
4. Nilbert M, Therkildsen C, Nissen A, Akerman M, Bernstein I. Sarcomas associated with hereditary nonpolyposis colorectal cancer: broad anatomical and morphological spectrum. Fam Cancer. 2009;8(3):209–13.
5. Walsh MD, Buchanan DD, Cummings MC, Pearson SA, Arnold ST, Clendenning M, Walters R, McKeone DM, Spurdle AB, Hopper JL, et al. Lynch syndrome-associated breast cancers: clinicopathologic characteristics of a case series from the colon cancer family registry. Clin Cancer Res. 2010; 16(7):2214–24.
6. van der Post RS, Kiemeney LA, Ligtenberg MJ, Witjes JA, Hulsbergen-van de Kaa CA, Bodmer D, Schaap L, Kets CM, van Krieken JH, Hoogerbrugge N. Risk of urothelial bladder cancer in Lynch syndrome is increased, in particular among MSH2 mutation carriers. J Med Genet. 2010;47(7):464–70.
7. da Silva FC, de Oliveira LP, Santos EM, Nakagawa WT, Aguiar Junior S, Valentin MD, Rossi BM, de Oliveira Ferreira F. Frequency of extracolonic tumors in Brazilian families with Lynch syndrome: analysis of a hereditary colorectal cancer institutional registry. Fam Cancer. 2010;9(4):563–70.
8. Rosty C, Walsh MD, Lindor NM, Thibodeau SN, Mundt E, Gallinger S, Aronson M, Pollett A, Baron JA, Pearson S, et al. High prevalence of mismatch repair deficiency in prostate cancers diagnosed in mismatch repair gene mutation carriers from the colon cancer family registry. Fam Cancer. 2014;13(4):573–82.
9. Haraldsdottir S, Hampel H, Wei L, Wu C, Frankel W, Bekaii-Saab T, de la Chapelle A, Goldberg RM. Prostate cancer incidence in males with Lynch syndrome. Genet Med. 2014;16(7):553–7.
10. Joost P, Therkildsen C, Dominguez-Valentin M, Jonsson M, Nilbert M. Urinary Tract Cancer in Lynch Syndrome; Increased Risk in Carriers of MSH2 Mutations. Urology. 2015.
11. Ferlay J, Shin HR, Bray F, Forman D, Mathers C, Parkin DM. Estimates of worldwide burden of cancer in 2008: GLOBOCAN 2008. Int J Cancer. 2010; 127(12):2893–917.
12. Engholm G, Ferlay J, Christensen N, Bray F, Gjerstorff ML, Klint A, Kotlum JE, Olafsdottir E, Pukkala E, Storm HH. NORDCAN–a Nordic tool for cancer information, planning, quality control and research. Acta Oncol. 2010;49(5): 725–36. Available from http://www.ancr.nu, accessed on 02/12/2015.
13. Ryan S, Jenkins MA, Win AK. Risk of prostate cancer in Lynch syndrome: a systematic review and meta-analysis. Cancer Epidemiol Biomarkers Prev. 2014;23(3):437–49.
14. Langeberg WJ, Kwon EM, Koopmeiners JS, Ostrander EA, Stanford JL. Population-based study of the association of variants in mismatch repair genes with prostate cancer risk and outcomes. Cancer Epidemiol Biomarkers Prev. 2010;19(1):258–64.
15. Tanaka Y, Zaman MS, Majid S, Liu J, Kawakami K, Shiina H, Tokizane T, Dahiya AV, Sen S, Nakajima K. Polymorphisms of MLH1 in benign prostatic hyperplasia and sporadic prostate cancer. Biochem Biophys Res Commun. 2009;383(4):440–4.
16. Hirata H, Hinoda Y, Kawamoto K, Kikuno N, Suehiro Y, Okayama N, Tanaka Y, Dahiya R. Mismatch repair gene MSH3 polymorphism is associated with the risk of sporadic prostate cancer. J Urol. 2008;179(5):2020–4.
17. Jafary F, Salehi M, Sedghi M, Nouri N, Jafary F, Sadeghi F, Motamedi S, Talebi M. Association between mismatch repair gene MSH3 codons 1036 and 222 polymorphisms and sporadic prostate cancer in the Iranian population. Asian Pac J Cancer Prev. 2012;13(12):6055–7.
18. Baca SC, Prandi D, Lawrence MS, Mosquera JM, Romanel A, Drier Y, Park K, Kitabayashi N, MacDonald TY, Ghandi M, et al. Punctuated evolution of prostate cancer genomes. Cell. 2013;153(3):666–77.
19. Pritchard CC, Morrissey C, Kumar A, Zhang X, Smith C, Coleman I, Salipante SJ, Milbank J, Yu M, Grady WM, et al. Complex MSH2 and MSH6 mutations in hypermutated microsatellite unstable advanced prostate cancer. Nat Commun. 2014;5:4988.

20. Taylor BS, Schultz N, Hieronymus H, Gopalan A, Xiao Y, Carver BS, Arora VK, Kaushik P, Cerami E, Reva B, et al. Integrative genomic profiling of human prostate cancer. Cancer Cell. 2010;18(1):11–22.

21. Young J, Simms LA, Biden KG, Wynter C, Whitehall V, Karamatic R, George J, Goldblatt J, Walpole I, Robin SA, et al. Features of colorectal cancers with high-level microsatellite instability occurring in familial and sporadic settings: parallel pathways of tumorigenesis. Am J Pathol. 2001;159(6):2107–16.

22. Win AK, Lindor NM, Young JP, Macrae FA, Young GP, Williamson E, Parry S, Goldblatt J, Lipton L, Winship I, et al. Risks of primary extracolonic cancers following colorectal cancer in lynch syndrome. J Natl Cancer Inst. 2012; 104(18):1363–72.

23. Goecke T, Schulmann K, Engel C, Holinski-Feder E, Pagenstecher C, Schackert HK, Kloor M, Kunstmann E, Vogelsang H, Keller G, et al. Genotype-phenotype comparison of German MLH1 and MSH2 mutation carriers clinically affected with Lynch syndrome: a report by the German HNPCC Consortium. J Clin Oncol. 2006;24(26):4285–92.

24. Grindedal EM, Moller P, Eeles R, Stormorken AT, Bowitz-Lothe IM, Landro SM, Clark N, Kvale R, Shanley S, Maehle L. Germ-line mutations in mismatch repair genes associated with prostate cancer. Cancer Epidemiol Biomarkers Prev. 2009;18(9):2460–7.

25. Pande D, Negi R, Karki K, Dwivedi US, Khanna RS, Khanna HD. Simultaneous progression of oxidative stress, angiogenesis, and cell proliferation in prostate carcinoma. Urol Oncol. 2013;31(8):1561–6.

26. Engel C, Loeffler M, Steinke V, Rahner N, Holinski-Feder E, Dietmaier W, Schackert HK, Goergens H, von Knebel Doeberitz M, Goecke TO, et al. Risks of less common cancers in proven mutation carriers with lynch syndrome. J Clin Oncol. 2012;30(35):4409–15.

27. Bauer CM, Ray AM, Halstead-Nussloch BA, Dekker RG, Raymond VM, Gruber SB, Cooney KA. Hereditary prostate cancer as a feature of Lynch syndrome. Fam Cancer. 2011;10(1):37–42.

28. Vasen HF, Stormorken A, Menko FH, Nagengast FM, Kleibeuker JH, Griffioen G, Taal BG, Moller P, Wijnen JT. MSH2 mutation carriers are at higher risk of cancer than MLH1 mutation carriers: a study of hereditary nonpolyposis colorectal cancer families. J Clin Oncol. 2001;19(20):4074–80.

29. Kastrinos F, Stoffel EM, Balmana J, Steyerberg EW, Mercado R, Syngal S. Phenotype comparison of MLH1 and MSH2 mutation carriers in a cohort of 1,914 individuals undergoing clinical genetic testing in the United States. Cancer Epidemiol Biomarkers Prev. 2008;17(8):2044–51.

30. Ahman AK, Jonsson BA, Damber JE, Bergh A, Gronberg H. Low frequency of microsatellite instability in hereditary prostate cancer. BJU Int. 2001;87(4): 334–8.

31. Chen Y, Wang J, Fraig MM, Metcalf J, Turner WR, Bissada NK, Watson DK, Schweinfest CW. Defects of DNA mismatch repair in human prostate cancer. Cancer Res. 2001;61(10):4112–21.

32. Ness N, Andersen S, Valkov A, Nordby Y, Donnem T, Al-Saad S, Busund LT, Bremnes RM, Richardsen E. Infiltration of CD8+ lymphocytes is an independent prognostic factor of biochemical failure-free survival in prostate cancer. Prostate. 2014;74(14):1452–61.

33. Flammiger A, Bayer F, Cirugeda-Kuhnert A, Huland H, Tennstedt P, Simon R, Minner S, Bokemeyer C, Sauter G, Schlomm T, et al. Intratumoral T but not B lymphocytes are related to clinical outcome in prostate cancer. APMIS. 2012;120(11):901–8.

34. Karja V, Aaltomaa S, Lipponen P, Isotalo T, Talja M, Mokka R. Tumour-infiltrating lymphocytes: A prognostic factor of PSA-free survival in patients with local prostate carcinoma treated by radical prostatectomy. Anticancer Res. 2005;25(6C):4435–8.

35. Castro E, Goh C, Olmos D, Saunders E, Leongamornlert D, Tymrakiewicz M, Mahmud N, Dadaev T, Govindasami K, Guy M, et al. Germline BRCA mutations are associated with higher risk of nodal involvement, distant metastasis, and poor survival outcomes in prostate cancer. J Clin Oncol. 2013;31(14):1748–57.

25

Immunohistochemical analysis of ezrin-radixin-moesin-binding phosphoprotein 50 in prostatic adenocarcinoma

Tanner L Bartholow[1*†], Michael J Becich[2], Uma R Chandran[2] and Anil V Parwani[3†]

Abstract

Background: Ezrin-radixin-moesin-binding phosphoprotein 50 (EBP50) is an adapter protein which has been shown to play an active role in a wide variety of cellular processes, including interactions with proteins related to both tumor suppression and oncogenesis. Here we use immunohistochemistry to evaluate EBP50's expression in normal donor prostate (NDP), benign prostatic hyperplasia (BPH), high grade prostatic intraepithelial neoplasia (HGPIN), normal tissue adjacent to prostatic adenocarcinoma (NAC), primary prostatic adenocarcinoma (PCa), and metastatic prostatic adenocarcinoma (Mets).

Methods: Tissue microarrays were immunohistochemically stained for EBP50, with the staining intensities quantified using automated image analysis software. The data were statistically analyzed using one-way ANOVA with subsequent Tukey tests for multiple comparisons. Eleven cases of NDP, 37 cases of NAC, 15 cases of BPH, 35 cases of HGPIN, 103 cases of PCa, and 36 cases of Mets were analyzed in the microarrays.

Results: Specimens of PCa and Mets had the lowest absolute staining for EBP50. Mets staining was significantly lower than NDP ($p = 0.027$), BPH ($p = 0.012$), NAC ($p < 0.001$), HGPIN ($p < 0.001$), and PCa ($p = 0.006$). Additionally, HGPIN staining was significantly higher than NAC ($p < 0.009$) and PCa ($p < 0.001$).

Conclusions: To our knowledge, this represents the first study comparing the immunohistochemical profiles of EBP50 in PCa and Mets to specimens of HGPIN, BPH, NDP, and NAC and suggests that EBP50 expression is decreased in Mets. Given that PCa also had significantly higher expression than Mets, future studies are warranted to assess EBP50's potential as a prognostic biomarker for prostate cancer.

Background

Prostate cancer is currently the second leading cause of cancer death in males[1]. Despite this, in the era of prostate specific antigen (PSA) screening, researchers have now estimated that clinically insignificant prostate cancer is actually overdiagnosed at a rate of 29% for whites and 44% for blacks, the PSA screen resulting in the detection of cancers that otherwise would only have been detected during autopsy in up to 15% and 37% of tumors in whites and blacks, respectively[2].

There is currently a limited amount of information in the literature on biomarkers with the potential to discern which cases of prostate cancer have the greatest potential to metastasize versus remain latent[3]. Evaluating the expression of tumor suppressor proteins that have been previously examined in other cancers may indicate novel biomarkers for prostate cancer that have the potential to assess individual patient prognosis and guide therapy selection.

One such biomarker is ezrin-radixin-moesin-binding phosphoprotein 50 (EBP50), which is also known as Na+/H+ exchanger regulatory factor 1, or NHERF1. A 50 kDa, 358 amino acid adaptor protein whose gene is located at 17q25.1, it consists of two PSD-95/Discs Large/ZO-1 (PDZ) domains and a carboxyl-terminal region that is capable of binding members of the ezrin-radixin-moesin (ERM) protein family[4-6]. With its multiple domains, it has been described as a participant in at least 30 unique cellular interactions, including those involving ion transport, secondarily coupled signaling

* Correspondence: bartholow.tanner@medstudent.pitt.edu
† Contributed equally
[1]University of Pittsburgh School of Medicine, Pittsburgh, PA, USA
Full list of author information is available at the end of the article

receptors, and tyrosine kinase receptors[5]. Among the oncologically relevant functions for the protein that have been demonstrated are its ability to recruit the tumor suppressor PTEN for inactivation of the phosphatidylinositol-3-OH kinase (PI3K)/Akt signaling pathway in glioblastoma multiforme[5,7], as well as an ability to provide cortical stabilization of β-catenin at cellular junctions in murine embryonic fibroblast models[8], both indicative of a tumor suppressor function.

Further supporting this notion, additional work has shown that an allele for EBP50 was deleted in 28 of 48 examined breast cancer cell lines[9]. Knocking-out existing EBP50 expression in T47D and MCF7 breast cancer cell lines has also been shown to lead to increased cell proliferation[10]. Zheng et al. have additionally noted that restoring EBP50 expression to a MDA-MB-231 breast cancer line, originally deficient in EBP50, inhibited cell growth and increased apoptosis[11]. Subsequent to this, the same group prepared a stably transfected HeLa-EBP50 clone, which also demonstrated decreased cell growth, suggesting a tumor suppressor role for EBP50 in cervical cancer as well.

In spite of this, a universal tumor suppressor function for EBP50 has not been observed. EBP50 has been shown to be overexpressed in hepatocellular carcinoma [12]. Cytoplasmic over expression has also been linked to the progression of colorectal carcinoma[13]. Furthermore, in contrast to the previously described work, Song et al. have reported that EBP50 immunoreactivity in breast cancer was positively associated with tumor stage and lymph node involvement[14], prompting others to suggest that its role in oncogenesis or tumor suppression may vary with cellular location, with a membranous or apical distribution supporting a tumor suppressor function and a cytoplasmic distribution conferring oncogenic properties [5].

To our knowledge, the expression of EBP50 has never been studied in prostate cancer. Here, we compare the immunohistochemical profiles in a series of 11 cases of normal donor prostate (NDP), 37 cases of normal tissue adjacent to prostatic adenocarcinoma (NAC), 15 cases of benign prostatic hyperplasia (BPH), 35 cases of high-grade prostatic intraepithelial neoplasia (HGPIN), 103 cases of primary prostatic adenocarcinoma (PCa), and 36 cases of metastatic prostatic adenocarcinoma (Mets) in order to examine if either a tumor suppressor or oncogenic function for EBP50 can be suggested in prostate cancer, providing further information about its potential as a diagnostic and/or prognostic biomarker.

Methods
Tissue Microarray Block Preparation
Tissue microarray (TMA) blocks were constructed using specimens obtained from the Health Sciences Tissue Bank at the University of Pittsburgh Medical Center, with the tissue bank rendering the honest broker services. All specimens were originally obtained with informed consent. Cores from the appropriate case specific paraffin-embedded tissue blocks were assembled into TMAs as described in a previous protocol[15]. The final TMAs consisted of 11 cases of NDP, 37 cases of NAC, 15 cases of BPH, 35 cases of isolated HGPIN (no accompanying cancer diagnosed), 103 cases of PCa, and 36 cases of Mets. No specimens of HGPIN included in this study were diagnosed at the time as containing PCa. All cases were initially prepared so that each one would be represented at least in triplicate. Due to variations in TMA processing, however, some cases were only able to be represented in duplicate. This occurred for three cases of the HGPIN, three cases of the Mets, three cases of the NAC, two cases of the BPH, and eight cases of the PCa. In such instances, these cases were still scored and included as a part of the final analysis.

Immunohistochemistry
Each TMA block was deparaffinized and then rehydrated with incremental ethanol concentrations. Decloaker was then used for heat induced epitope retrieval, followed by a 5 minute TBS buffer rinse. A Dako autostainer was then used to stain the TMAs with anti-EBP50 (working dilution 1:400), a mouse monoclonal antibody (Catalogue # MA1-19291) from Thermo Scientific (Waltham, MA). Immunolabeling was conducted using Dako Dual Envision + Polymer (Catalogue # K4061) from Dako (Carpinteria, CA). The slides were counterstained with hematoxylin and coverslipped.

Scoring of Slides
All slides for this project were scanned as digital whole slides images (WSI) using ScanScope XT (by Aperio, Vista, CA). The individual tissue cores for each WSI were viewed using Aperio ImageScope (Version 11.0.2.716) and scored by applying the Positive Pixel Count Algorithm to each one. In order to detect the EBP50 staining, a hue value of 0.1 and hue width of 0.5 was chosen for the algorithm, corresponding to the suggested range for the detection of brown immunostaining using the software (Aperio Positive Pixel Count Algorithm instruction manual). By analyzing the average pixel intensity with a predetermined hue value and width, the stromal tissue and cell nuclei that appear blue and do not feature the immunostain are negated by the software and excluded from the final analysis that determines the average staining intensity. This, in effect, controls for the glandular to stromal tissue ratio present in the TMA cores.

The validity of using Aperio software for quantitative immunohistochemistry has been previously documented in other studies[16,17]. The average staining intensity was then determined by the software for each core, utilizing a formula that sums the intensities of weak, moderate, and strong staining pixels and divides this value by the total number of weak, moderate, and strong pixels. Staining intensities for the software are reported on a scale of 0-255, corresponding to light transmission through the specimen. Therefore, higher staining intensities correspond with lower scores on the light transmissibility scale. Scores in the range of 220-175 are classified as weak staining, 175-100 are classified as moderate staining, and 0-100 are classified as strong staining. In order to make staining scores more intuitive in our figures, our results are reported as the difference between no stain detection (255) and the average staining intensity as reported by the software, so that higher values correspond with the higher staining intensities. This value is referred to as the "staining intensity" throughout the rest of the manuscript.

The means for each case, and subsequently for each tissue type were then determined. For the specimens of adenocarcinoma, the Gleason score and tumor stage, where available, were also reported. The Clinical TNM, as opposed to the Pathologic TNM, staging classification was used to assess the specimens. All means were reported with standard errors.

One-way ANOVA with subsequent Tukey tests for multiple comparisons (α = 0.05) were used to compare the tissue types, PCa carcinoma stages, and PCa Gleason scores. Graphical analysis was conducted using Microsoft Excel 2007 (by Microsoft Corporation, Redmond, WA) and R: A Language and Environment for Statistical Computing (R Development Core Team. R Foundation for Statistical Computing Vienna, Austria. 2011. ISBN 3-900051-07-0, <http://www.R-project.org>).

Photomicrographs of tissue cores were taken using an Olympus BX51 microscope using Spot Advanced V4.6 (Diagnostic Instruments, Inc.) software. All images were taken at 20×.

This study received exempt approval (PRO08040368) from the University of Pittsburgh Institutional Review Board.

Results

Patient Ages

The average patient ages with standard deviations for the tissue types in this study are NDP 32 ± 13 years, NAC 63 ± 6 years, BPH 67 ± 9 years, PIN 63 ± 8 years, PCa 64 ± 9 years, and Mets 70 ± 10 years.

Staining Intensities

The mean staining scores for NDP, BPH, NAC, HGPIN, PCa, and Mets were 141.23 ± 2.43, 140.66 ± 2.42, 139.91 ± 2.52, 151.76 ± 2.88, 135.72 ± 1.45, 125.55 ± 2.63 (Figure 1A). Box plots showing the individual staining scores are featured in Figure 1B. A one-way ANOVA (p < 0.001), with subsequent Tukey tests for multiple comparisons, showed significant differences between Mets and NDP (p = 0.027), NAC (p < 0.001), BPH (p = 0.012), HGPIN (p < 0.001), and PCa (p = 0.006). Differences were also seen between HGPIN and PCa (p < 0.001) and NAC (p < 0.009).

Five out of thirty-seven specimens of NAC (13.5%), 1/15 specimens of BPH (6.7%), 17/35 specimens of

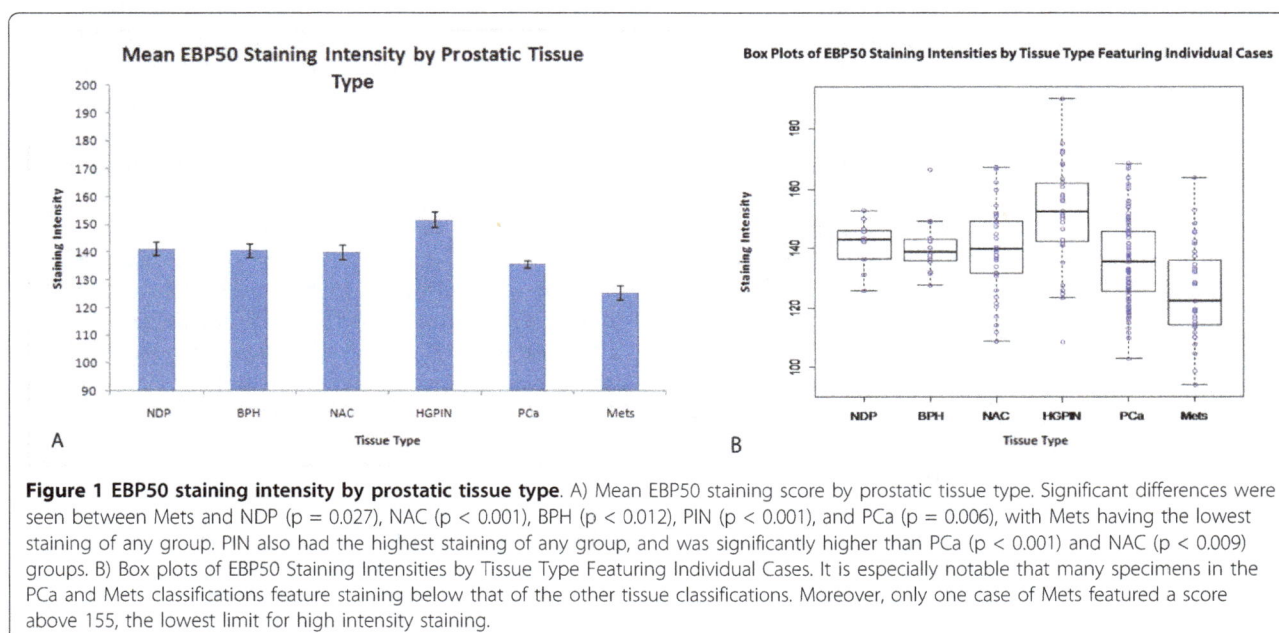

Figure 1 EBP50 staining intensity by prostatic tissue type. A) Mean EBP50 staining score by prostatic tissue type. Significant differences were seen between Mets and NDP (p = 0.027), NAC (p < 0.001), BPH (p < 0.012), PIN (p < 0.001), and PCa (p = 0.006), with Mets having the lowest staining of any group. PIN also had the highest staining of any group, and was significantly higher than PCa (p < 0.001) and NAC (p < 0.009) groups. B) Box plots of EBP50 Staining Intensities by Tissue Type Featuring Individual Cases. It is especially notable that many specimens in the PCa and Mets classifications feature staining below that of the other tissue classifications. Moreover, only one case of Mets featured a score above 155, the lowest limit for high intensity staining.

HGPIN (48.6%), 10/103 specimens of PCa (9.7%), and 1/36 specimens of Mets (2.8%) had staining scores in the highest intensity category. Although 0/11 specimens of NDP had staining in the highest intensity category, 4/11 specimens were less than 10 intensity scale points below the threshold for highest intensity category (36.4%).

When classified by tumor stage, the mean scores were stage 2, 139.60 ± 2.43 (n = 39), stage 3, 130.66 ± 2.29 (n = 37), and stage 4, 137.03 ± 2.61 (n = 27). A resultant one-way ANOVA (p = 0.024) with subsequent Tukey tests for multiple comparisons showed significant differences between stage 2 and stage 3 (p = 0.021).

When classified by Gleason score, the average staining score was 133.13 ± 3.52 (n = 15) for those with a score of 6 or less, 135.69 ± 2.06 (n = 49) for those with a score of 7, and 137.13 ± 2.54 (n = 38) for those with a score of 8 or more. No significant differences were seen between the Gleason score classifications (p = 0.672).

Staining Patterns

Representative photomicrographs of the TMA cores are shown in Figure 2. Across most specimens, a cytoplasmic EBP50 staining pattern was noted. However, in many specimens, more prevalent amongst the benign and pre-cancerous tissues, a membranous or apical staining pattern was distinctly notable as more predominant than co-accompanying cytoplasmic staining. Such cores were noted in 3/11 cases of NDP (27.3%), 11/15 cases of BPH (73.3%), 12/37 cases of NAC (32.4%), 12/35 cases of HGPIN (34.8%), 10/103 cases of PCa (9.7%), and 0/36 cases of Mets.

Discussion

In the EBP50 stained specimens, the average staining intensities were highest in the specimens of HGPIN, and lowest in the specimens of PCa and Mets. HGPIN had significantly higher staining than Mets, NAC, and PCa. Despite the fact that HGPIN was significantly different than the BPH and NDP groups but not the NAC group, the means were relatively similar between BPH, NDP, and NAC, suggesting that the staining intensity does not vary greatly between these classifications.

Previous work has shown that radixin, an ERM protein and binding partner of EBP50 that is responsible for linking F-actin to plasma membrane proteins[5,18], also demonstrated higher absolute staining in specimens of HGPIN than in other prostatic tissue types, including PCa and NAC [19]. This finding may indicate that the higher expression of both proteins in HGPIN may reflect a unique feature of the pre-cancerous tissue physiology, and that both may be down regulated in specimens of prostatic adenocarcinoma.

Mets tissue had significantly lower staining than all other tissue types, including PCa, indicating that loss of EPB50 expression may play a role in select cases of prostate cancer metastasis. This is further echoed by the fact that only 1/36 cases of metastatic tissue showed high intensity range staining for EBP50. Given that EBP50 has been previously shown in murine fibroblast models to promote adherens junction stabilization through mediating the interaction of β-catenin with E-cadherin, its loss of expression is plausible with tumor dissemination[8].

Despite this, however, it is important to note that these findings may also contain a correlative component that is not prognostic in nature. While all of the tumors in this study were primary tumors at the time of specimen retrieval, definitive follow-up information on these patients was not available. In this sense, from this study it is not possible to rule out that the decreased EBP50 expression, at least in part, may be due to the metastatic location itself. The current results, however, indicate and warrant later phase biomarker studies[20] that will longitudinally correlate EBP50 expression directly with patient outcomes to further evaluate its potential to predict metastatic risk in prostate cancer.

A significant increase in EBP50 staining between Stage 2 and 3 PCa specimens was also observed. It is possible that this finding represents a change in tumor physiology between the two stages, however, given that this trend was not noted in Stage 4 PCa specimens, it is also possible that this represents a spurious finding, and should be further evaluated before definitive conclusions are reached. No differences were seen between the Gleason score classifications.

In general, EBP50's expression is increased in polarized epithelial cells, such as the liver, kidney, pancreas, small intestine, and the prostate[5]. Considering the diverse intracellular roles that have been proposed for EBP50, it may be difficult to elucidate a clear, singular mechanism whereby it may promote oncogenesis or tumor suppression within individual tissue types.

Differing hypotheses to explain to the behavior of EBP50 in cancer have been proposed, especially given the multiple studies that seem to support two opposing functions for EBP50 in cancer [9-11,21]. Zheng, et al have suggested that in many cases of breast cancer where EBP50 is expressed, it may not be expressed in sufficient quantities to halt tumor progression[11]. Others have demonstrated that the hypoxia associated with tumor necrosis can increase EBP50 (NHERF1), which increases Na+/H+ activity, in turn decreasing local pH and promoting tumor dissemination[4,21]. And while it has been shown that EBP50 can cluster with EGFR, PDGFR, and the tumor suppressor NF2 to halt cell signaling and hence cancer progression[11,22-24], others have posited that EBP50's PDZ domains may actually allow for new tumor-specific interactions[4].

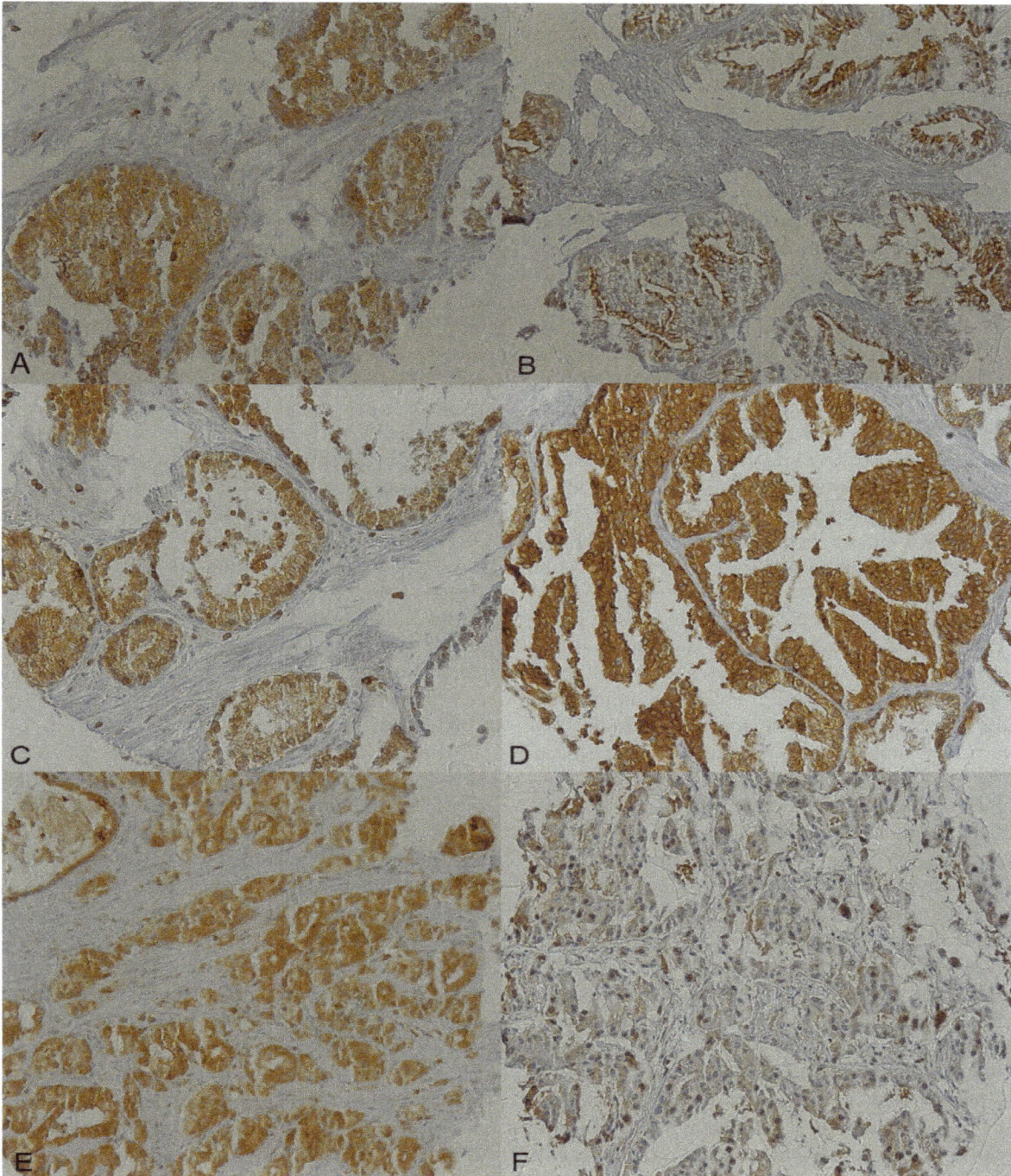

Figure 2 Photomicrographs of TMA cores. Photomicrographs of TMA cores (20×). A) NDP, B) BPH, C) NAC, D) HGPIN, E) PCa, and F) Mets. Note the predominantly membranous pattern in BPH, which was noted in cores from 11/15 cases. To a lesser degree, this is also noted in the depicted specimen of HGPIN, although the cytoplasmic staining is also intense, which partially obscures the distinction. In the remainder of depicted cores, the staining is largely cytoplasmic. No membranous staining was noted in any of the metastatic cores.

These different findings, in part, have been reconciled with the hypothesis that EBP50 may have different functions by cellular location, with a tumor suppressor function associated with a membranous/apical distribution, and an oncogenic function promoted by a cytoplasmic location[5]. In support of this hypothesis, previous work has demonstrated a progression from luminal to cytoplasmic EBP50 expression occurs across normal to ductal carcinoma in-situ to invasive and metastatic breast cancer tissues[25]. While membranous EBP50 has been shown to stabilize β-catenin at cell membranes[8], non-stabilized β-catenin is also capable of forming growth-promoting transcription complexes in the nucleus and has been prominently associated with hepatocellular carcinoma[26]. Hence, it is interesting that an overexpression of EBP50 with a focal nuclear localization has been documented in hepatocellular carcinoma[12]. A similar phenomenon has been noted in colorectal cancer, where membranous EBP50 loss and increased cytoplasmic expression has been noted in the colorectal adenoma-to-carcinoma transition, with subsequent increases in cellular invasion and epithelial-to-mesenchymal transition, processes that demonstrated reversibility when EBP50 was reexpressed at the apical membrane of intestinal epithelium[13]. Additionally, in normal astrocytes, EBP50 has demonstrated a membranous distribution, while it has demonstrated a cytoplasmic distribution in many cases of glioblastoma multiforme [7]. This corresponds with the absence of the EBP50-binding tumor suppressor PTEN and the activation of the growth-promoting Akt pathway, which is traditionally silenced by PTEN through recruitment to the plasma membrane by EBP50[7].

Relating these examples specifically to prostate cancer, it has been demonstrated that β-catenin can interact with androgen receptor and increase its transcriptional activity, hence contributing to prostate cancer progression[27,28]. Moreover, the tumor suppressor PTEN is frequently found mutated in prostate cancer, with subsequent PI3K/Akt signaling shown to promote cell survival[27,29]. Interestingly, the PI3K/Akt pathway also increases the stability of β-catenin in prostate cancer [30]. Based on these findings, it is possible to suggest that EBP50, under the appropriate circumstances, may possess a tumor suppressor function in prostate cancer similar to those described above in other cancer types.

While a cytoplasmic staining pattern for EBP50 was noted across most specimens examined in this study, a membranous/apical staining pattern was clearly more prominent than cytoplasmic staining in many cores, most commonly in the benign and pre-neoplastic specimens (Figure 2). While cores with clearly more prominent membranous staining were found in 73.3% of BPH cases studied (Figure 2B), this finding was only noted in

9.7% of cases of PCa and not in any specimens of Mets. Although an overlap between the expression patterns still existed between many of the benign and cancerous specimens, this trend concurs with the above hypothesis regarding strong membranous expression and tumor suppression and warrants further study to determine its potential to assess metastatic risk.

As a final note of interest, in one model of EBP50 function, its PDZ-2 domain has been shown to bind to the C-terminal ERM-binding domain, inhibiting the binding of other proteins to the PDZ domains, such as PTEN and B-catenin[31]. In this same model, when ezrin, an ERM protein, binds the C-terminal domain, the PDZ domains are freed up for additional binding partners. In the intestinal epithelium of ezrin knock-out mice, EBP50 has been shown to be displaced to the cytoplasm[5,32]. In light of this, it is an interesting finding that ezrin expression has been inversely correlated with tumor differentiation in prostate cancer[33], and that moesin, another ERM protein, showed higher incidences of lymph node metastases when it was associated with a cytoplasmic distribution as opposed to a membranous one in oral squamous cell carcinoma[34]. Hence, EBP50's location and function may also be directly linked to the location and presence of the ERM proteins that ultimately enable PDZ domain interactions.

Conclusions

These results provide a basis for the characterization of the staining patterns and intensities of EBP50 in PCa and Mets in comparison to benign prostate tissue. The immunostaining was highest in specimens of HGPIN. Its expression was lowest in Mets, with the expression in Mets significantly lower than that of all other tissue groups, including PCa (p = 0.006). As a significant decrease between Stage 2 and 3 cancer was observed (p = 0.021), it is also possible that EBP50 expression is altered with carcinoma stage, although significant differences were not seen when Stages 2 and 3 were compared to Stage 4. No differences were seen when comparing the Gleason scores of the PCa specimens.

EBP50 staining was a combination of membranous/apical and cytoplasmic in the prostatic tissues examined. Although a clear distinction would not be made in all cases, a predominant membranous staining pattern was more commonly observed in benign specimens than in malignant ones. As an example, 11/15 cases of BPH featured cores with a readily apparent predominant membranous staining pattern compared to the adjacent cytoplasm, while this was only observed in 10/103 cases of PCa and was not seen in any cases of Mets.

It is also important to note, however, as this membranous/cytoplasmic distinction was not noted in all comparisons between benign and cancerous specimens, that an alternate explanation may account for these findings. As a general decrease in overall staining intensity was observed between the benign specimens and the cancerous/metastatic specimens, this lack of membranous staining may simply reflect an overall staining decrease, making it difficult to appreciate the true ratio of membranous to cytoplasmic staining from a visual examination. This is especially true in the cases of metastatic cancer, where the overall staining is very faint across all specimens in the first place.

Given that a significant decrease in staining was noted between specimens of PCa and Mets, further studies of EBP50 are justified to assess its potential for clinical usage in prognosis assessment of patients with prostate cancer.

Acknowledgements

This work was supported by the Clinical and Translational Science Institute Multidisciplinary Predoctoral Fellowship program, awarded through the Clinical and Translational Science Institute and the Institute for Clinical Research Educational Education at the University of Pittsburgh (grant 5TL1RR024155-02 and grant 5TL1RR024155-05) to Tanner L. Bartholow. Additional funds were provided by the Doris Duke Charitable Foundation, and the Departments of Pathology and Biomedical Informatics at the University of Pittsburgh.
The authors of this paper would like to thank Marianne Notaro for assistance with TMA preparation, Marie Acquafondata for assistance with immunohistochemical staining, Kevin McDade with assistance in graphical design, and the Clinical Scientist Training Program, funded by the Office of the Dean at the University of Pittsburgh School of Medicine.

Author details

[1]University of Pittsburgh School of Medicine, Pittsburgh, PA, USA. [2]Department of Biomedical Informatics, University of Pittsburgh School of Medicine, Pittsburgh, PA, USA. [3]Department of Pathology, University of Pittsburgh School of Medicine, Pittsburgh, PA, USA.

Authors' contributions

TB assisted in scoring tissue microarrays under the direct supervision of an attending pathologist, performed the statistical calculations, and drafted the manuscript. UC assisted with statistical calculations and reviewed the manuscript. AP conceived of the study, developed and approved the study protocol, approved all tissue microarray scoring, and revised the manuscript. MB also conceived of the study, developed and approved the protocol, and revised the manuscript. All authors have read and approved the final manuscript.

Competing interests

The authors declare that they have no competing interests.

References

1. Jemal A, Siegel R, Xu J, Ward E: **Cancer statistics, 2010.** *CA Cancer J Clin* 2010, **60**:277-300.
2. Etzioni R, Penson DF, Legler JM, di Tommaso D, Boer R, Gann PH, Feuer EJ: **Overdiagnosis due to prostate-specific antigen screening: lessons from U.S. prostate cancer incidence trends.** *J Natl Cancer Inst* 2002, **94**(13):981-990.
3. Chandran UR, Dhir R, Ma C, Michalopoulos G, Becich M, Gilbertson J: **Differences in gene expression in prostate cancer, normal appearing prostate tissue adjacent to cancer and prostate tissue from cancer free organ donors.** *BMC Cancer* 2005, **5**:45.
4. Bellizzi A, Malfettone A, Cardone RA, Mangia A: **NHERF1/EBP50 in Breast Cancer.** *Clinical Perspectives Breast Care (Basel)* 2010, **5**(2):86-90.
5. Georgescu MM, Morales FC, Molina JR, Hayashi Y: **Roles of NHERF1/EBP50 in cancer.** *Curr Mol Med* 2008, **8**(6):459-468.
6. Morales FC, Takahashi Y, Kreimann EL, Georgescu MM: **Ezrin-radixin-moesin (ERM)-binding phosphoprotein 50 organizes ERM proteins at the apical membrane of polarized epithelia.** *Proc Natl Acad Sci USA* 2004, **101**(51):17705-17710.
7. Molina JR, Morales FC, Hayashi Y, Aldape KD, Georgescu MM: **Loss of PTEN binding adapter protein NHERF1 from plasma membrane in glioblastoma contributes to PTEN inactivation.** *Cancer Res* 2010, **70**(17):6697-6703.
8. Kreimann EL, Morales FC, de Orbeta-Cruz J, Takahashi Y, Adams H, Liu TJ, McCrea PD, Georgescu MM: **Cortical stabilization of beta-catenin contributes to NHERF1/EBP50 tumor suppressor function.** *Oncogene* 2007, **26**(36):5290-5299.
9. Dai JL, Wang L, Sahin AA, Broemeling LD, Schutte M, Pan Y: **NHERF (Na+/H + exchanger regulatory factor) gene mutations in human breast cancer.** *Oncogene* 2004, **23**(53):8681-8687.
10. Pan Y, Wang L, Dai JL: **Suppression of breast cancer cell growth by Na +/H+ exchanger regulatory factor 1 (NHERF1).** *Breast Cancer Res* 2006, **8**(6):R63.
11. Zheng JF, Sun LC, Liu H, Huang Y, Li Y, He J: **EBP50 exerts tumor suppressor activity by promoting cell apoptosis and retarding extracellular signal-regulated kinase activity.** *Amino Acids* 2010, **38**(4):1261-1268.
12. Shibata T, Chuma M, Kokubu A, Sakamoto M, Hirohashi S: **EBP50, a beta-catenin-associating protein, enhances Wnt signaling and is over-expressed in hepatocellular carcinoma.** *Hepatology* 2003, **38**(1):178-186.
13. Hayashi Y, Molina JR, Hamilton SR, Georgescu MM: **NHERF1/EBP50 is a new marker in colorectal cancer.** *Neoplasia* 2010, **12**(12):1013-1022.
14. Song J, Bai J, Yang W, Gabrielson EW, Chan DW, Zhang Z: **Expression and clinicopathological significance of oestrogen-responsive ezrin-radixin-moesin-binding phosphoprotein 50 in breast cancer.** *Histopathology* 2007, **51**(1):40-53.
15. Kajdacsy-Balla A, Geynisman JM, Macias V, Setty S, Nanaji NM, Berman JJ, Dobbin K, Melamed J, Kong X, Bosland M, Orenstein J, Bayarl J, Becich M, Dhir R, Datta MW: **Practical aspects of planning, building, and interpreting tissue microarrays: the Cooperative Prostate Cancer Tissue Resource experience.** *J Mol Histol* 2007, **38**(2):113-121.
16. Lloyd MC, Allam-Nandyala P, Purohit CN, Burke N, Coppola D, Bui MM: **Using image analysis as a tool for assessment of prognostic and predictive biomarkers for breast cancer: How reliable is it?** *J Pathol Inform* 2010, **1**:29.
17. Bolton KL, Garcia-Closas M, Pfeiffer RM, Duggan MA, Howat WJ, Hewitt SM, Yang XR, Cornelison R, Anzick SL, Meltzer P, Davis S, Lenz P, Figueroa JD, Pharoah PD, Sherman ME: **Assessment of automated image analysis of breast cancer tissue microarrays for epidemiologic studies.** *Cancer Epidemiol Biomarkers Prev* 2010, **19**(4):992-999.
18. Louvet-Vallee S: **ERM proteins: from cellular architecture to cell signaling.** *Biol Cell* 2000, **92**(5):305-316.
19. Bartholow TL, Chandran UR, Becich MJ, Parwani AV: **Immunohistochemical staining of radixin and moesin in prostatic adenocarcinoma.** *BMC Clin Pathol* 2011, **11**:1.
20. Pepe MS, Etzioni R, Feng Z, Potter JD, Thompson ML, Thornquist M, Winget M, Yasui Y: **Phases of biomarker development for early detection of cancer.** *J Natl Cancer Inst* 2001, **93**(14):1054-1061.
21. Cardone RA, Bellizzi A, Busco G, Weinman EJ, Dell'Aquila ME, Casavola V, Azzariti A, Mangia A, Paradiso A, Reshkin SJ: **The NHERF1 PDZ2 domain regulates PKA-RhoA-p38-mediated NHE1 activation and invasion in breast tumor cells.** *Mol Biol Cell* 2007, **18**(5):1768-1780.
22. Curto M, Cole BK, Lallemand D, Liu CH, McClatchey AI: **Contact-dependent inhibition of EGFR signaling by Nf2/Merlin.** *J Cell Biol* 2007, **177**(5):893-903.
23. James MF, Beauchamp RL, Manchanda N, Kazlauskas A, Ramesh V: **A NHERF binding site links the betaPDGFR to the cytoskeleton and regulates cell spreading and migration.** *J Cell Sci* 2004, **117**(Pt 14):2951-2961.
24. Maudsley S, Zamah AM, Rahman N, Blitzer JT, Luttrell LM, Lefkowitz RJ, Hall RA: **Platelet-derived growth factor receptor association with Na(+)/H (+) exchanger regulatory factor potentiates receptor activity.** *Mol Cell Biol* 2000, **20**(22):8352-8363.

25. Mangia A, Chiriatti A, Bellizzi A, Malfettone A, Stea B, Zito FA, Reshkin SJ, Simone G, Paradiso A: **Biological role of NHERF1 protein expression in breast cancer.** *Histopathology* 2009, **55**(5):600-608.

26. Yam JW, Wong CM, Ng IO: **Molecular and functional genetics of hepatocellular carcinoma.** *Front Biosci (Schol Ed)* 2010, **2**:117-134.

27. Verras M, Sun Z: **Roles and regulation of Wnt signaling and beta-catenin in prostate cancer.** *Cancer Lett* 2006, **237**(1):22-32.

28. Truica CI, Byers S, Gelmann EP: **Beta-catenin affects androgen receptor transcriptional activity and ligand specificity.** *Cancer Res* 2000, **60**(17):4709-4713.

29. Steck PA, Pershouse MA, Jasser SA, Yung WK, Lin H, Ligon AH, Langford LA, Baumgard ML, Hattier T, Davis T, Fyre C, Hu R, Swedlund B, Teng OH, Tavtigian SV: **Identification of a candidate tumour suppressor gene, MMAC1, at chromosome 10q23.3 that is mutated in multiple advanced cancers.** *Nat Genet* 1997, **15**(4):356-362.

30. Sharma M, Chuang WW, Sun Z: **Phosphatidylinositol 3-kinase/Akt stimulates androgen pathway through GSK3beta inhibition and nuclear beta-catenin accumulation.** *J Biol Chem* 2002, **277**(34):30935-30941.

31. Morales FC, Takahashi Y, Momin S, Adams H, Chen X, Georgescu MM: **NHERF1/EBP50 head-to-tail intramolecular interaction masks association with PDZ domain ligands.** *Mol Cell Biol* 2007, **27**(7):2527-2537.

32. Saotome I, Curto M, McClatchey AI: **Ezrin is essential for epithelial organization and villus morphogenesis in the developing intestine.** *Dev Cell* 2004, **6**(6):855-864.

33. Musial J, Sporny S, Nowicki A: **Prognostic significance of E-cadherin and ezrin immunohistochemical expression in prostate cancer.** *Pol J Pathol* 2007, **58**(4):235-243.

34. Kobayashi H, Sagara J, Kurita H, Morifuji M, Ohishi M, Kurashina K, Taniguchi S: **Clinical significance of cellular distribution of moesin in patients with oral squamous cell carcinoma.** *Clin Cancer Res* 2004, **10**(2):572-580.

26

Overall and worst gleason scores are equally good predictors of prostate cancer progression

Teemu T Tolonen[1,2], Paula M Kujala[2], Teuvo LJ Tammela[3], Vilppu J Tuominen[1], Jorma J Isola[1] and Tapio Visakorpi[1*]

Abstract

Background: Gleason scoring has experienced several modifications during the past decade. So far, only one study has compared the prognostic abilities of worst (WGS) and overall (OGS) modified Gleason scores after the ISUP 2005 conference. Prostatic needle biopsies are individually paraffin-embedded in 57% of European pathology laboratories, whereas the rest of laboratories embed multiple (2 - 6) biopsies per one paraffin-block. Differences in the processing method can have a far-reaching effect, because reporting of the Gleason score (GS) is different for individually embedded and pooled biopsies, and GS is one of the most important factors when selecting treatment for patients.

Methods: The study material consisted of needle biopsies from 236 prostate cancer patients that were endocrine-treated in 1999-2003. Biopsies from left side and right side were embedded separately. Haematoxylin-eosin-stained slides were scanned and analyzed on web-based virtual microscopy. Worst and overall Gleason scores were assessed according to the modified Gleason score schema after analyzing each biopsy separately. The compound Gleason scores (CGS) were obtained from the original pathology reports. Two different grade groupings were used: GS 6 or less vs. 7 vs. 8 or above; and GS 7(3 + 4) or less vs. 7(4 + 3) and 8 vs. 9-10. The prognostic ability of the three scoring methods to predict biochemical progression was compared with Kaplan-Meier survival analysis and univariate and multivariate Cox regression analyses.

Results: The median follow-up time of the patients was 64.5 months (range 0-118). The modified GS criteria led to upgrading of the Gleason sums compared to the original CGS from the pathology reports 1999-2003 (mean 7.0 for CGS, 7.5 for OGS, 7.6 for WGS). In 43 cases WGS was > OGS. In a univariate analysis the relative risks were 2.1 (95%-confidence interval 1.8-2.4) for CGS, 2.5 (2.1-2.8) for OGS, and 2.6 (2.2-2.9) for WGS. In a multivariate analysis, OGS was the only independent prognostic factor.

Conclusions: All of the three Gleason scoring methods are strong predictors of biochemical recurrence. The use of modified Gleason scoring leads to upgrading of GS, but also improves the prognostic value of the scoring. No significant prognostic differences between OGS and WGS could be shown, which may relate to the apparent narrowing of the GS scale from 2-10 to 5-10 due to the recent modifications.

Background

Grading of prostatic needle biopsies has undergone several refinements in the last decade. First, Epstein suggested that a diagnosis of Gleason score (GS) 2 + 2 = 4 cancer should not be made on the needle biopsies, because subsequent radical specimens showed upgrading in virtually all cases [1]. Next, worst Gleason score

(WGS) was shown superior to overall Gleason score (OGS) in predicting the final GS of the radical specimen, yielding fewer cases of unwanted upgrading events [2]. The third major adaptation was made in the consensus conference of International Society of Urological Pathology 2005, leading to a refinement called modified GS [3]. In that scheme, any aggressive cancer seen on the needle biopsies should be recorded and incorporated to the GS, even if present in small amount.

Worst Gleason score (WGS) is recommended for individually processed biopsies by ISUP 2005 consensus

* Correspondence: tapio.visakorpi@uta.fi
[1]Institute of Medical Technology, University of Tampere and Tampere University Hospital, Tampere, Finland
Full list of author information is available at the end of the article

conference [3]. In the case of pooled biopsies, the exact number of biopsies is sometimes difficult to know due to tissue fragmentation and/or overlapping of the biopsies, and thus, WGS cannot be reliably assessed [3].

According to a recent survey among European pathology laboratories, approximately one half of the participants use individually processed biopsies, while the others immerse multiple biopsies per formalin container without special identification tags (Lars Egevad, personal communication). Individually processed biopsies allow clinicians to localize the histopathological findings to the anatomic biopsy site. In addition, when the biopsy cores are individually embedded in paraffin blocks, a separate GS can be assessed for each biopsy, and the worst of them is usually reported to the clinicians to guide the treatment. Instead, the uropathologists did not reach consensus whether to use worst or overall GS in the case when multiple cancer-containing biopsies are pooled to one formalin container without identification tags [3].

A few studies comparing OGS and WGS have been published and only one of them after the ISUP conference [4]. In three studies WGS at any biopsy site was better than OGS at predicting the pathological T-stage and GS in radical prostatovesiculectomy specimens [2,4,5] whereas in one study, OGS performed better in predicting progression-free survival in patients treated with radiotherapy [6].

Our earlier study analyzing biopsies from endocrine-treated patients indicated that OGS was the strongest independent prognosticator of all histopathological parameters [7]. Gleason score assessment according to ISUP 2005, using the most aggressive pattern as a secondary Gleason grade even when it is present in only a small area, yielded the best prognostic classification using groupings < 7(4 + 3), 7(4 + 3)-8, and 9-10. In the present study, we examined whether the WGS in a single biopsy core would improve prognostic accuracy when compared with OGS. We also evaluated the prognostic value of compound Gleason score from the original pathology reports before the ISUP 2005 era.

Methods
Material
The study was approved by the Ethical Committee of Tampere University Hospital (TAUH) and the National Authority for Medicolegal Affairs. From 1999 to 2003, 295 consecutive new prostate cancer patients, diagnosed from core biopsies, were primarily hormonally treated in the TAUH. Representative formalin-fixed, paraffin-embedded samples were available from 236 (80%) cases. Of these, clinical follow-up data were available for 233/236 (99%) cases. The end-point, biochemical progression, was defined as a ≥ 25% rise in PSA, with a PSA

value ≥ 2.0 ng/ml above the nadir in two consecutive measurements, as recommended by The Prostate Cancer Clinical Trials Working Group (PCWG2) guidelines [8]. The median PSA value at the time of diagnosis was 15.5 ng/ml (mean 144 ng/ml, S.D. 772). Tumors were organ-confined (clinical T1-2) in 126 patients and advanced (cT3-4) in 107 patients. Bone scintigraphy was done in all symptomatic patients and in asymptomatic patients when PSA was ≥ 20 ng/ml or they had aggressive (original compound GS > 7) prostate cancer. Based on bone scintigraphy, metastasis was detected in 40 (17%) patients. The primary hormonal treatments were luteinizing-hormone releasing-hormone (LHRH) analog (n = 169), surgical castration (n = 43), antiandrogen bicalutamide (n = 21), and maximal androgen blockade (n = 3).

Two slides from each patient were analyzed. The most representative hematoxylin and eosin (H&E)-stained slide, consisting of biopsies from the left or right lobe, was selected and scanned with Aperio ScanScope® XT (software version 9; Aperio Technologies, USA) and viewed in JPEG2000 format using JVSview virtual microscopy software (version 1.2) [9].

The WGS and OGS were evaluated according to the recommendations of the International Society of Urological Pathologists 2005 by one pathologist (T.T.T.) [3]. The evaluation was performed on the scanned images of the most representative side of the prostate on a virtual microscope. The overall Gleason score was derived as a sum of the predominant and the most aggressive (or secondary) patterns of all the biopsy cores, treated as one long core. The worst Gleason score in a single biopsy core was assessed in cases for which one biopsy contained a higher Gleason grade (e.g., 4 + 4 cancer) and other cores a lower grade (e.g. 3 + 4). In the cases in which all positive biopsy cores contained same Gleason grade (e.g., 3 + 3) or there was only one core positive for cancer, the WGS was equal to the OGS. A Gleason score of 7 was considered as two separate grades (e.g., the WGS could equal 4 + 3 and the OGS 3 + 4). The evaluation of CGS was originally made by several pathologists, mainly by two uropathologists, who assessed CGS as sum of the predominant and the second most common Gleason patterns based on the evaluation of needle biopsy specimens from both lobes. In this study the CGS was obtained directly from the original pathology reports.

Two different grade groupings were used: GS 6 or less vs. 7 vs. 8 or above; and GS 7(3 + 4) or less vs. 7(4 + 3) and 8 vs. 9-10.

Statistical analysis
The agreement between Gleason scoring methods was analyzed with the κ-coefficient method. A survival analysis with PSA progression as end-point was performed

using the Kaplan-Meier method, and the statistical significance of survival differences between patient groups was determined with a Mantel-Cox test. The univariate and multivariate Cox regression analyses were performed to calculate the relative risk estimates (RR) and to evaluate the independence of the prognostic grading methods. No clinicopathologic data other than the different Gleason scoring methods were included in the multivariate analysis. However, these data had been analyzed by us previously [7].

Results

Basic characteristics

The median age of the patients was 73.8 years (range 52.7-88.8). The median PSA at the time of diagnosis was 15.7 ng/ml (range 2.4-10750.0 ng/ml). The median follow-up time was 64.5 months (range 0-118). The distribution of numbers of biopsy cores per side is provided in Table 1. The differences in progression-free survival between different treatment forms were not assessed because patients were not randomized, and due to bias that LHRH analogue was used in 72.5% of cases.

Needle biopsy findings

The average number of positive biopsy sites was 3.1 (median 3, range 1-7). The number of cases with multiple positive biopsy sites was 191/236 (80.9%). Worst GS was higher than OGS in 43/236 (18.2%) cases. In general, the modified GS system yielded higher Gleason scores. The average GS was 7.6 (median 8, 95%-confidence interval 5.0-10.3) for WGS, 7.5 (7.0, 5.0-10.0) for OGS, and 7.0 (7, 4.5-9.6) for CGS. The distribution of Gleason scores according to grading method is shown in Figure 1. The number of cases with OGS = 7 was 65. In 14 (22%) cases of them there was at least one positive biopsy core containing higher-grade cancer (WGS 4 + 4 = 8). In 12 (31%) of 39 cases with OGS 3 + 4 = 7, a positive biopsy core with the highest score showed WGS 4 + 3. Overall GS = 9 was encountered in 52 cases of which the biopsy core with highest GS showed

Table 1 Distribution of needle biopsy cores

No. cores/lobe[1]	No. cases (n = 236)
1	2
2	7
3	52
4	60
5	50
6	56
7	7
8	1
9	1

[1]The average number of cores per lobe 4.5 (median 4, range 1-9).

WGS = 10 in 10 (19%) cases. In three cases the difference between WGS and OGS was 2; in all of them OGS = 8 (3 + 5 or 5 + 3) and WGS = 10 (5 + 5).

Statistical analyses

The agreement between WGS and OGS was high (κ-coefficient = 0.82). A significantly lower concordance was found between WGS and CGS (κ = 0.48) and OGS and CGS (κ = 0.44). All Gleason scoring methods provided prognostically highly significant information (Figure 2A, B, C, D, E, and 2F).

The univariate analyses of OGS and WGS yielded similar relative risks (Figure 2). Re-classification of the Gleason score groups to < 7(4 + 3), 7(4 + 3)-8, 9-10 improved slightly prognostic value of the scoring. In the multivariate analysis of the six different Gleason grading methods, OGS reclassified as < 7(4 + 3), 7(4 + 3)-8, 9-10 was the strongest (and only) independent prognostic factor (RR 2.6, 95% confidence interval 2.0-3.5).

Discussion

The refinements of the ISUP 2005 consensus conference on Gleason scoring of needle biopsies have generally yielded better prognostic accuracy [10]. Our results indicate that modified Gleason scores according to the ISUP 2005 system are higher than compound GS's from 1999-2003, and this upgrading is associated with improved prognostic accuracy. Moreover, the results suggest, that OGS may be a slightly stronger or at least equally adequate predictor of PSA progression than WGS, when assessed from pooled biopsies.

A major implication of the revised 2005 ISUP guidelines has been the mandate to integrate the most aggressive tertiary patterns to secondary in needle biopsy scoring, even when the pattern is limited to a small area. A recent webmicroscope-based concordance study about Gleason grading of GS 6-8 by the European Network of Uropathologists suggested that general pathologists are starting to overgrade the experts (Lars Egevad, personal communication). Because Gleason grading is subjective, it is not difficult to detect some glandular fusion, and to interpret them as secondary Gleason pattern 4. Due to aforementioned issues, a fraction of cancers previously graded as GS 3 + 3 = 6 would nowadays end up with GS 3 + 4 = 7. Thus, it has been suggested that changing definitions shift the cut-off between low-grade and high grade cancers from 3 + 4 to 4 + 3 [11,12]. The results of the present study are consistent with that.

According to the 2005 ISUP consensus conference, the highest (worst) GS should not be assessed from biopsies immersed in the same formalin container ("pooled biopsies") due to tissue fragmentation [3]. When all six biopsies from one lobe are formalin-fixed

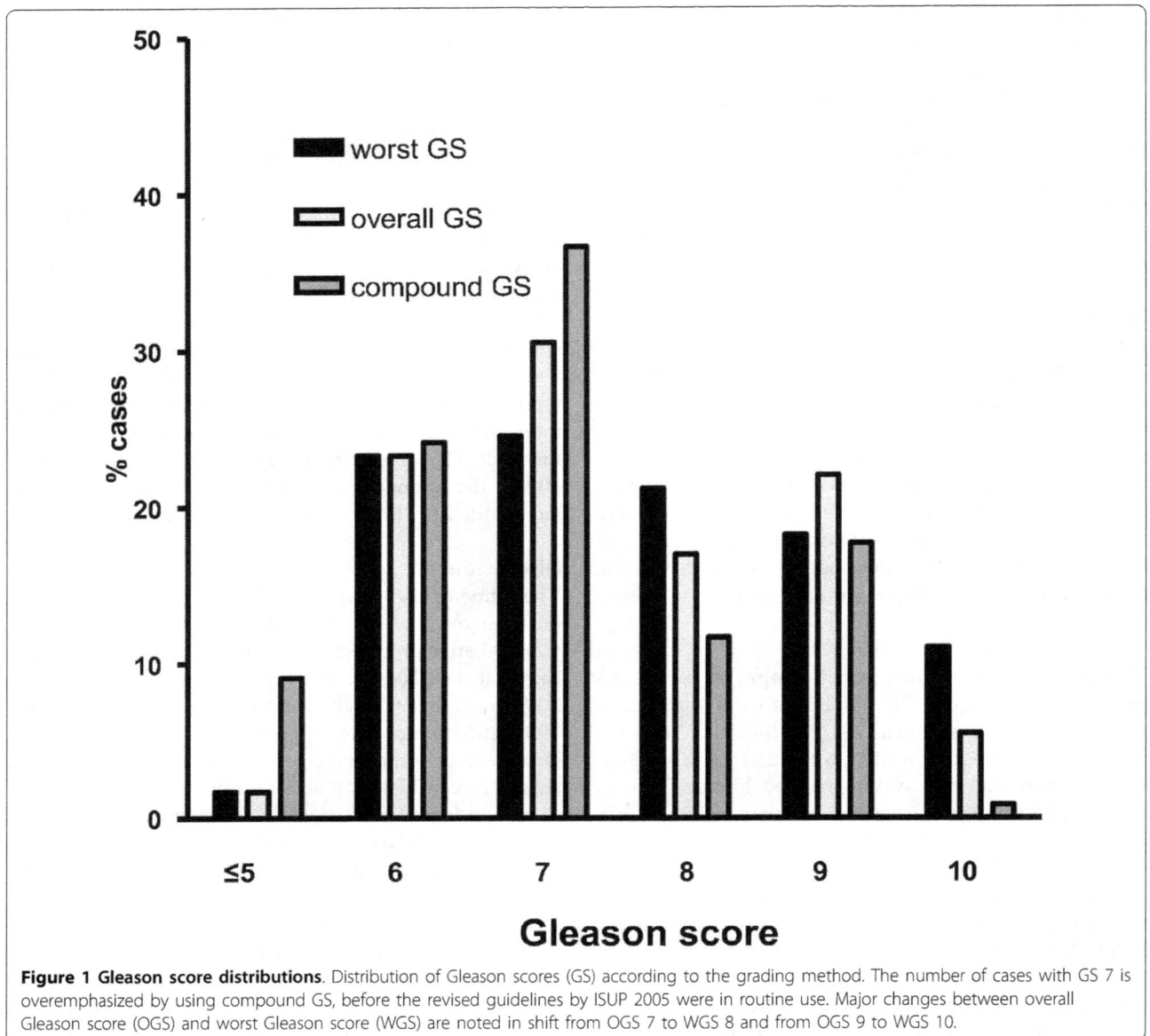

Figure 1 Gleason score distributions. Distribution of Gleason scores (GS) according to the grading method. The number of cases with GS 7 is overemphasized by using compound GS, before the revised guidelines by ISUP 2005 were in routine use. Major changes between overall Gleason score (OGS) and worst Gleason score (WGS) are noted in shift from OGS 7 to WGS 8 and from OGS 9 to WGS 10.

in the same container, they may become fragmented or overlap when embedded, disturbing the attempt to assess the WGS of the individual needle biopsies. To avoid this, some laboratories choose to ink pooled cores different colors and thus be more specific about sites and fragmentation. On the other hand, WGS was recently shown to be a better predictor of the histopathological findings from subsequent radical prostatectomy specimens [4]. In our study, the WGS was assessed from the needle biopsies of one prostate lobe embedded in one paraffin block. Because of this, it is possible that our WGS results were biased by tissue fragmentation. However, in the majority of the cases (n = 193/236, 82%), the WGS was equal to the OGS. If there were a

bias due to fragmentation, we should expect more cases with WGS > OGS.

A major problem when multiple biopsies are stored in one container is that the exact locus information of the biopsies is lost unless site identifiers are used. Another disadvantage is that it is harder to keep all the biopsies in the same plane of section, but this can be avoided in eg. by using foam plastic inside the cassettes. The locus information is essential when considering targeted brachytherapy or cryotherapy in focal carcinomas. Moreover, the anatomic localization of carcinoma foci is useful when planning nerve-sparing radical prostatectomy and to avoid side effects from external-beam radiotherapy. The problems associated

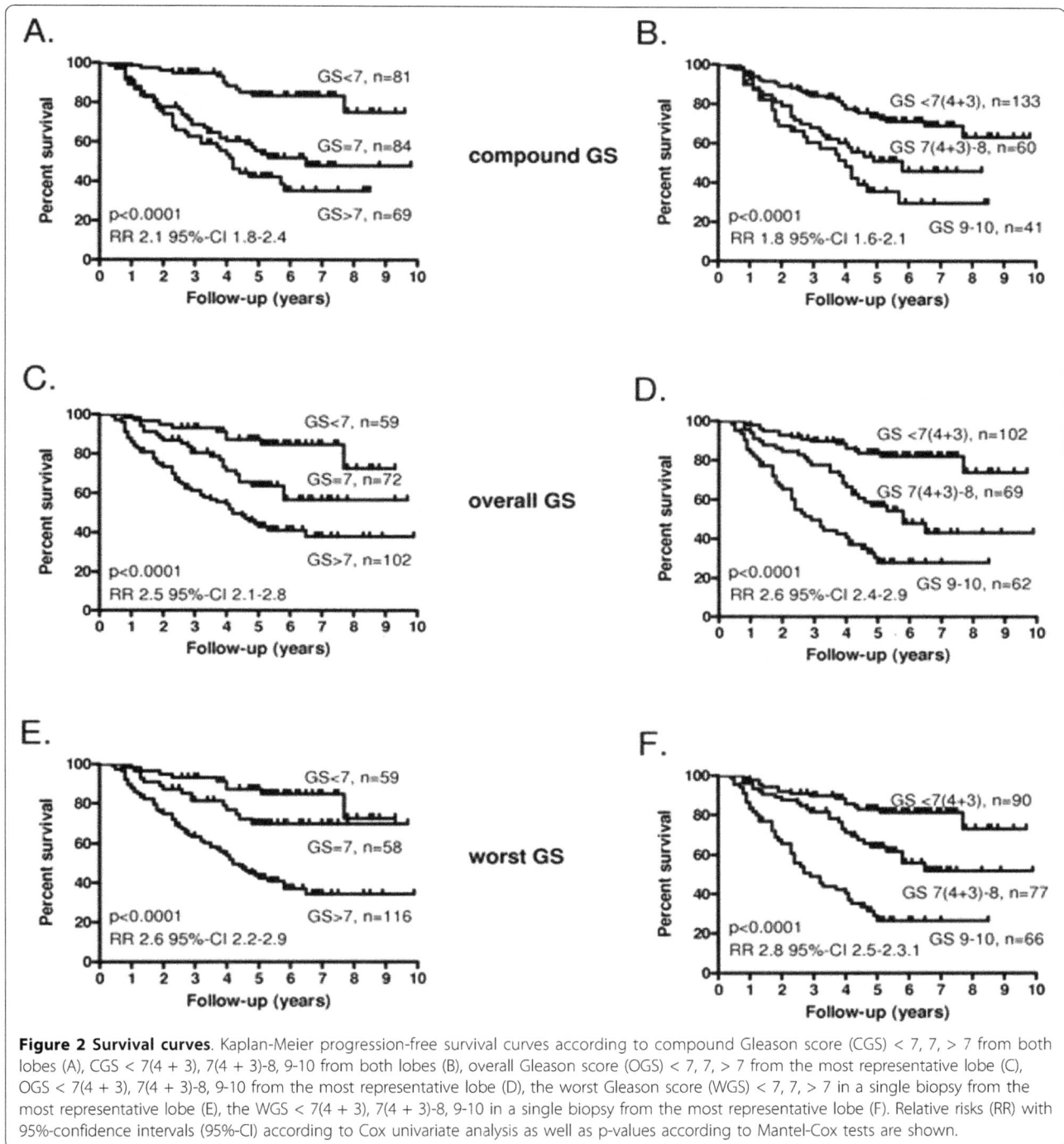

Figure 2 Survival curves. Kaplan-Meier progression-free survival curves according to compound Gleason score (CGS) < 7, 7, > 7 from both lobes (A), CGS < 7(4 + 3), 7(4 + 3)-8, 9-10 from both lobes (B), overall Gleason score (OGS) < 7, 7, > 7 from the most representative lobe (C), OGS < 7(4 + 3), 7(4 + 3)-8, 9-10 from the most representative lobe (D), the worst Gleason score (WGS) < 7, 7, > 7 in a single biopsy from the most representative lobe (E), the WGS < 7(4 + 3), 7(4 + 3)-8, 9-10 in a single biopsy from the most representative lobe (F). Relative risks (RR) with 95%-confidence intervals (95%-CI) according to Cox univariate analysis as well as p-values according to Mantel-Cox tests are shown.

with placing multiple biopsies in one container can be overcome by immersing one core biopsy per formalin-container, which is quite laborious for all the participants: the urologist, laboratory technicians, and pathologist. Two major advantages of embedding multiple needle biopsy cores in one paraffin block are the reduced workload and the ability to analyze

immunohistochemical stainings from all the biopsies at once, when deemed necessary.

There are a few limitations in the present study. First, although PSA progression works as a surrogate endpoint for progressive prostate cancer, it does not necessarily correlate specifically with cancer or overall survival. Due to the small number of deaths in our series, we cannot conclude that OGS was a better prognostic factor in terms of death as a hard end-point. To address this question, a longer follow-up is needed. Second, CGS was not re-evaluated in the present study; instead it was obtained from the original pathology reports, which limits the value of this comparison. Third, the study contained a limited number of cores and the number of cases in which WGS > OGS was rather low (n = 43). Therefore, it is not surprising that the WGS and OGS yield similar results.

Conclusions

Overall and worst Gleason scores provide comparable prognostic information. We conclude that clinicopathological practice using one container per lobe (six biopsies) and yielding an overall Gleason score is a straightforward and cost-effective procedure that correlates well to prognosis in hormone-treated patients. Therefore, the use of individually embedded biopsies should be dictated by the need for anatomic site information and weighed against the increased workload for the pathology laboratory.

Acknowledgements
We wish to thank Ms. Mariitta Vakkuri and Ms. Riitta Vaalavuo for their skillful technical assistance. The work was supported by the Academy of Finland, the Cancer Society of Finland, the Reino Lahtikari Foundation, the Sigrid Juselius Foundation and the Competitive Research Funding of the Pirkanmaa Hospital District.

Author details
[1]Institute of Medical Technology, University of Tampere and Tampere University Hospital, Tampere, Finland. [2]Department of Pathology, Centre for Laboratory Medicine, Tampere University Hospital, Tampere, Finland. [3]Department of Urology, University of Tampere and Tampere University Hospital, Tampere, Finland.

Authors' contributions
This study has been designed by PK, TV, and TTT. The needle biopsy samples have been analyzed by TTT. Manuscript has been written by TTT, PK and JI. VT is responsible for the digitalization of the images and virtual microscope system. TLJT has acquired the clinical database of the patients. TV is responsible for the statistical analyses and finalization of the manuscript. Conclusions have been drawn mainly by TTT, JI, TV and PK. All authors read and approved the final manuscript.

Competing interests
The authors declare that they have no competing interests.

References
1. Epstein JI: Gleason Score 2-4 Adenocarcinoma of the Prostate on Needle Biopsy: A Diagnosis That Should Not Be Made. Am J Surg Pathol 2000, 24:477-478.
2. Kunz GM Jr, Epstein JI: Should each core with prostate cancer be assigned a separate Gleason score? Hum Pathol 2003, 34:911-914.
3. Epstein JI, Allsbrook WC Jr, Amin MB, Egevad L, The ISUP Grading Committee: The 2005 International Society of Urological Pathology (ISUP) Consensus Conference on Gleason Grading of Prostatic Carcinoma. Am J Surg Pathol 2005, 29:228-242.
4. Kunju LP, Daignault S, Wei JT, Shah RB: Multiple prostate cancer cores with different Gleason grades submitted in the same specimen container without specific site designation: should each core be assigned an individual Gleason score? Hum Pathol 2009, 40:558-564.
5. Poulos CK, Daggy JK, Cheng L: Preoperative prediction of Gleason grade in radical prostatectomy specimens: the influence of different Gleason grades from multiple positive biopsy sites. Mod Pathol 2005, 18:228-234.
6. Forman JD, DeYoung C, Tekyi-Mensah S, Bolton S, Grignon D: The prognostic significance of the worst vs. overall gleason score in patients with multiple positive prostate needle biopsies. Int J Radiat Oncol Biol Phys 2000, 48(3 suppl):206.
7. Tolonen TT, Tammela TLJ, Kujala PM, Tuominen VJ, Isola J, Visakorpi T: Histopathological variables and biomarkers enhancer of zeste homologue 2, Ki-67 and minichromosome maintenance protein 7 as prognosticators in primarily endocrine-treated prostate cancer. BJU Int [http://dx.doi.org/10.1111/J.1464-410X.2011.10253.x].
8. Scher HI, Halabi S, Tannock I, Morris M, Sternberg CN, Carducci MA, Eisenberger MA, Higano C, Bubley GJ, Dreicer R, Petrylak D, Kantoff P, Basch E, Kelly WK, Figg WD, Small EJ, Beer TM, Wilding G, Martin A, Hussain M, Prostate Cancer Clinical Trials Working Group: Design and end points of clinical trials for patients with progressive prostate cancer and castrate levels of testosterone: recommendations of the Prostate Cancer Clinical Trials Working Group. J Clin Oncol 2008, 26:1148-1159.
9. Tuominen V, Isola J: The application of JPEG2000 in virtual microscopy. J Digit Imaging 2009, 22:250-258.
10. Billis A, Guimaraes MS, Freitas LL, Meirelles L, Magna LA, Ferreira U: The impact of the 2005 international society of urological pathology consensus conference on standard Gleason grading of prostatic carcinoma in needle biopsies. J Urol 2008, 180:548-552.
11. Lotan TL, Epstein JI: Clinical applications of changing definitions within the Gleason grading system. Nat Rev Urol 2010, 7:136-142.
12. Thompson IM, Canby-Hagino E, Lucia MS: Stage migration and grade inflation in prostate cancer: Will Rogers meets Garrison Keillor. J Natl Cancer Inst 2005, 97:1236-1237.

27

Impact of seminal trace element and glutathione levels on semen quality of Tunisian infertile men

Fatma Atig[1,3*], Monia Raffa[2], Ben-Ali Habib[1], Abdelhamid Kerkeni[2], Ali Saad[1] and Mounir Ajina[1]

Abstract

Background: Growing evidence indicates that oxidative stress can be a primary cause of male infertility. Non-enzymatic antioxidants play an important protective role against oxidative damages and lipid peroxidation. Human seminal plasma is a natural reservoir of antioxidants. The aim of this study was to determine glutathione (GSH) concentrations, trace element levels (zinc and selenium) and the lipid peroxidation end product, malondialdehyde (MDA), in the seminal plasma of men with different fertility potentials.

Methods: Semen samples from 60 fertile men (normozoospermics) and 190 infertile patients (74 asthenozoospermics, 56 oligozoospermics, and 60 teratozoospermics) were analyzed for physical and biochemical parameters. Zinc (Zn) and selenium (Se) levels were estimated by atomic absorption spectrophotometry. Total GSH (GSHt), oxidized GSH (GSSG), reduced GSH (GSHr) and MDA concentrations were measured spectrophotometrically.

Results: Zn and Se concentrations in seminal plasma of normozoospermics were more elevated than the three abnormal groups. Nevertheless, only the Zn showed significant differences. On the other hand, Zn showed positive and significant correlations with sperm motility (P = 0.03, r = 0.29) and count (P < 0.01, r = 0.49); however Se was significantly correlated only with sperm motility (P < 0.01, r = 0.36). GSHt, GSSG and GSHr were significantly higher in normozoospermics than in abnormal groups. We noted a significant association between seminal GSHt and sperm motility (P = 0.03). GSSG was highly correlated to sperm motility (P < 0.001) and negatively associated to abnormal morphology (P < 0.001). GSHr was significantly associated to total sperm motility (P < 0.001) and sperm count (P = 0.01). MDA levels were significantly higher in the three abnormal groups than in normozoospermics. Rates of seminal MDA were negatively associated to sperm motility (P < 0.01; r = -0.24) and sperm concentration (P = 0.003; r = -0.35) Meanwhile, there is a positive correlation between seminal lipid peroxidation and the percentage of abnormal morphology (P = 0.008).

Conclusions: This report revealed that decreased seminal GSH and trace element deficiencies are implicated in low sperm quality and may be an important indirect biomarker of idiopathic male infertility. Our results sustain that the evaluation of seminal antioxidant status in infertile men is necessary and can be helpful in fertility assessment from early stages.

Keywords: Antioxidants, Idiopathic oligoasthenoteratozoospermia, Male infertility, Oxidative stress, Reactive oxygen species, Spermatozoa, Seminal plasma

Background

It is increasingly recognized that reactive oxygen species (ROS) are of significant pathophysiological importance in the etiology of male infertility [1]. ROS are highly reactive oxidizing agents belonging to the class of free radicals containing one or more unpaired electrons which are continuously being generated through metabolic and pathophysiologic processes [2]. It has been postulated that oxidants interfere with normal sperm function via membrane lipid peroxidation and fragmentation of nucleic acids, which result in sperm dysfunction [3]. Due to their abundance of membrane polyunsaturated fatty acids (PUFAs) and their capacity to generate ROS, human spermatozoa are highly

---

* Correspondence: atigfatma@hotmail.fr
[1]Unit of Reproductive Medicine, University Farhat Hached Hospital, 4000 Soussa, Tunisia
Full list of author information is available at the end of the article

susceptible to oxidative stress [3]. The more important marker of lipid peroxidation is MDA. This by-product has been used in biochemical assays to monitor the degree of peroxidative damage sustained by spermatozoa. The results of such assay exhibit an excellent correlation with the degree to which sperm function is impaired [4]. High levels of seminal MDA represent increased lipid peroxidation rates, which diminishes fertility [3,4].

Hence, human spermatozoa are known to possess all of the major antioxidant defensive systems' including catalase, superoxide dismutase (SOD), glutathione peroxidase (GPX) and glutathione reductase (GRD) [5], their effectiveness is impaired by their limited concentrations and distribution. Interestingly, the seminal plasma is well equipped with an array of antioxidant defence mechanisms to protect the spermatozoa against oxidants. Antioxidants that are present in the seminal plasma compensate for the deficiency in cytoplasmic enzymes in the spermatozoa [4]. The activities of seminal antioxidant enzymes like SOD and GPX, has been measured in several studies [5]. Additionally, low molecular weight scavengers from seminal plasma appeared to be more important than enzymes, for example, trace elements and GSH [1,5].

Trace elements in human semen comprising Zn and Se have been shown to be essential for testicular development and spermatogenesis [6-9]. Zn is one of the primary factors responsible for deoxyribonucleic acid (DNA) transcription and protein synthesis which are major parts of sperm development [8]. Its concentrations are very high in the male genital organs, particularly in the prostate gland [7]. Zn can oppose the oxidation by binding sulphydryl groups in proteins and by occupying binding sites for copper in lipids and DNA [8]. It can also be a cofactor of Copper/Zn-SOD [6]. Recent studies hypothesized that insufficient intake of Zn impairs antioxidant defences. This may be an important risk factor in oxidant release and makes the spermatozoa more susceptible to lipid peroxidation [6].

Se, in particular, is an essential element for normal testicular development, spermatogenesis, and spermatozoa motility and function [9]. Se may protect against oxidative DNA damage in human sperm cells. However, the exact mechanism by which Se eliminates oxidative stress to improve male fertility and semen quality in humans is still controversial. The role of Se could be mediated via selenoenzymes, such as GPX [10]. The best-characterized spermatozoal effects of Se deficiency are: important loss of motility, breakage at the midpiece level [9,10] and increased incidence of sperm-shape abnormalities, mostly of the sperm head [10].

One more important antioxidant in humans is GSH [3]. It serves as a cofactor for GPX and reacts directly with

ROS by its free sulphydryl groups. When present in extracellular space, GSH is able to react directly with cytotoxic aldehydes produced during lipid peroxidation and thus protects the sperm plasma membrane [11]. GSHt is an imperative antioxidant via its ability to cycle between GSHr and GSSG. GSHt scavenges excess ROS and oxidized to GSSG, which is subsequently converted back to GSHr via GRD. The fertility promoting role of GSH has been established through different studies where GSH has been found to be reduced in oligozoospermics and azoospermics compared to normozoospermics [12].

Keeping in view the main protection provided by seminal plasma antioxidants against oxidative damages, the purpose of our present study was to (1) evaluate the non-enzymatic antioxidant profiles of idiopathic infertile men and to (2) assess their impact on semen parameters. In order to fulfil this goal, we measured the concentrations of Zn, Se, GSH and MDA in the seminal plasma of 250 infertile men. To our knowledge, this report which investigated the repercussions of human seminal antioxidants on sperm quality constitutes the first one conducted in Tunisia.

Methods
Study design and subject selection
A prospective controlled study was employed, involving 250 men (22-50 years) consulting for infertility evaluation in our laboratory of Cytogenetic and Reproductive Biology, Farhat Hached University Hospital, Sousse (Tunisia). Inclusion and exclusion criteria for selection of idiopathic infertile males were as follows:

Inclusion criteria
Males of couples living together with regular unprotected coitus for a reasonable period of time but not less than 1 year without conception.

Exclusion criteria
A detailed medical history was performed for all studied cases. Subjects currently on any medication or antioxidant supplementation were not included. In addition, subjects with testicular varicocele, genital infection, leukocytospermia, chronic illness and serious systemic diseases, smokers and alcoholic men were excluded from the study because of their well-known high seminal ROS levels and decreased antioxidant activity.

Study consent
A written consent of each subject was taken after explaining the aims and objectives of the study and its benefits on individual and society. Also, the study was approved by the Local Ethic Committee of the Farhat Hached University Hospital, Sousse (Tunisia).

Semen analysis
Semen samples were collected by masturbation into sterile cups following 3 days of sexual abstinence. After

30 minutes of liquefaction, standard semen parameters (Volume, motility, concentration and morphology) were immediately evaluated according to the World Health Organization guidelines (1999) [13]. Sperm motility was classified into four categories: rapid progressive motile (Type a), slow progressive motile (Type b), non-progressive motile and immotile spermatozoa, and was assayed at exactly 0.5 and 2 hours after liquefaction.

Total progressive motility was defined as the combination of type a rapid motility and type b slow progressive (At least 30% of sperm should have normal motility (categories a + b)). Sperm concentration was determined with an improved Neubauer Hemacytometer® counting chamber and normal values of concentration were " > 20×106 sperm/ml". Morphology was measured by recording the percentage of abnormal forms in the sample based on the classification of "David" [14] and at least 30% of sperm should have normal morphology.

After semen analysis, selected subjects were divided into four categories (Details of groups and semen characteristics were described in Tables 1 and 2):

a. **Normozoospermics-Normo [60 cases]:** Subjects of this group represent fertile men (controls). They are characterized by normal values for sperm motility (> 30%), sperm concentration (> 20×106 sperm/ml) and normal sperm morphology (> 30%).

b. **Asthenozoospermics-Astheno [74 cases]:** This study group consists of isolated asthenozoospermic men whose infertility is determined mainly by less than normal levels for sperm motility (< 30%), with normal values of morphologically normal sperm (< 30%) and sperm concentration (> 20×106 sperm/ml).

c. **Oligozoospermics-Oligo [56 cases]:** Infertility of this group is defined mainly by an isolated oligozoospermia (< 20×106 sperm/ml), with normal levels for sperm motility (> 30%) and morphologically normal sperm (> 30%)

d. **Teratozoospermics-Terato [60 cases]:** This category of patients consists of isolated teratozoospermic men whose infertility is determined essentially by less than normal levels for morphologically normal sperm (< 30%), with normal values of sperm concentration (> 20×106 sperm/ml) and motility (> 30%).

After semen analysis, seminal plasma was separated from spermatozoa by centrifugation at 3500 rpm for 15 minutes and stored at -80°C until antioxidant analysis.

Chemicals

All reagents and chemicals were of analytical grade or higher purity and obtained from standard commercial suppliers. Ultra-pure water was received from water purification Milli-Q system (Millipore Corporation, USA).

Biochemical Procedures

a. **Analytical methods for determination of Zn and Se levels**

For all the experiment, flame atomic absorption spectrophotometry (AAS) was adopted for Zn determination and furnace AAS for Se measurement. The measures were implemented using a Zeenit 700-Analytik-Jena, Germany, equipped with deuterium and Zeeman background correction, respectively, as recommended by the manufacturer. Detection limits for these microelements were as follows: Zn (0.47 µg/l) and Se (0.78 µg/l).

b. **Determination of GSHt and GSSG contents**

GSHt and GSSG levels were measured spectrophotometrically in deproteinized seminal plasma samples, by the method of Akerboom & Sies, (1981) [15], using 5,5'-

Table 1 General characteristics of the studied population

parameters	Characteristics	Number(n)	Percentage (%)
Age (Years)	≤ 35	105	42
	> 35	145	58
Duration of infertility	≤ 10	183	72.2
	> 10	67	28.8
Type of infertility	Primary	191	76.4
	Secondary	59	32.6
Area	Rural	94	37.6
	Urban	156	62.4
Diet	Vegetarian	138	55.2
	Mixed	112	54.8
Sperm criteria	Fertile	60	24
	Asthenozoospermics	74	29.6
	Oligozoospermics	56	22.4
	Teratozoospermics	60	24
Duration of sexual abstinence (Days)	3	250	100

Table 2 Descriptive statistics and comparison of conventional semen parameters fertile and the three infertile groups

Parameters	Fertile (n = 60)	Astheno (n = 74)	Oligo (n = 56)	Terato (n = 60)	P-Value		
					Fertile Vs Astheno	Fertile Vs Oligo	Fertile Vs Terato
Age (years)	33.43 ± 4.40	34.95 ± 4.20	40.27 ± 4.50	39.00 ± 5.01	NS	NS	NS
Mean ± SD Min-Max	22.00-41.00	29.00-42.00	30.00-50.00	28.00-50.00			
Volume (ml)	3.89 ± 1.48	3.34 ± 1.67	4.21 ± 2.44	3.65 ± 1.73	NS	NS	NS
Mean ± SD Min-Max	2.00-5.56	2.00-7.58	2.00-8.23	2.00-6.34			
Sperm motility (%)	48.72 ± 14.22	18.40 ± 9.62	45.72 ± 13.42	44.32 ± 12.45	P < 0.001	NS	NS
Mean ± SD Min-Max	43.00-100	1.00-30.00	40.00-99.00	40.00-97.00			
Sperm Count (x10^6/ml)	75.86 ± 23.83	46.21 ± 24	9.56 ± 6.51	54.00 ± 26.23	P < 0.001	P < 0.001	0.001
Mean ± SD Min-Max	30.00-100	20.00-100	1.00-15.00	26.00-100			
Abnormal morphology (%)	60.90 ± 13.28	60.42 ± 11.85	65.24 ± 16.36	81.79 ± 11.49	NS	NS	P < 0.001
Mean ± SD Min-Max	39.00-65.00	41.00-72.00	41.00-69.00	77.00-98.00			

Note: Astheno = Asthenozoospermics, Oligo = Oligozoospermics, Terato = Teratozoospermics, Max = maximum, Min = minimum, ml = milliliter, SD = Standard Deviation. Data are expressed as means ± SD. NS = Not significant. P ≤ 0.05 = significant.

dithiobis (2-nitrobenzoic acid). Absorbance values were compared with standard curves from known amounts of GSH standards.

c. Assessment of oxidative stress by measurement of Lipid Peroxidation

Lipid peroxidation was measured by determining the MDA production, using the Thiobarbituric Acid (TBA) method (Yagi, (1976)) [16]. After liquefaction, semen samples were centrifuged at 3500 rpm for 15 min to get seminal plasma. Then, 0.1 ml of seminal plasma was added to 0.75 ml of TBA reagent (0.8 g of 2-TBA dissolved in 80 ml of distilled water with 0.5 ml of NaOH. Perchloric acid (7%) was added to this mixture in order to adjust the pH = 7.4). This mixture was heated for 1 hour at 95°C in a warm water bath. After cooling, the tube was centrifuged for 10 min at 4000 rpm and the supernatant's absorbance was read on a spectrophotometer at 535 nm.

Statistical analysis

The Windows computing program Statistical Package for the Social Sciences "SPSS 11.0" (SPSS, Chicago, IL, USA) was used for analyzing the data. All data were expressed as mean ± standard deviation (S.D.). The differences that existed between the evaluated study groups were assessed by performing an analysis of variance (One-way ANOVA) and the post hoc test (Tukey test) to conduct pair-wise comparisons. The differences were considered to be significant at values of P ≤ 0.05. Finally, Pearson's correlation was performed to examine the correlation between trace elements, MDA and semen quality. All hypothesis testing were two-sided with a probability value of 0.05 deemed as significant (P < 0.05 = significant*; P < 0.001 = highly significant**).

Results

As shown in Table 2 the mean of age of the fertile group (33.4 ± 4.4 years) was decreased when compared to asthenozoospermics (34.9 ± 4.2 years), oligozoospermics (40.2 ± 4.5 years) and teratozoospermics (39 ± 5 years), but the difference was not significant. There was no significant correlation between patient's age and seminal antioxidant status. The mean values of the examined sperm parameters in controls and infertile groups are shown in Table 2. Sperm count, motility and the percentage of normal morphology were significantly higher in normozoospermics than the three abnormal groups.

Trace element and GSH levels

In this study and as shown in Table 3, concentrations of seminal trace elements "Zn and Se" were more elevated in the control group than the three abnormal groups. However, only the Zn showed significantly differences after comparison between controls and asthenozoospermics (P = 0.02), oligozoospermics (P = 0.008) and teratozoospermics (P = 0.04). Moreover, a significant increase of mean GSHt were found in normozoospermics (57.00 ± 19.54 µmol/l) compared to asthenozoospermics (38.41 ± 23.92 µmol/l P < 0.001) and teratozoospermics (45.77 ± 17.62 µmol/l P = 0.002). Also, a highly significant decline in GSSG concentration was detected in the seminal plasma of teratozoospermics compared to the fertile group (P < 0.001) (Table 3). GSHr showed an increased concentration in normozoospermic group compared to Asthenozoospermics (P < 0.001); however, there was no significant difference observed when compared with oligozoospermics and teratozoospermics.

Seminal MDA content

Lipid peroxidation as expressed by MDA level in the seminal plasma was found to be significantly higher in the three abnormal groups than in fertile group. Mean

Table 3 Seminal antioxidant status and MDA concentrations of the different studied groups

Parameters	Fertile (n = 60)	Astheno (n = 74)	Oligo (n = 56)	Terato (60)	P-Value		
					Fertile Vs. Astheno	Fertile Vs. Oligo	Fertile VS. Terato
Zinc (mg/l)	144 ± 42.13	122 ± 34.69	120.51 ± 25.33	126 ± 24.82	0.02	0.008	0.04
Mean ± SD Min-Max	49.00-239	54.00-190	46.52-94.55	52-200			
Selenium (µg/l)	64 ± 20.64	56.00 ± 22.81	55.00 ± 21.44	57.00 ± 24.31	NS	NS	NS
Mean Min-Max	44.00-84.00	30.00-72.00	41.00-69.00	36.00-76.00			
GSHt (µmol/l)	57.00 ± 19.54	38.41 ± 23.92	52.86 ± 7.08	45.77 ± 17.62	< 0.001	NS	0.002
Mean ± SD Min-Max	25.63-99.55	7.18-96.84	43.88-60.86	14.22-68.45			
GSSG (µmol/l)	22.81 ± 13.38	21.89 ± 12.67	24.84 ± 11.75	9.74 ± 5.82	NS	NS	< 0.001
Mean ± SD Min-Max	0.00-55.19	2.63-79.07	8.82-43.86	2.27-35.53			
GSHr	34.27 ± 14.91	16.63 ± 12.83	28.00 ± 14.22	36.00 ± 16.71	< 0.001	NS	NS
Mean ± SD Min-Max	19.00-55.00	13.00-31.00	13.85-43.00	19.00-42.00			
MDA (µmol/l)	2.30 ± 0.94	3.52 ± 1.93	3.21 ± 1.37	3.64 ± 1.73	0.002	0.004	< 0.001
Mean ± SD Min-Max	1.37-2.33	2.21-4.83	2.28-4.29	2.66-4.68			

Note: Astheno = Asthenozoospermics, Oligo = Oligozoospermics, Terato = Teratozoospermics, GSHt = Total glutathione, GSSG = Oxidized glutathione, GSHr = reduced glutathione, MDA = Malondialdehyde acid, Max = maximum, Min = minimum, ml = millilitre, SD = Standard Deviation, NS = Not significant. Data are expressed as means ± SD. P ≤ 0.05 = significant.

MDA levels in abnormal groups were found to be 3.52 ± 1.93 µmol/l in the asthenozoospermic group, 3.21 ± 1.37 µmol/l in the oligozoospermic group and 3.64 ± 1.73 µmol/l in the teratozoospermic group (Table 3). In effect, rates of seminal MDA were negatively associated to sperm motility (P < 0.01; r = -0.24) and sperm concentration (P = 0.003; r = -0.35) Meanwhile, there was a positive correlation between seminal lipid peroxidation and the percentage of abnormal morphology (P = 0.008; r = 0.19) (Table 4).

Correlations between seminal antioxidant status and sperm parameters

Significant positive correlations were detected between seminal Zn concentrations and sperm motility (P = 0.03, r = 0.29) and sperm concentration (P < 0.01, r = 0.49). Seminal Se showed a highly significant relationship only with sperm motility (P < 0.01, r = 0.36) (Table 4).

As shown in Table 4 we noted a significant association between seminal GSHt and sperm motility (P = 0.03, r = 0.13). However, seminal GSSG was highly correlated to sperm motility (P < 0.001, r = 0.22) and negatively associated to the percentage of sperm atypical forms (P < 0.001, r = -0.39) Seminal GSHr was significantly associated to sperm motility (P < 0.001, r = 0.42) and sperm concentration (P = 0.01, r = 0.11).

Discussion

The key results in this study were: *(1)* An impaired antioxidant status was observed in seminal plasma of infertile men. *(2)* The fertile group showed a significant decrease in seminal lipid peroxidation levels compared to the three abnormal groups. *(3)* Positive correlations

exist between enhanced seminal antioxidant status and good semen quality. Total sperm motility was significantly correlated to the seminal trace elements and different forms of GSH. The sperm concentration was positively associated to the seminal Zn and seminal GSHr amounts. However, the percentage of atypical sperm forms showed a significantly negative relationship to seminal GSSG. *(4)* Inversely to the non-enzymatic antioxidants, seminal MDA levels were negatively correlated to the sperm parameters. These findings indicated that some idiopathic infertile men may be poorly equipped to deal with oxidative stress due to the impaired seminal antioxidant defences. As a consequence, we suggest such a possibility and call for more systematic research on the role of oxidative stress in idiopathic male infertility.

The detailed biochemical mechanisms underlying the physiopathology of male infertility are not clearly understood. There has been evidence supporting the notion

Table 4 The value of Pearson's correlation coefficients calculated between the antioxidant parameters and sperm criteria

Elements	Motility	Sperm count	Atypical forms
Zinc	0.29*	0.49**	NS
Selenium	0.36**	NS	NS
GSHt	0.13*	NS	NS
GSSG	0.22**	NS	-0.39*
GSHr	0.42**	0.11*	NS
MDA	-0.24*	-0.35*	0.19*

Note: GSHt = Total glutathione, GSSG = Oxidized glutathione, MDA = Malondialdehyde acid, NS = Not significant. * Significant correlation P < 0.05, ** Correlation strongly significant P ≤ 0.001.

that major changes in seminal antioxidants could be related to abnormal spermatozoa function and fertilization capacity [9]. Hence, seminal plasma is considered to be the central source of antioxidants that protect sperm cells against oxidative damages. The antioxidant system eliminates ROS to maintain a reduced environment in cells through enzymatic and non-enzymatic approaches. The most studied antioxidants are the SOD, GPX and catalase enzymes. Information about seminal non-enzymatic antioxidants and male fertility potential is quite inadequate till date. Moreover, it is important to underline the contradictions and the controversial outcomes found in the literature. In fact, these differences can be due to several variables among which are inclusion and exclusion criteria for patient selection, analytical methodologies, sperm anomalies (in our study, each patient group has a single sperm anomaly; whether asthenozoospermia, or oligozoospermia or teratozoospermia), lifestyle or dietary pattern and the patient's origin.

In our study, we tried to explore the concentrations of Zn, Se and GSH in the seminal plasma of our patient groups and controls in order to estimate their contribution to maintain a good quality of sperm.

The mean seminal Zn concentrations in control and abnormal groups were between 120 and 144 mg/l. These values were comparable with a few similar studies reported by Lewis Jones et al. (118 mg/l) [17] and Kruse et al. (123 mg/l) [18]. However, the reported Zn levels in other studies were considerably higher than our findings; Omu et al. (171 mg/l) [19] and Chia et al. (183 mg/l) [7]. These differences may be due to the slightly different techniques used in the measurement of Zn concentrations and the difference in cigarette-smoking habits. In comparison with the control group, our infertile patients showed decreased seminal Zn concentrations; however these differences were not significant. Inflammatory conditions, prostatitis, accumulation of toxic heavy metals and frequent ejaculation can negatively influence the secretory function of the prostate and lead to a drop in seminal Zn content [7,20]. Nevertheless, these factors were excluded from our investigation and reduced Zn amounts of infertile patients can be explained by other mechanisms. Increased sperm ROS in infertile men explain the decrease of seminal Zn concentrations, arising the harmful effects of ROS to sperm cells which are associated with abnormal sperm parameters [8]. Powell [21] supports this hypothesis, noting that reduction in Zn concentration can lead to an increase in oxidation of membrane lipids, DNA and proteins; which can provoke the loss of membrane integrity. In our study, the negative and not significant correlation between Zn and MDA confirmed that reduction in seminal Zn levels is associated to the decline of its antioxidant capacity and the increase of lipid peroxidation and low sperm quality.

Additionally, seminal Zn concentrations demonstrated significant differences between fertile and infertile men, which corroborated with the findings of Colagar et al. [6]. Furthermore, like Zaho et al. [22] we observed positive relationships between good sperm production, motility and increased seminal Zn content. With these findings we can support the extensive evidence defending the antioxidant capacity of seminal Zn to yield various benefits in sperm including reduction of MDA and decreasing of DNA fragmentation [10]. Therefore, Zn may be useful in idiopathic oligoasthenoteratozoospermia in reducing oxidative stress and the associated sperm membrane and DNA damage [10].

Se is also an essential trace element that plays an important role in a number of physiological processes including human reproduction [22]. This element becomes crucial for maintaining normal spermatogenesis and male fertility [23]. In our study, we reported a slight increase of seminal Se in controls compared to infertile groups. This was in agreement with the observations of Saaranen et al. [24] and Akinloye et al. [9] who showed a significant decrease of seminal Se levels in asthenozoospermics and oligozoospermics. Takasaki et al. [25] did not find any difference in seminal Se amounts between fertile and infertile men. Meanwhile, a follow-up study 4.5-5 years after the initial assay revealed that low Se levels (< 35 ng/ml) were associated with male infertility.

Our findings sustain the data supporting the negative influence of low seminal Se levels on the number of spermatozoa and sperm motility [9,10]. This evidence can be confirmed by the correlation of the seminal Se and sperm motility observed in our investigation. The association of Se with a protein present in the tail of spermatozoa isolated from bulls and rats [26] and its localization in the mitochondria capsule protein of the midpiece [27] of spermatozoa are possible indications of its importance in sperm motility and male infertility.

Decreased Se concentrations in seminal plasma of infertile men were accompanied by increased levels of seminal MDA of the same patients. In this respect, the diminution of Se activity as an antioxidant can explain the elevated lipid peroxidation in infertile patients. In effect, the only biochemical role of Se in mammals depends on its presence as a seleno-cysteine residue at each of the four catalytic site of the enzyme "GPX" [9]. GPX plays a crucial role in the antioxidant defences of the epididymis and the ejaculated spermatozoa [27].

In addition to the impaired Zn and Se concentrations in seminal plasma of infertile men, we reported also decreased seminal GSHt, GSSG and GSHr levels in the three abnormal groups. Oshendorf et al. [28] found a moderate reduction of GSH in oligozoospermic compared to normozoospermic men, while other studies found GSH levels below the limit of detection (< 2.5 µM) in seminal plasma of oligozoospermics, or GSH levels to be significantly reduced in seminal plasma of infertile males compared to those of fertile ones [1,3]. Even GSH therapy was found to improve the semen quality [29]. Our results provide evidence that higher levels of GSH in seminal plasma seem to play a role in protection against oxidative damage and to improve the sperm motility and morphology. While stating that, other studies could not observe any difference in GSH concentration between fertile and infertile men [8] and this may be due to the contribution of spermatozoal ROS leading to the up-regulation of thiol synthesis in order to protect sperm from oxidative damage. Raijmakers et al. [30] also reported that median levels of seminal GSH were significantly lower in infertile males as compared to normozoospermics, and found a positive association between seminal GSH level and sperm morphology and motility. In our investigation, we found that higher GSHt, GSSG and GSHr levels in seminal plasma were associated with a higher quality of sperm motility and count, however lower GSSG levels were associated with a higher degree of spermatozoa with abnormal morphology and immobility. These findings were compatible with that observed by Bhardwaj A et al. [12] and Eskiocak S et al. [31].

Accordingly; we can suggest that the loss of sperm motility in asthenozoospermic samples may result from the over-oxidation of sperm sulphydryl. GSH displays maximal staining in the mid-piece and tail region, which are important regions for motility of spermatozoa [31]. These results imply that seminal plasma GSH levels may play a role in the protection against oxidative damage by reducing lipid peroxidation on sperm membrane. It could therefore be proposed that the concentration of GSH could be used as a chemical parameter to assess male fertility. The beneficial role of GSH to minimize oxidative damage to the spermatozoa can make it a suitable candidate for therapeutic usage in the treatment of male infertility.

Altered antioxidant status was observed in the seminal plasma, which was collected during our study from infertile men. This might cause oxidative damage and makes the sperm highly susceptible to lipid peroxidation. MDA production reflects the peroxidation of membrane polyunsaturated phospholipids [32,33]. Our results established a significant increase in the amount of seminal MDA in abnormal groups compared to normozoospermics. Accordingly, lipid peroxidative degradation of sperm membrane integrity may be held responsible for abnormal sperm motility, concentration and morphology. Our results were corroborative with Hesham et al. [3] and Ben Abdallah F et al. [34] who reported that MDA content was elevated in oligozoospermic and

asthenozoospermic groups. However, there was controversy about seminal MDA activity and sperm quality. We showed that higher seminal MDA levels were negatively associated with sperm motility and sperm count. Nevertheless, a positive relationship was observed between increased lipid peroxidation and the abnormal sperm morphology, which was compatible with the findings of Suleiman et al. [35]. Increased MDA levels in seminal plasma of abnormal groups could represent the pathological effects lipid peroxidation has on the spermatozoa membrane and consequently on sperm motility and viability.

Conclusions

In summary, associations of seminal Zn, Se and GSH with other parameters of semen quality indicate that the decrease of seminal antioxidants can be a risk factor for sperm abnormality and idiopathic male infertility. It was also shown that increased MDA levels in the abnormal groups could represent the pathological effects of lipid peroxidation on sperm function. These data suggested that routine determination of antioxidant status during infertility investigation is recommended. Furthermore, future research should focus on enzymatic and non-enzymatic antioxidants; genetic susceptibility and their repercussions on semen quality.

Abbreviations

ROS: Reactive Oxygen Species; PUFAs: Polyunsaturated Fatty Acids; MDA: Malondialdehyde Acid; SOD: Superoxide Dismutase; GPX: Glutathione peroxidase; GRD: Glutathione peroxidase; GSH: Glutathione; Zn: Zinc; DNA: Desoxirubonucleic Acid; Se: Selenium; GSHt: Total glutathione; GSHr: Reduced glutathione; GSSG: Oxidized glutathione; Normo: Normozoospermic men; Astheno: Asthenozoospermic men; Oligo: Oligozooseprmic men; Terato: Teratozoospermic men; AAS: Atomic Absorption Spectroscopy; TBA: Thiobarbituric Acid; SD: Standard Deviation; Max: Maximum; Min: Minimum; NS: Not Significant.

Acknowledgements

We want to thank Dr. Monia Raffa (Research Laboratory of "Trace elements, free radicals and antioxidants", Biophysical Department, Faculty of Medicine, Monastir, Tunisia) for her help and assistance during biochemical analysis.

Author details

[1]Unit of Reproductive Medicine, University Farhat Hached Hospital, 4000 Soussa, Tunisia. [2]Research Laboratory of "Trace elements, free radicals and antioxidants", Biophysical Department, Faculty of Medicine, University of Monastir, 5000 Monastir, Tunisia. [3]Department of Cytogenetic and Reproductive Reproduction, Farhat Hached, University Teaching Hospital, 4000 Sousse, Tunisia.

Authors' contributions

All the authors made substantial contributions to the design and conception of the study. Particularly, FA wrote the manuscript, contributed to the analysis and interpretation of the data. AK conceived of the study, and participated in its design and coordination and helped to draft the manuscript. MA contributed to the development of the protocol and study instruments. All the authors have been involved in drafting and revising the manuscript, have read, and approved the final manuscript.

Competing interests

The authors declare that they have no competing interests.

References

1. Chaudhari AR, Das P, Singh R: **Study of oxidative stress and reduced glutathione levels in seminal plasma of human subjects with different fertility potential.** *Biomed Res* 2008, 19:207-210.

2. Agarwal A, Sharma R, Nalella KP, Thomas AJ, Alvarez JG, Sikka SC: **Reactive oxygen species as an independent marker of male factor infertility.** *Fertil Steril* 2006, 86:878-885.

3. Hesham N, Moemen LA, Abu Elela MH: **Studying the levels of malondialdehyde and antioxidant parameters in normal and abnormal human seminal plasma.** *Aust J Basic Appl Sci* 2008, 2:773-778.

4. Agarwal A, Saleh RA, Bedaiwy MA: **Role of reactive oxygen species in the pathophysiology of human reproduction.** *Fertil Steril* 2003, 79:829-843.

5. Potts RJ, Notarianni LJ, Jefferies TM: **Seminal plasma reduces exogenous oxidative damage to human sperm, determined by the measurement of DNA strand breaks and lipid peroxidation.** *Mutat Res* 2000, 447:249-256.

6. Colagar AH, Marzony ET, Chaichi MJ: **Zinc levels in seminal plasma are associated with sperm quality in fertile and infertile men.** *Nutr Res* 2009, 29:82-88.

7. Chia SE, Ong CN, Chua LH, Ho LM, Tay SK: **Comparison of zinc concentrations in blood and seminal plasma and the various sperm parameters between fertile and infertile men.** *J Androl* 2000, 21:53-57.

8. Ebisch IMW, Thomas CMG, Peters WHM, Braat DDM, Steegers-Theunissen RPM: **The importance of folate, zinc and antioxidants in the pathogenesis and prevention of subfertility.** *Hum Reprod Update* 2007, 13:163-174.

9. Akinloye O, Arowojolu O, Shittu B, Adejuwon CA, Osotimehin B: **Selenium Status of Idiopathic Infertile Nigerian Males.** *Biol Trace Elem Res* 2005, 104:9-18.

10. Agarwal A, Sekhon LH: **Oxidative stress and antioxidants for idiopathic oligoasthenoteratospermia: Is it justified?** *Indian J Urol* 2011, 27:74-85.

11. Sørensen MB, Stoltenberg M, Danscher G, Ernst E: **Chelation of intracellular zinc ions affects human sperm cell motility.** *Mol Hum Reprod* 1999, 5:338-341.

12. Bhardwaj A, Verma A, Majumdar S, Khanduja KL: **Status of Vitamin E and reduced glutathione in semen of Oligozoospermic & azoospermic patients.** *Asian J Androl* 2000, 2:225-228.

13. World Health Organization: *WHO laboratory manual for the examination of human semen and semen-cervical mucus interaction.* 4 edition. Cambridge, UK: Published on behalf of the World Health Organization by Cambridge University Press; 1999, 1-86.

14. David G: **Editorial: sperm banks in France.** *Arch Fr Pediatr* 1975, 5:401-404.

15. Akerboom TPM, Sies H: **Assay of glutathione disulfide and glutathione mixed disulfides in biological samples.** *Methods Enzymol* 1981, 77:373-378.

16. Yagi K: **A simple fluorometric assay for lipoperoxide in blood plasma.** *Biochem Med* 1976, 5:212-216.

17. Lewis-Jones DL, Aird IA, Biljan MM, Kingsland CR: **Effects of sperm activity on zinc and fructose concentrations in seminal plasma.** *Hum Reprod* 1996, 11:2465-2467.

18. Kruse WE, Zwick EM, Batschulat K, Rohr G, Ambruster FP, Petzoldt D, *et al*: **Are zinc levels in seminal plasma associated with seminal leukocytes and other determinants of semen quality?** *Fertil Steril* 2002, 77:260-269.

19. Omu AE, Dashti H, Al-Othman S: **Treatment of asthenozoospermia with zinc sulphate: andrological, immunological and obstetric outcome.** *Eur J Obstet Gynecol Reprod Biol* 1998, 79:179-184.

20. Dissanayake D, Wijesinghe P, Ratnasooriya W, Wimalasena S: **Relationship between seminal plasma zinc and semen quality in a sub-fertile population.** *J Hum Reprod* 2010, 3:124-128.

21. Powell SR: **Antioxidant properties of zinc.** *J Nutr* 2000, 130:1447-1454.

22. Zhao RP, Xiong CL: **Zinc content analysis in serum, seminal plasma and spermatozoa of asthenozoospermic and oligoasthenozoospermic patients.** *Zhonghua Nan Ke Xue* 2005, 11:680-682.

23. Boitani C, Puglisi R: **Selenium, a Key Element in Spermatogenesis and Male Fertility.** *Adv Exp Med Biol* 2008, 636:65-73.

24. Saaranen M, Suistomaa U, Vanha-Perttula T: **Semen selenium content and sperm mitochondrial volume in human and some animal's species.** *Hum Reprod* 1989, 4:504-508.

25. Takasaki N, Tonami H, Simizu A, Ueno N, Ogita T, Okada S, *et al*: **Semen selenium and infertility.** *Bull Osaka Med Sch* 1987, 33:87-96.

26. Bedwal RS, Bahuguna A: **Zinc, copper and selenium in reproduction.** *Experientian* 1994, 50:626-640.

27. Sunde RA: **The biochemistry of selenoproteins.** *J Am Oil Chem Soc* 1984, 61:1891-1900.

28. Ochsendorf FR, Buhl R, Bästlein A, Beschmann H: **Glutathione in spermatozoa and seminal plasma of infertile men.** *Hum Reprod* 1998, 13:353-359.

29. Lenzi A, Gandini L, Picardo M: **A rationale for glutathione therapy.** *Hum Reprod* 1998, 13:1419-1422.

30. Raijmakers MT, Roelofs HM, Steegers EA, Steegers-Theunissen RRP, Mulder TP, Knapen MF, *et al*: **Glutathione and glutathione S-transferases A1-1 and P1-1 in seminal plasma may play a role in protecting against oxidative damage to spermatozoa.** *Fertil Steril* 2003, 79:169-172.

31. Eskiocak S, Gozen AS, Yapar SB, Tavas F, Kilic AS, Eskiocak M: **Glutathione and free sulphydryl content of seminal plasma in healthy medical students during and after exam stress.** *Hum Reprod* 2005, 9:2595-6000.

32. Storey BT: **Biochemistry of the induction and prevention of lipo-peroxidative mechanisms damage in human spermatozoa.** *Mol Hum Reprod* 1997, 3:203-213.

33. Agarwal A, Allamaneni SS: **Free radicals and male reproduction.** *J Indian Med Assoc* 2011, 109:184-187.

34. Ben Abdallah F, Dammak I, Attia H, Hentati B, Ammar-Keskes L: **Lipid peroxidation and antioxidant enzyme activities in infertile men: correlation with semen parameter.** *J Clin Lab Anal* 2009, 23:99-104.

35. Suleiman SA, Ali ME, Zaki ZM, El Malik EM, Nasr MA: **Lipid peroxidation and human sperm motility: protective role of vitamin E.** *J Androl* 1996, 17:530-537.

28

Minimal percentage of dose received by 90% of the urethra (%UD90) is the most significant predictor of PSA bounce in patients who underwent low-dose-rate brachytherapy (LDR-brachytherapy) for prostate cancer

Nobumichi Tanaka[1*], Isao Asakawa[2], Kiyohide Fujimoto[1], Satoshi Anai[1], Akihide Hirayama[1], Masatoshi Hasegawa[2], Noboru Konishi[3] and Yoshihiko Hirao[1]

Abstract

Background: To clarify the significant clinicopathological and postdosimetric parameters to predict PSA bounce in patients who underwent low-dose-rate brachytherapy (LDR-brachytherapy) for prostate cancer.

Methods: We studied 200 consecutive patients who received LDR-brachytherapy between July 2004 and November 2008. Of them, 137 patients did not receive neoadjuvant or adjuvant androgen deprivation therapy. One hundred and forty-two patients were treated with LDR-brachytherapy alone, and 58 were treated with LDR-brachytherapy in combination with external beam radiation therapy. The cut-off value of PSA bounce was 0.1 ng/mL. The incidence, time, height, and duration of PSA bounce were investigated. Clinicopathological and postdosimetric parameters were evaluated to elucidate independent factors to predict PSA bounce in hormone-naïve patients who underwent LDR-brachytherapy alone.

Results: Fifty patients (25%) showed PSA bounce and 10 patients (5%) showed PSA failure. The median time, height, and duration of PSA bounce were 17 months, 0.29 ng/mL, and 7.0 months, respectively. In 103 hormone-naïve patients treated with LDR-brachytherapy alone, and univariate Cox proportional regression hazard model indicated that age and minimal percentage of the dose received by 30% and 90% of the urethra were independent predictors of PSA bounce. With a multivariate Cox proportional regression hazard model, minimal percentage of the dose received by 90% of the urethra was the most significant parameter of PSA bounce.

Conclusions: Minimal percentage of the dose received by 90% of the urethra was the most significant predictor of PSA bounce in hormone-naïve patients treated with LDR-brachytherapy alone.

Keywords: Prostate cancer, Brachytherapy, PSA bounce, Post-dosimetry, UD90 (%)

* Correspondence: sendo@naramed-u.ac.jp
[1]Department of Urology, Nara Medical University, 840 Shijo-cho, Kashihara, Nara 634-8522, Japan
Full list of author information is available at the end of the article

Background

Several investigators have reported PSA (prostate-specific antigen) bounce, a transient PSA elevation that is frequently observed after low-dose-rate brachytherapy (LDR-brachytherapy) [1-10]. Although the factors that affect PSA fluctuation after LDR-brachytherapy are unclear, multiple factors including age, prostatitis due to radiation or urinary tract infection, acute urinary retention, laboratory error, instrumentation, ejaculation, radiation proctitis, and testosterone recovery after androgen deprivation therapy (ADT) are currently considered as etiologies of PSA bounce. Most importantly, it is difficult to differentiate between PSA bounce and biochemical failure, and this situation produces a dilemma for patients and physicians to determine whether the treatment has failed or not. Several cut-off values of PSA, such as 0.1, 0.2, and 0.4 ng/mL, have been used to define PSA bounce. Seventeen to 62% of patients who underwent LDR-brachytherapy showed a PSA bounce during the first 3 years after LDR-brachytherapy [1-10]. The incidence of PSA bounce in Japanese patients is reportedly similar to that in American patients [8,9].

We investigated PSA bounce rates after LDR-brachytherapy to elucidate independent predictors of PSA bounce in our series of patients.

Methods

Two hundred patients who were clinically diagnosed with localized prostate cancer (cT1c-2cN0M0) and underwent LDR-brachytherapy between July 2004 and November 2008 and a minimum follow-up of 18 months were enrolled in this prospective study. The patients' characteristics are shown in Table 1. The median age, PSA value at diagnosis, and follow-up period were 70 years (range: 51–80), 7.6 ng/mL (range: 3.1-32.1), and 38 months (range: 18–65), respectively. One pathologist (NK) with expertise in prostate cancer diagnosis reviewed the Gleason score of all biopsy specimens centrally. The PSA values (PSA; ST AIA-PACK PSA II) were measured at 1, 3, and 6 months after LDR-brachytherapy, and then every 6 months.

The institutional review board of Nara Medical University approved this study, and informed consent was obtained from all patients after explaining the aim and methods of this study.

Treatment

Among the 200 patients, 137 did not receive neoadjuvant or adjuvant androgen deprivation therapy (ADT), and 4 received both neoadjuvant and adjuvant ADT. The median period of neoadjuvant ADT was 6.0 months (range: 1 to 54 months), and the scheduled period of adjuvant ADT was 2 years. Of the remaining patients, 55 received only neoadjuvant ADT and 4 received only

Table 1 Patients' characteristics

	Bounce (-) (n = 150)	Bounce (+) (n = 50)	p value
Age (year)			
mean, median (range)	69.2, 70.0 (55-80)	67.4, 68.5 (51-79)	0.132§
PSA at diagnosis (ng/mL)			
mean, median (range)	9.1, 7.8 (3.1-32.1)	7.8, 6.7 (3.7-16.7)	0.029§
10 or less	106	41	
10-20	37	9	
greater than 20	7	0	0.156*
biopsy Gleason score			
6 or less	91	37	
7	53	11	
8-10	6	2	0.210*
clinical T stage			
T1c	88	32	
T2a	50	15	
T2b	7	2	
T2c	5	1	0.904*
neo-Adjuvant/ Adjuvant			
none	102	35	
neo-Ad (+)	40	15	
Ad (+)	4	0	
neo-Ad (+), Ad (+)	4	0	0.417*
Combined EBRT			
yes	49	9	
no	101	41	0.050*
biochemical recurrence			
yes	10	0	
no	140	50	0.069*
Number of PSA measurement			
mean, median (range)	8.5, 8.0 (5-15)	10.3, 10.5 (6-14)	< 0.001§
Follow-up period (month)			
mean, median (range)	36.7, 36.0 (18-64)	46.0, 47.0 (20-65)	< 0.001§

*Chi-square test and §student t-test.

adjuvant ADT. One hundred and forty-two patients were treated with LDR-brachytherapy alone and 58 patients were treated with LDR-brachytherapy in combination with external beam radiation therapy (EBRT) (Table 1).

From July 2004 to April 2007, LDR-brachytherapy alone was performed at the prescribed dose of 145 Gy in 93 patients, and after May 2007 it was performed at the prescribed dose of 160 Gy in 49 patients. The prescribed dose was 110 Gy for the patients who received LDR-brachytherapy in combination with EBRT. The target portion of EBRT was determined one month after LDR-brachytherapy, and the patients received 45 Gy (in 25 fractions of 1.8 Gy per fraction) using a four-field box technique via 6–10 MV photon energy. The clinical target volume included both the whole prostate and one third of the proximal seminal vesicle.

From July 2004 to April 2007, LDR-brachytherapy was performed after preplanning by modified peripheral loading techniques using Mick's applicator [11]. From May 2007 to October 2008, we introduced an intraoperative planning method, and thereafter used real-time planning and peripheral loading.

Postdosimetric evaluation

The therapeutic planning and post-implant dosimetric evaluation were performed using the planning system, Interplant Version 3.3 (CMS, Inc., St. Louis, USA) from July 2004 to October 2008, and thereafter Variseed 8.0 (Varian Medical Systems, Palo Alto, CA, USA).

Post-implant CT scanning and post-implant dosimetric study was performed by one radio-oncologist (AI) at 1 month after LDR-brachytherapy. The dosimetric parameters analyzed in this study were minimal percentage of the dose received by 90% of the prostate gland (%D90), minimal dose (Gy) received by 90% of the prostate gland (D90), percentage prostate volume receiving 100% and 150% of the prescribed minimal peripheral dose (V100/150), minimal percentage of the dose received by 30% and 90% of the urethra (%UD30 and %UD90), minimal dose (Gy) received by 30% and 90% of the urethra (UD30 and UD90), and rectal volume (mL) receiving 100% of the prescribed dose (R100).

Statistic analysis

To elucidate independent factors to predict PSA bounce in hormone-naïve patients who underwent LDR-brachytherapy alone, prostate volume at implantation, prostate volume at postdosimetry, %D90, D90, V100, V150, R100, %UD90, UD90, %UD30, and biologically effective dose (BED) were evaluated. The BED was calculated to evaluate an independent factor to predict PSA bounce, and an α/β ratio of 2 was used [12].

In this study, PSA bounce was defined as an elevation in the PSA value of 0.1 ng/mL or more compared to the previous lowest value (excluding the 1 month PSA value), followed by a decline to a level at or below the pre-bounce value. We used Phoenix definition (nadir + 2 ng/mL) as the definition of PSA failure [13]. Estimated PSA bounce-free rate was calculated by the Kaplan-Meier method. Cox proportional hazards model was used to determine predictive parameters of PSA bounce both in univariate and multivariate analysis (backward stepwise selection method). To analyze the differences in categorical parameters, the chi-square test was employed. Student's t-test was used to evaluate the differences in continuous variables. ANOVA by

Bonferroni's procedure and Dunnett's procedure were applied to intergroup comparisons of the incidence of PSA elevation of ≥0.1 ng/mL, as well as the incidence, time, height, and duration of PSA bounce among the 4 groups treated with monotherapy with or without neoadjuvant ADT and combination therapy with or without neoadjuvant ADT. All statistical analyses were performed using PASW Statistics 17.0 (SPSS Inc., Chicago, IL, USA). All p values below 0.05 were considered statistically significant.

Results

Of all patients, 92 (46%) showed PSA elevation of 0.1 ng/mL or greater from a PSA nadir during the follow-up period. The mean duration from LDR-brachytherapy to the PSA elevation was 17.4 months (median: 17 months). Of these 92 patients, 10 showed PSA failure and 50 showed PSA bounce (54%). The mean time to PSA bounce was 16.4 months (median: 17 months). The mean height and duration of PSA bounce were 0.49 ng/mL (median: 0.29 ng/mL) and 9.8 months (median: 7.0 months), respectively. The estimated 3-year PSA bounce-free rate was 72.4%. The mean number of PSA measurements in patients without PSA bounce was 8.5 (median: 8) while that in patients with PSA bounce was 10.3 (median: 10.5). PSA was more frequently measured in patients with PSA bounce than in those without it ($p < 0.001$) (Table 1). Of these 50 patients with PSA bounce, 8 (16%) showed a second PSA bounce. The mean duration from LDR-brachytherapy to the second PSA bounce was 29.3 months (median: 29.5 months). The mean height and duration of the second PSA bounce were 0.47 ng/mL (median: 0.18 ng/mL) and 6.8 months (median: 6.0 months), respectively.

The mean PSA value at diagnosis was significantly higher in patients without PSA bounce than in patients with PSA bounce. The mean follow-up period and the number of PSA measurements in patients without PSA bounce were significantly shorter and smaller than those in patients with PSA bounce. There was no significant difference in the prostate volume at postdosimetry between patients with and without PSA bounce (Table 1).

Regarding postdosimetric parameters, %D90, V100, V150, and R100 showed no significant differences between patients with and without PSA bounce, while UD90 (%) and UD90 (Gy), showed a significantly higher value in patients with PSA bounce. Patients without PSA bounce showed a significantly higher BED (Table 2).

The incidence of PSA elevation of ≥0.1 ng/mL, the incidence of PSA bounce, the mean time to PSA bounce, the mean height of PSA bounce, and the estimated 3-year PSA bounce-free rate of each treatment group are summarized in Table 3. The incidence of PSA elevation of >0.1 ng/mL was significantly higher

Table 2 Postdosimetric parameters (all patients: n = 200)

	Bounce (-) (n=150)	Bounce (+) (n=50)	P value
	(mean ± SD)	(mean ± SD)	(t-test)
Prostate volume at postdosimetry (mL)	27.3 ± 8.7	29.0 ± 8.9	0.233
%D90 (%)	110.6 ± 9.9	109.7 ± 9.1	0.577
D90 (Gy)	152.3 ± 24.5	153.3 ± 19.4	0.772
V100 (%)	93.7 ± 3.6	93.5 ± 3.6	0.700
V150 (%)	62.3 ± 10.4	62.1 ± 10.3	0.881
R100 (mL)	0.10 ± 0.19	0.08 ± 0.10	0.668
Urethral volume (mL)	0.53 ± 0.28	0.41 ± 0.23	0.004
%UD90 (%)	97.6 ± 12.8	101.8 ± 12.7	0.049
UD90 (Gy)	134.1 ± 24.5	142.5 ± 23.6	0.035
%UD30 (%)	140.2 ± 18.0	143.8 ± 22.3	0.256
Minimal urethral dose (Gy)	100.9 ± 21.6	111.3 ± 22.2	0.004
BED (Gy2)	188.5 ± 25.2	177.0 ± 23.2	0.005

in the monotherapy with neoadjuvant ADT group than in the combination therapy without neoadjuvant ADT group (ANOVA; $p = 0.006$), whereas the incidence of PSA bounce showed no significant difference between the groups. The mean height of PSA bounce in the monotherapy without neoadjuvant ADT group was significantly higher than that in the monotherapy with neoadjuvant ADT group (ANOVA; $p = 0.005$), whereas the time to PSA bounce and PSA bounce duration showed no significant difference between the two groups. The estimated 3-year bounce-free rate of the monotherapy without neoadjuvant ADT, combination therapy without neoadjuvant ADT, monotherapy with neoadjuvant ADT, and combination therapy with neoadjuvant ADT groups were 68.8%, 80.6%, 66.7%, and 80.9%, respectively. Patients who underwent adjuvant ADT (n = 8) showed no PSA bounce during the follow-up periods (Figure 1). There were no significant

differences in the estimated 3-year PSA bounce-free rates among the 4 groups (log-rank test).

Subgroup analysis in hormone-naïve patients who underwent LDR-brachytherapy alone
The mean %UD90, UD90 and %D30% in patients who showed PSA bounce were significantly higher than those in patients without PSA bounce (Table 4). A univariate Cox proportional regression hazard model showed that age, %UD30, and %UD90 were independent predictors of PSA bounce after LDR-brachytherapy. Finally, %UD90 was the most significant parameter of PSA bounce in the multivariate Cox proportional regression hazard model (Table 5).

Discussion
PSA bounce, which is frequently observed after LDR-brachytherapy, is a curious phenomenon caused by an

Table 3 PSA bounce in each group

	Hormone naive		Neo-adjuvant ADT	
	monotherapy	Combined EBRT	monotherapy	Combined EBRT
	(n=103)	(n=38)	(n=34)	(n=17)
PSA elevation rate of 0.1 ng/mL or greater	51 (50%)	25 (66%)	9 (27%)	6 (35%)
Frequency of PSA bounce	29 (28%)	12 (32%)	3 (18%)	15 (18%)
Time to bounce (mos)	17.4, 17, (5-36)	14.8, 11.5 (5-35)	13.7, 8.5, (5-26)	18.3, 15, (14-26)
Mean, median, (range)				
Height (ng/mL)	0.51, 0.34, (0.13-1.74)	0.48, 0.26, (0.12-1.85)	0.19, 0.16, (0.10-0.40)	0.90, 0.68, (0.16-1.87)
Mean, median, (range)				
Duration (mos)	9.1, 6.0, (3-36)	11.8, 11.5, (2-31)	6.0, 6.0, (3-9)	15.3, 17.0, (7-22)
Mean, median, (range)				
3-yr bounce free rate (%)	68.8	80.6	66.7	80.9

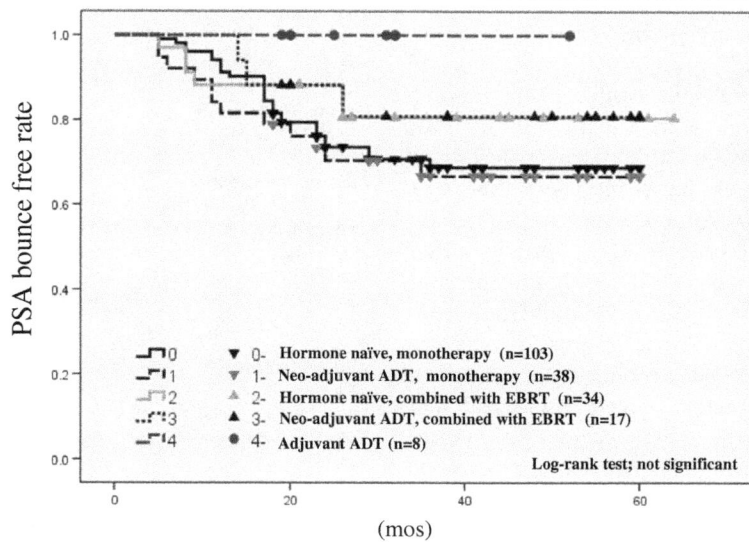

Figure 1 PSA bounce (0.1 ng/mL)-free rate in all patients stratified by treatment procedure (neoadjuvant/ adjuvant ADT and monotherapy/ combination with EBRT).

unknown mechanism. Reportedly, 17% to 62% of patients are diagnosed with PSA bounce using several definitions [1-10]. The median time to PSA bounce varied from 15 months to 26 months [1,2,4,6,7,9,10]. The median height of PSA bounce was 0.4 ng/mL to 0.8 ng/mL [1,2,4,6-9]. The median duration of PSA bounce was 6.8 months to 22.5 months [2,3,6,7]. In daily practice, doctors and patients are annoyed when PSA elevation shows biochemical recurrence or PSA bounce due to the comparatively high incidence and long duration of PSA bounce. In the present study, the incidence of PSA

bounce, the median time to PSA bounce, the median height of PSA bounce, and the median duration of PSA bounce were 25%, 17 months, 0.29 ng/mL, and 7.0 months, respectively. The median height in our series was lower than that in previous studies. Presumably, it was caused by the definition of PSA bounce (cut-off value of 0.1 ng/mL).

In the subgroup analysis, the incidence of PSA elevation of ≥0.1 ng/mL was significantly higher in the monotherapy with neoadjuvant ADT group than the combination therapy without neoadjuvant ADT ($p = 0.006$) group. However, the incidence of PSA bounce was not significantly different in these four groups. This result was comparable to that of previous reports [5,6,10]. Moreover, the estimated 3-year bounce-free rates in these four groups showed no significant differences in this study.

The present study showed that %UD90, UD90, and BED were significantly different between patients with PSA bounce and those without PSA bounce, whereas age and prostate volume showed no significant difference among all patients. To avoid the influence of neoadjuvat/adjuvant ADT and EBRT, we evaluated the

Table 4 Postdosimetric parameters (hormone-naïve, monotherapy: n = 103)

	Bounce (-) (n=74)	Bounce (+) (n=29)	P value
	(mean ± SD)	(mean ± SD)	(t-test)
Age (year)	68.8 ± 6.1	66.1 ± 7.7	0.060
PV at postdosimetry (mL)	27.9 ± 8.0	30.8 ± 8.2	0.109
%D90 (%)	110.1 ± 10.4	112.1 ± 8.0	0.338
D90 (Gy)	167.6 ± 17.6	164.3 ± 12.5	0.360
V100 (%)	93.6 ± 3.8	94.4 ± 2.7	0.272
V150 (%)	62.7 ± 8.9	65.5 ± 8.8	0.163
R100 (mL)	0.10 ± 0.20	0.10 ± 0.10	0.936
Urethral volume (mL)	0.55 ± 0.26	0.42 ± 0.23	0.019
%UD90 (%)	95.6 ± 12.1	104.7 ± 11.3	0.001
UD90 (Gy)	145.3 ± 18.2	153.3 ± 16.2	0.041
%UD30 (%)	140.2 ± 16.1	151.5 ± 21.8	0.005
Minimal urethral dose (Gy)	107.5 ± 19.3	119.1 ± 16.6	0.006
BED (Gy2)	177.5 ± 19.7	173.7 ± 13.9	0.354

Table 5 Univariate and multivariate analyses to predict PSA bounce (Cox proportional regression hazard model)

	Univariate	Multivariate	p - value	95% C.I.
	p - value	Hazard ratio		
Age	0.044			
%UD90(%)	0.004	1.037	0.007	1.010-1.064
%UD30 (%)	0.011			

C.I confidence interval.

predictive parameters of PSA bounce in patients treated with LDR-brachytherapy alone without neoadjuvant/adjuvant ADT. In this group, %UD90, UD90 and %UD30 showed a significant difference between patients with PSA bounce and those without PSA bounce, while age showed a marginal difference ($p = 0.06$). Previous studies have reported that age, D90, isotope, and prostate volume were the significant predictive factors of PSA bounce [3-9]. On the other hand, age, %UD90 and %UD30 were significant predictive parameters of PSA bounce by univariate analysis using a Cox proportional regression hazard model in this study. Multivariate analysis indicated % UD90 as predictive parameters. The pathological reason why %UD90 affects the incidence of PSA bounce is unknown. It is most probable that a higher dose to the urethra causes a higher incidence of radiation-induced urethritis and prostatitis.

Various factors including age, radiation-induced proctitis, prostatitis (radiation-induced or infection), ejaculation, laboratory error, urinary retention, testosterone recovery after ADT, and instrumentation, are considered as etiologies of PSA bounce. Assessment strongly suggests that sexual activity, inflammatory stimulation and androgen manipulation are associated with PSA bounce. It is necessary to investigate the correlation between PSA bounce and the data of urine analysis, urodynamics study, and serum androgen level in the future.

Our present study has some limitations such as a small number of patients and a short follow-up period. Indeed, there were only 50 patients who showed PSA bounce out of the 82 patients with PSA elevation of ≥ 0.1 ng/mL after LDR-brachytherapy without PSA failure. The other 32 patients with PSA elevation did not reach the PSA nadir level during the follow-up period. Longer follow-up is necessary to confirm PSA bounce in this patient group. The difference in the prescribed monotherapy dose (145 Gy vs. 160 Gy) may also influence the incidence of PSA bounce. In this study, we did not evaluate this matter because the follow-up period of the patients who received a prescribed dose of 160 Gy was significantly shorter than that of the patients who received 145 Gy (data not shown). The definition of PSA bounce is also controversial. In this study, we adopted a cut-off value of 0.1 ng/mL. The results of studies with a longer follow-up period and a different cut-off value of PSA bounce are expected in the near future.

Conclusions

There is no significant difference in the prevalence of PSA bounce between groups treated with LDR-brachytherapy alone and those treated with LDR-brachytherapy in combination with EBRT, regardless of neoadjuvant ADT. In hormone-naïve patients treated with LDR-brachytherapy alone, %UD90 was the most significant predictor of PSA bounce.

Competing interests
The authors declare that they have no conflict of interest.

Authors' contributions
All authors made substantial contributions to the acquisition and interpretation of data, critical revision of the manuscript for important intellectual content, and approved the final version for publication. YH, NK and MH made substantial contributions to the conception and design of the study. NT performed the statistical analysis. All authors read and approved the final manuscript.

Author details
[1]Department of Urology, Nara Medical University, 840 Shijo-cho, Kashihara, Nara 634-8522, Japan. [2]Department of Radiation Oncology, Nara Medical University, Nara, Japan. [3]Department of Pathology, Nara Medical University, Nara, Japan.

References
1. Critz FA, Williams WH, Benton JB, Levinson AK, Holladay CT, Holladay DA: Prostate specific antigen bounce after radioactive seed implantation followed by external beam radiation for prostate cancer. *J Urol* 2000, 163(4):1085–1089.
2. Das P, Chen MH, Valentine K, Lopes L, Cormack RA, Renshaw AA, Tempany CM, Kumar S, D'Amico AV: Using the magnitude of PSA bounce after MRI-guided prostate brachytherapy to distinguish recurrence, benign precipitating factors, and idiopathic bounce. *Int J Radiat Oncol Biol Phys* 2002, 54(3):698–702.
3. Stock RG, Stone NN, Cesaretti JA: Prostate-specific antigen bounce after prostate seed implantation for localized prostate cancer: descriptions and implications. *Int J Radiat Oncol Biol Phys* 2003, 56(2):448–453.
4. Critz FA, Williams WH, Levinson AK, Benton JB, Schnell FJ, Holladay CT, Shrake PD: Prostate specific antigen bounce after simultaneous irradiation for prostate cancer: the relationship to patient age. *J Urol* 2003, 170(5):1864–1867.
5. Toledano A, Chauveinc L, Flam T, Thiounn N, Solignac S, Timbert M, Rosenwald JC, Cosset JM: PSA bounce after permanent implant prostate brachytherapy may mimic a biochemical failure: a study of 295 patients with a minimum 3-year followup. *Brachytherapy* 2006, 5(2):122–126.
6. Bostancic C, Merrick GS, Butler WM, Wallner KE, Allen Z, Galbreath R, Lief J, Gutman SE: Isotope and patient age predict for PSA spikes after permanent prostate brachytherapy. *Int J Radiat Oncol Biol Phys* 2007, 68(5):1431–1437.
7. Crook J, Gillan C, Yeung I, Austen L, McLean M, Lockwood G: PSA kinetics and PSA bounce following permanent seed prostate brachytherapy. *Int J Radiat Oncol Biol Phys* 2007, 69(2):426–433.
8. Satoh T, Ishiyama H, Matsumoto K, Tsumura H, Kitano M, Hayakawa K, Ebara S, Nasu Y, Kumon H, Kanazawa S, Miki K, Egawa S, Aoki M, Toya K, Yorozu A, Nagata H, Saito S, Baba S: Prostate-specific antigen 'bounce' after permanent 125I-implant brachytherapy in Japanese men: a multi-institutional pooled analysis. *BJU Int* 2009, 103(8):1064–1068.
9. Kanai K, Nakashima J, Sugawara A, Shigematsu N, Nagata H, Kikuchi E, Miyajima A, Nakagawa K, Kubo A, Oya M: Prediction of PSA bounce after permanent prostate brachytherapy for localized prostate cancer. *Int J Clin Oncol* 2009, 14(6):502–506.
10. McGrath SD, Antonucci JV, Fitch DL, Ghilezan M, Gustafson GS, Vicini FA, Martinez AA, Kestin LL: PSA bounce after prostate brachytherapy with or without neoadjuvant androgen deprivation. *Brachytherapy* 2010, 9(2):137–144.
11. Tanaka N, Asakawa I, Kondo H, Tanaka M, Fujimoto K, Hasegawa M, Konishi N, Hirao Y: Technical acquisition and dosimetric assessment of iodine-125 permanent brachytherapy in localized prostate cancer: our first series of 100 patients. *Int J Urol* 2009, 16(1):70–74.

12. Stock RG, Stone NN, Cesaretti JA, Rosenstein BS: **Biologically effective dose values for prostate brachytherapy: effects on PSA failure and posttreatment biopsy results.** *Int J Radiat Oncol Biol Phys* 2006, **64**(2):527–533.

13. Roach M 3rd, Hanks G, Thames H Jr, Schellhammer P, Shipley WU, Sokol GH, Sandler H: **Defining biochemical failure following radiotherapy with or without hormonal therapy in men with clinically localized prostate cancer: recommendations of the RTOG-ASTRO Phoenix Consensus Conference.** *Int J Radiat Oncol Biol Phys* 2006, **65**(4):965–974.

29

Improving prostate cancer detection in veterans through the development of a clinical decision rule for prostate biopsy

Owen T Hill[1*], Thomas J Mason[2], Skai W Schwartz[3] and Philip R Foulis[4]

Abstract

Background: We sought to improve prostate cancer (PC) detection through developing a prostate biopsy clinical decision rule (PBCDR), based on an elevated PSA and laboratory biomarkers. This decision rule could be used after initial PC screening, providing the patient and clinician information to consider prior to biopsy.

Methods: This case–control study evaluated men from the Tampa, Florida, James A. Haley (JH) Veteran's Administration (VA) (N = 1,378), from January 1, 1998, through April 15, 2005. To assess the PBCDR we did all of the following: 1) Identified biomarkers that are related to PC and have the capability of improving the efficiency of PC screening; 2) Developed statistical models to determine which can best predict the probability of PC; 3) Compared each potential model to PSA alone using Receiver Operator Characteristic (ROC) curves, to evaluate for improved overall effectiveness in PC detection and reduction in (negative) biopsies; and 4) Evaluated dose–response relationships between specified lab biomarkers (surrogates for extra-prostatic disease development) and PC progression.

Results: The following biomarkers were related to PC: hemoglobin (HGB) (OR = 1.42 95% CI 1.27, 1.59); red blood cell (RBC) count (OR = 2.52 95% CI 1.67, 3.78); PSA (OR = 1.04 95% CI 1.03, 1.05); and, creatinine (OR = 1.55 95% CI 1.12, 2.15). Comparing all PC stages versus non-cancerous conditions, the ROC curve area under the curve (AUC) enlarged (increasing the probability of correctly classifying PC): PSA (alone) 0.59 (95% CI 0.55, 0.61); PBCDR model 0.68 (95% CI 0.65, 0.71), and the positive predictive value (PPV) increased: PSA 44.7%; PBCDR model 61.8%. Comparing PC (stages II, III, IV) vs. other, the ROC AUC increased: PSA (alone) 0.63 (95% CI 0.58, 0.66); PBCDR model 0.72 (95% CI 0.68, 0.75), and the PPV increased: 20.6% (PSA); PBCDR model 55.3%.

Conclusions: These results suggest evaluating certain common biomarkers in conjunction with PSA may improve PC prediction prior to biopsy. Moreover, these biomarkers may be more helpful in detecting clinically relevant PC. Follow-up studies should begin with replicating the study on different U.S. VA patients involving multiple practices.

Background

The number of men who undergo prostate biopsies to rule out prostate cancer (PC) increases annually (estimated at over one million per year) [1]. This is in large part a result of elevated serum prostate specific antigen (PSA) values identified during routine PC screening [2,3]. Debate over the appropriateness of PC screening continues [1-7]. In addition, there is considerable controversy over the course one should take upon detecting PSA elevations [2-5].

Moreover, it is inconclusive whether early PC detection results in lower morbidity and mortality for the men identified [3-6].

PC screening has been fraught with controversy and the overtreatment of low-risk PC is considered a major public health problem [8,9]. The U.S. Preventive Services Task Force (USPSTF), National Cancer Institute (NCI), World Health Organization (WHO), and other international agencies do not recommend PC screening [7]. Conversely, the American Cancer Society (ACS), American College of Radiology (ACR), and the American Urological Association (AUA) recommend screening men above the age of 50 with a routine serum PSA and digital rectal exam

* Correspondence: owen.hill@us.army.mil
[1]Injury Epidemiology Research Section, Military Performance Division, United States Army Institute of Environmental Medicine, Natick, MA, USA
Full list of author information is available at the end of the article

(DRE) [7]. Proponents for routine PC screening argue that it is a valuable early detection tool as it can identify PC in asymptomatic men prior to clinical presentation. In theory, earlier identified PC should be at a less advanced stage, which implies a more treatable state. This is controversial, as PC is heterogeneous, in some cases indolent (never becoming clinically evident), while in other cases PC can be aggressive, rapidly advancing from a pre-clinical state to distant metastases [8].

An easy to implement screening tool that detects 'aggressive' PC is needed. The primary goal of PC screening is to detect cancer before it is too advanced for treatment, and to bypass the tumors that are not destined to shorten a man's life [9]. With that stated, delineation between different types of PC is difficult, but of paramount importance. PSA research over the last two decades has improved our ability to identify PC [2,3,8,10]. However; this has resulted in needless biopsies and treatments and is a reason for the protracted debate over the PSA utility as a PC screening tool [3].

Despite a wealth of published literature that has evaluated PSA and argued against its use, it remains a mainstay for patients and clinicians. Prior attempts at improving PC screening have focused on replacing PSA with a new test. Tools such as PSA velocity, PSA density, Free/Total PSA ratio, and PCA3 testing have all shown promise for improving PC screening, but difficult implementation and a lack of universal acceptance among clinicians have hindered incorporation into daily clinical practice [2,3,5]. Clearly, PC screening is in need of improvement. Therefore, the purpose of this investigation was to improve the efficiency of PC detection through the development of a novel clinical decision rule. We investigated and propose the prostate biopsy clinical decision rule (PBCDR) that implements both elevated PSA and readily available laboratory biomarkers. If accurate, the PBCDR could be used as an advanced screening tool after PSA as it provides additional clinically significant information to assist the clinician and patient in reaching a decision regarding the urgency of a prostate biopsy.

To develop and validate this advanced screening tool we did all of the following: (1) Identified biomarkers that are related to PC and have the capability of improving the efficiency of PC screening; (2) Developed statistical models to determine which can best predict the probability of PC; (3) Compared each potential model to the current screening tool (PSA only) using ROC curves, to evaluate for improved overall effectiveness in PC detection and reduction in (negative) biopsies; (4) Evaluated dose–response relationships between specified lab biomarkers (surrogates for extra-prostatic disease development) and PC progression. If present, the degree of change between the reference 'normal' value and the

observed lab value could provide valuable insight for differentiating between indolent and clinically relevant PC.

Methods

Population, inclusion/exclusion criteria, and data sources

This study was a case–control analysis, evaluating 1,378 prior military servicemen (40–90 years of age), from the James A. Haley Veteran's Administration (VA) hospital from January 1, 1998 through April 15, 2005 who had undergone prostate biopsy. Only patients with a PSA value of 4 ng/dL (or higher), with laboratory data obtained at the time of the PSA sample, and an initial diagnosis of PC, prostatic interstitial neoplasm (PIN), benign prostatic hypertrophy (BPH), or prostatitis were included in the analysis. Patients with history of prior genital urinary malignancy, and those with inadequate biopsy specimens were excluded from analysis. Subjects meeting inclusion criteria were classified into one of four 'histology' groups. The cases consist of biopsy-confirmed PC. The non-PC cases were classified into three groups: (1) PIN, (2) BPH, or (3) prostatitis. Biopsies with isolated atypical small acinar proliferation were included in the PIN group. This study was approved by the Institutional Review Board at the University of South Florida and James A. Haley VA hospital.

Case identification/data collection methods

A case of PC is defined by prostate tissue that demonstrates cells of adenocarcinoma on histologic evaluation [11]. With that, identification of study subjects was accomplished through searching the Anatomic Pathology portion of VisTa (Systematized Nomenclature of Medicine (SNOMED) finalized accession logs) to find all cases coded as 'prostate disease' (SNOMED codes: 77220, 77103, 77102, 77101, 77110, 77105, 77350, 77230, 77210, 77300, 77200, 77240, 77104, 77100, 77000, 77900, 77250). SNOMED is a classification system of the College of American Pathologists, and is the standard tool used by pathologists to create, share, and retrieve pathology information. The patient's identification number, date of the specimen, diagnosis text code, and accompanying narrative text description were captured through this VISTA search. The collection of both the diagnosis text code and accompanying text description was performed intentionally as a way to validate the histologic diagnosis. For instance, if the diagnosis code was 'adenocarcinoma of the prostate' (SNOMED code 77220); the corresponding narrative text description would provide the same diagnosis. The goal of this initial search was to capture all prostate related cases; hence the large number of SNOMED codes used.

The James Haley VA electronic medical records (EMR) were then accessed for all of the potential PC cases to validate the diagnosis. This was accomplished by confirming the International Classification of Diseases, ninth revision (ICD–9) PC codes and capturing basic demographic, laboratory biomarkers, and any previous pathology results.

Data reduction strategies were employed which ultimately left 1,378 participants available (from 2,575 potential subjects) for statistical analysis. Over 500 prostate biopsies (541) did not meet inclusion criteria because they were performed on men who did not have a PSA test value of 4.0 ng/dL or greater. Typical situations that would result in this scenario include biopsies secondary to suspicious DRE or Transrectal ultrasound (TRUS), or other reasons (e.g. positive family history). There were 321 biopsies identified as "repeat biopsies", which were then dropped from the study. Next, biopsies performed as a result of other genital urinary malignancies (i.e. bladder, renal, ureter, and penile cancer) (N=260) were excluded. It is important to note that the specific prompting for all prostate biopsies was confirmed through a detailed record review of each prostate biopsy report within the VISTA system. These notes were in narrative form and were validated by confirming the ICD-9 code for that event. Lastly, participants without a full complement of laboratory biomarkers were excluded from the study (N=75). Thus our final analysis was based on 1,378 patients.

Outcomes - PC classification

PC classification was based on Stage and Gleason sum for each patient with histologic confirmation of PC. The Stages were categorized as follows: Stage I for non-palpable, prostate contained cancer (analogous to T1 non-palpable PC); Stage II for palpable prostate contained cancer (analogous to T2 palpable PC); Stage III for locally spread PC (analogous to T3/T4 PC); and Stage IV for metastatic PC (analogous to M1 PC). To determine the Gleason sum, the two most prominent areas of PC activity (as identified by the evaluating pathologist on histologic examination) were identified. Each prominent area was given a score of 1–5, with 1 being well differentiated, and 5 being poorly differentiated (implying a more aggressive appearance). The two scores are added together, and this number was the recorded Gleason sum for all subsequent analyses.

Statistical analysis

Univariate, bivariate, logistic regression, linear regression, and receiver operator characteristic (ROC) curves were utilized. Data were analyzed utilizing SAS statistical software. Descriptive analysis allowed for careful review of data frequencies, measures of central tendency, and distribution shapes. Bivariate analysis tested all identified biomarkers to determine the statistical significance and degree of correlation between these independent variables and PC. Multivariate logistic regression was utilized to

evaluate which statistical model can best predict the probability of PC.

We first defined a "Case" as any stage of PC and a "Control" as any non-cancerous prostate condition (PIN, BPH, and prostatitis). In a secondary analysis, we redefined a "Case" as PC stages (II, III, IV) and "Control" as stage I PC, or any non-cancerous prostate condition. Our reasoning was that as Stage 1 cancer is localized, it may be unlikely to progress to advanced disease.

A complete model (including age, ethnicity, biomarkers, and any interaction terms) was established initially. Exclusion of each covariate was performed, looking for a change in the overall – 2 Log Likelihood Ratio. A potential covariate was permanently removed from the model development process if there was no effect on the overall – 2 Log Likelihood value. This lack of change indicates the variable is not contributing to the prediction of the outcome, and conversely, if there was a change of statistical significance, the variable was included in the final model. To test for differences between the full model and the final model, evaluation of the likelihood ratio p-value was performed, in which a value greater than 0.05 indicated a satisfactory fit of the smaller model. Regression diagnostic techniques were employed to increase the reliability of the data.

ROC curves were used to address which statistical models could best predict the probability of PC and if a dose–response relationship existed between specified lab biomarkers and PC progression. ROC curves are graphical tools, which plot the sensitivity vs. 1- the specificity for a binary classification system (as a function of changes in the cut-off value threshold). This analysis technique was used to judge the validity of proposed model. Mean and median values of all significant biomarkers were determined for each PC stage subset to determine if a gradient exists between advancing PC severity and laboratory biomarkers.

Results

Table 1 outlines the demographics of the study participants. The mean age of the subjects was 68 years (SD=8.5). Most of the men had either prostatitis, BPH, or stage I PC (79.4%). Stage II, III and IV PC accounted for 20.6% of all diagnoses. The study population was largely Caucasian (study total=70.75%, PC=69.4%, PIN=71.73%, BPH=74.82%, prostatitis=69.29%). Age at diagnosis (PC stage I group=68.37, PC stage II group=69.73, PC stage III group=67.73, stage IV group 67.88, PIN group=67.75, BPH group=67.83, prostatitis group=68.17) was comparable across all diagnosis groups.

Table 2 outlines the mean value and standard deviation of all continuous laboratory biomarkers by the prostate biopsy results. The mean values of albumin, hemoglobin (HGB), RBC count, creatinine, and folate all

Table 1 Demographics of study particpants by prostate biopsy results

	Prostatitis N=342	BPH N=282	PIN N=138	PC stage I N=332	PC stage II N=220	PC stage III N=48	PC stage IV N=16
Ethnicity*							
Caucasian	237(69%)	211(75%)	99 (72%)	238 (72%)	149 (68%)	31(65%)	10 (63%)
Black	18 (5%)	19 (7%)	13 (9%)	34 (10%)	22 (10%)	7 (15%)	4 (25%)
Hispanic	22 (6%)	14 (5%)	7 (5%)	15 (5%)	11 (5%)	1 (2%)	1 (6%)
Other	65 (20%)	38 (14%)	19 (14%)	45 (13%)	38 (17%)	9 (18%)	1 (6%)
Mean Age**	68.17	67.83	67.75	68.37	69.73	67.73	67.88
SD Age	8.54	8.19	8.49	8.99	9.36	9.39	10.6

* P-value < 0.05.
** Not statistically significant.

decreased as the stage of PC increased. Conversely, the mean value of PSA increased as PC stage increased. No trends were observed for mean values of mean corpuscular volume (MCV), BUN, platelet count, WBC, LDH, and bilirubin. Trend significance tests revealed that as the prostate biopsy result increased from prostatitis to stage IV PC, the mean value of HGB, creatinine, PSA, and BUN varied from reference normal (p < 0.05). No trends were observed for the lab biomarkers RBC, MCV, albumin, WBC, bilirubin, and platelet count.

Crude Odds Ratios (with 95% CI) for the association of each laboratory biomarker with PC are presented in two ways:

Primary analysis: all PC stages vs. non-cancerous prostate conditions
Secondary analysis: PC (stages II, III, IV) vs. (PC stage I, PIN, BPH, and prostatitis)

Primary analysis

In this analysis, Hemoglobin, PSA, and serum BUN were related significantly to PC positive cases (when compared to non-cancerous prostate conditions) (Table 3).

Secondary analysis

When the stage I PC subjects were placed in the comparison group (leaving stage II, III, and IV PC subjects as the 'cases'), hemoglobin, age, PSA, hematuria, and RBC count demonstrated statistically significant relationships with the PC positive cases (when compared to the comparison group: stage I PC, PIN, BPH, and prostatitis) (Table 4).

Table 5 summarizes laboratory biomarkers, which demonstrate a statistically significant relationship with PC.

Table 6 outlines the PPV of PSA (> 4 ng/dL) alone for PC detection. This PPV was evaluated as method 1 and 2 (described above).

The positive predictive value was decreased significantly when stage I PC was not considered a case. In particular,

the PPV decreased by 24.1% when the stage I PC group was considered in the comparison group.

Multiple models were run, individually excluding each covariate, to assess the change of the −2 Log Likelihood value and the C-statistic. Analyses were terminated when the model with the lowest −2 Log Likelihood value and highest C-statistic was determined for each of the two analysis methods (Tables 7 and 8).

ROC curves (Figures 1, 2, 3 and 4) demonstrate the validity of analysis method 1 and 2, respectively and the difference between the existing PC screening test (PSA alone) and the PBCDR. Confidence intervals between PSA alone and PBCDR models (PSA + lab biomarkers) did not overlap and were statistically significantly different. **The ROC AUC: Method 1 PSA alone 0.59, (95% CI 0.55, 0.61) to PBCDR (PSA+ significant lab biomarkers) 0.68 (95% CI 0.65, 0.71); Method 2 PSA alone 0.63, (95% CI 0.58, 0.66) to PBCDR (PSA+ significant lab biomarkers) 0.72 (95% CI 0.68, 0.75).**

To determine the ideal cut-points for recommending prostate biopsy, four different cut-points where chosen, each providing either increased sensitivity or specificity. The cut-points are presented in four ways:

- *Cut-point 1* – The maximum likelihood ratio. This was determined by dividing the sensitivity by 1- the specificity (SEN/1-SPC), thus maximizing the quotient.
- *Cut point 2* – The probability that yielded a sensitivity of approximately 90% with the highest corresponding specificity.
- *Cut point 3* – The probability that yielded a sensitivity of approximately 80% with the highest corresponding specificity.
- *Cut point 4* – The probability that yielded a specificity of approximately 80% with the highest corresponding sensitivity (Table 9).

Table 2 Mean value and SD of Lab biomarkers by Prostate biopsy results

	Prostatitis	BPH	PIN	PC stage I	PC stage II	PC stage III	PC stage IV
	N=342	N=282	N=138	N=332	N=220	N=48	N=16
Albumin							
Mean	4	3.98	4.09	4.04	4	3.95	3.9
SD	0.38	0.37	0.37	0.38	0.42	0.39	0.42
HGB *							
Mean	14.27	14.24	14.3	14.17	13.7	12.59	12.84
SD	1.54	1.76	1.68	1.66	1.87	2.2	14.08
RBC							
Mean	4.67	4.65	4.76	4.69	4.63	4.58	4.5
SD	0.46	0.52	0.52	0.5	0.57	0.44	0.67
Creatinine							
Mean	1.25	1.16	1.2	1.16	1.15	1.14	1.13
SD	0.7	0.32	0.35	0.56	0.34	0.39	0.2
PSA*							
Mean	8.06	7.99	7.67	9.7	14.12	21.85	44.03
SD	6.74	11.2	4.58	11.66	29.27	30.21	48.71
MCV							
Mean	90.78	91.13	90.09	91.17	90.98	90.23	92.24
SD	4.65	5.35	5.79	5.05	6.11	4.18	4.99
Bilirubin							
Mean	0.66	0.65	0.6	0.66	0.67	0.65	0.6
SD	0.4	0.3	0.25	0.35	0.35	0.34	0.3
BUN*							
Mean	17.98	17.6	17.23	16.53	17.4	16	15.97
SD	6.93	7.9	6.5	6.56	6.73	6.74	4.54
Platlet							
Mean	230.45	227.63	240.81	226.54	232.5	234.3	235.44
SD	59.16	61.56	84.31	62.26	69.25	68.07	50.76
WBC							
Mean	7.24	7.11	7.42	7.19	7.13	10.41	7.37
SD	2.11	2.17	3.24	2.42	2.08	17.78	1.84
Folate							
Mean	12.93	12.56	12.31	13.37	11.92	10.71	10.03
SD	5.44	5.78	5.29	5.25	5.43	5.44	4.99
LDH							
Mean	426.91	424.78	371.84	404.6	406.41	392.11	393.33
SD	375.09	144.84	185.54	155.38	158.19	170.98	73.76

*Trend significance ($P<0.05$).

Table 10 summarizes the PPV between PSA alone and the PBCDR. Within each analysis method the PBCDR has increased PPV percentages, respectively.

To evaluate our hypothesis that there exists a gradient between specified lab biomarkers and increasing PC stage, the mean values of each specified laboratory biomarker (with accompanying 95% CI) was determined for each PC stage. In agreement with our hypothesis, we observed a change in the mean value of the biomarkers, HGB, RBC, Albumin and PSA, away from the normal reference levels as the PC stage increased (Table 11).

Table 3 Odds ratio and 95% CI for method 1: PC (all stages) vs. non-cancerous conditions, per laboratory unit

Covariates included	Odds ratio	OR 95% confidence interval
HGB *	0.872	(.821-.927)
Age	1.01	(.99-1.02)
PSA*	1.04	(1.02-1.06)
Hematuria	0.953	(0.86-1.06)
Proteinuria	0.943	(0.83-1.07)
Albumin	1.03	(0.78-1.36)
Creatinine	0.762	(0.76-1.01)
MCV	1.01	(0.99-1.03)
PLT	1	(0.99-1.00)
RBC	0.918	(0.75-1.13)
Total Bilirubin	1.14	(0.84-1.55)
BUN*	0.98	(0.96-0.99)
WBC	1.01	(0.98-1.05)

*P < 0.05.

A trend analysis was performed to determine whether or not the change seen with lab biomarkers HGB, RBC, Albumin, and PSA was statistically significant. Models were analyzed by first coding each continuous laboratory biomarkers as the criterion variable, with the PC stage coded as the predictor. The model results suggest that PC stage is a significant statistical predictor for gradient changes in HGB, RBC count, Albumin, and PSA.

A case example providing a glimpse of the real world application of the proposed PBCDR is outlined below (Table 12).

Patient's PBCDR Total Sum −2.68 <−0.16. <u>Recommendation</u>? No Biopsy for patient.

Table 4 Odds ratio and 95% CI for method2: PC (stage II, III, IV) vs. other (PC stage I, PIN, BPH, prostatitis), per laboratory unit

Covariates included	Odds ratio	OR 95% confidence interval
HGB *	0.79	(.738-.851)
AGE*	1.02	(1.01-1.03)
PSA*	1.04	(1.03-1.05)
Hematuria*	1.23	(1.10-1.38)
Proteinuria	1.16	(1.00-1.34)
Albumin	0.77	(0.55-1.08)
Creatinine	0.76	(0.52-1.12)
MCV	1	(0.97-1.03)
PLT	1	(0.99-1.00)
RBC*	0.76	(0.59-0.98)
Total Bilirubin	1.15	(0.80-1.66)
BUN	0.99	(0.98-1.01)
WBC	1.03	(0.99-1.06)

*P < 0.05.

Table 5 Summary table of independent variables that demonstrate statistically significant relations with PC (by analysis methods 1–2)

Independent variable	Method 1	Method 2
Hemoglobin (HGB)	**	**
RBC count		*
BUN	*	
Hematuria		*
PSA	**	**
Age		*

*P <0.05, ** P <0.001.

Discussion

The persistent inability to differentiate between indolent and aggressive PC has been one of the major limitations of PSA PC screening. To our knowledge, evaluating combinations of laboratory biomarkers, used concomitantly with an elevated PSA, has not been researched as a PSA augmentation strategy. Therefore, the key focus of this study was to determine if the laboratory biomarkers under evaluation were related to more advanced/aggressive PC stages. Our study found that HGB (OR=1.42 95% CI 1.27-1.59), RBC count (OR=2.52 95% CI 1.67-3.78), PSA (OR=1.04 95% CI 1.03-1.05), serum creatinine (OR=1.55 95% CI 1.12-2.15), and 'Black" ethnicity (OR=1.88 95% CI 1.25-2.85) were significantly related to the PC group (method 1 PC stages I-IV). RBC count (p < 0.0001), HGB (p < 0.0001) and creatinine (p < 0.05) demonstrated increased PC risk with a 1 unit negative change in their value; while age (p < 0.005), PSA value (p < 0.005), and MCV level (p < 0.0001) demonstrated increased PC risk with 1 unit positive increase in their respected values (consistent with what one would expect). Analysis method 2 (PC stage I in comparison group) demonstrated HGB (OR 1.47 95% CI 1.31, 1.61), RBC count (OR 2.15 95% CI 1.43, 3.23), serum creatinine (OR 1.83 95% CI 1.18, 2.85), PSA (OR 1.033 95% CI 1.02, 1.05), MCV (OR 1.05 95% CI 1.02, 1.08), and age (OR 1.018 95% CI 1.01, 1.04) were significantly related to PC stages II-IV. ROC curves were compared to address whether the addition of these significant lab biomarkers would improve PC prediction when compared to PSA alone. The AUC increased from: **Primary Analysis** PSA alone 0.59, (95% CI 0.55, 0.61) to PBCDR best fit model 0.68, (95% CI 0.65, 0.71); **Secondary Analysis** PSA alone 0.63, (95% CI 0.58, 0.66), to

Table 6 Positive predictive value of PSA > 4 ng/dL

Comparison groups	Method 1	Method 2
PC Cases/Total biopsies	616/1,378	284/1,378
Positive Predictive Value	44.70%	20.60%

Method 1: PC (all stages) vs. non-cancerous conditions (PIN, BPH, prostatitis).
Method 2: PC (stage II, III, IV) vs. other (stage I PC, PIN, BPH, prostatitis).

Table 7 Best fit logistical regression for method 1: risk of PC with lab biomarkers and 95% CI, per laboratory unit method 1: PC (all stages) vs. non-cancerous conditions (PIN, BPH, prostatitis)

Parameter	ML Est.	SE	OR	95% CI	C stat	−2 LL
Intercept	−7.9494	1.88	xx	xx	0.68	1777.339
HGB*	−0.3519	0.06	0.70	(0.63-.79)		
RBC*	−0.9227	0.21	0.40	(0.26-0.60)		
Hematuria*	−0.2874	0.15	0.75	(0.56-1.01)		
Creatinine*	−0.4393	0.17	0.65	(0.47-0.89)		
Black*	0.6336	0.21	1.89	(1.25-2.90)		
PSA*	0.0408	0.08	1.04	(1.03-1.06)		
AGE*	0.0196	0.01	1.02	(1.01-1.03)		
MCV*	0.0663	0.02	1.07	(1.04-1.10)		
Albumin	0.2871	0.16	1.33	(0.98-1.82)		

*P < 0.05.

PBCDR best fit model 0.72, (95% CI 0.68, 0.75). The differences between the models are statistically significant. In addition to the ROC curve, the validity (sensitivity/specificity) and positive/negative predictive values were determined. For the PSA only model, one can only determine the positive predictive value, given patients with a PSA less than 4 ng/dL are not routinely forwarded for prostate biopsy. The PPV of PSA alone (> = 4 ng/dL) decreased from 44.7% (method 1) to 20.6% (method 2). This indicates PSA is less effective as a tool for identifying the more clinically relevant PC (stages II-IV). Conversely, the PPV of the PBCDR method 2 (cut point 1) model was 55.3%, with a NPV of 81.9%, and specificity of 96.2%. These values demonstrate the PBCDR yielded significantly higher validity and predictive scores than that of PSA alone. In alignment with our hypothesis that there exists a gradient of change between the significant lab biomarkers and increasing levels of PC; HGB, RBC, PSA and Albumin demonstrated a significant gradient.

Table 8 Best fit logistical regression model for method 2: risk and 95% CI for PC with lab biomarkers, per laboratory unit

Parameter	ML Est.	SE	OR	95% CI	C Stat	−2 LL
Intercept	−5.1041	xx	xx	xx	0.713	1276.366
HGB*	−0.3784	0.05	0.69	(0.62, 0.76)		
RBC*	−0.7641	0.21	0.46	(0.30, 0.70)		
Creatinine*	−0.6069	0.23	0.55	(0.35, 0.85)		
PSA *	0.0325	0.01	1.03	(1.02, 1.05)		
Age*	0.0183	0.01	1.02	(1.01, 1.04)		
MCV*	0.0488	0.02	1.05	(1.02, 1.08)		
Black	0.3612	0.24	1.44	(0.90, 2.31)		

*P <0.001.

One important potential benefit of the PBCDR model is a reduction in prostate biopsies. In our study population, the PPV of PSA alone (in identifying stage II-IV PC) was 20.6% (284/1378). The PBCDR model (Method 2, cutpoint 1), yielded a positive predictive value of 55.3% (52/94), a specificity of 96.2%, and sensitivity of 18.3%. If this particular PBCDR model was employed (as opposed to PSA alone), the number of unnecessary biopsies (those that did not identify PC stage II-IV) would have been reduced from 1,092 to 92. Moreover, with a specificity of 96.2%, the PBCDR model would correctly identify greater than 9 out of every 10 men who do not have PC. In 1998, the JH VA performed 1,610 biopsies. If one were to apply the PBCDR (comparing PC stage II-IV vs. stage I PC, PIN, BPH, and prostatitis) to the 1,378 subjects within this study, 52 of the 92 total biopsies (PPV= 55.3%) would have been positive for PC versus the PSA alone (PPV 44.7%). In addition, if the PBCDR would have been employed, approximately 1,052 negative biopsies would not have been performed. This would have resulted in a substantial decrease in cost for the VA, as well as reduced anxiety for the patient, and a reduced risk of biopsy morbidity (given the biopsies would have never been performed).

Our study was consistent with previous published reports in many ways. The proportion of PC that was localized to the prostate is consistent with the screening stage shift phenomenon (increased amounts of pre-clinical disease are detected), with Stage I comprising 53.9% of all PC cases; Stage II 35.7%; Stage III 7.8%; and Stage IV 2.59% (data not shown).

Secondly, all laboratory biomarkers demonstrated 'movement' in the direction away from the 'normal' value that is consistent with previous literature and is biologically plausible.[15] For instance, the mean PSA value increased from 7.67 (prostatitis) to 44.03 (stage IV PC). Multiple published studies have reported that a low hemoglobin value is an independent risk factor for poor survival outcomes in patients with hormone refractory PC [11]. In addition; the correlation between PC and hematologic disorders has been long recognized for its clinical significance, with anemia a frequent clinical manifestation of advancing PC [9,11]. In this study, the laboratory parameters HGB, RBC count, and MCV (all indicators of hematologic state) demonstrated values below their normal reference range in patients with clinically relevant PC (stage II-IV). When comparing the subjects with histologically confirmed prostatitis to patients with histologically confirmed stage III PC, the difference becomes evident. HGB decreased from 14.27 to 12.59 (p < 0.05), RBC count decreased from 4.67 to 4.58 (p < 0.05). Lastly, there was an 83% increase in the risk of PC for African American (AA) men when compared to Caucasian men, which is consistent with AA ethnicity as being a major PC risk factor [8].

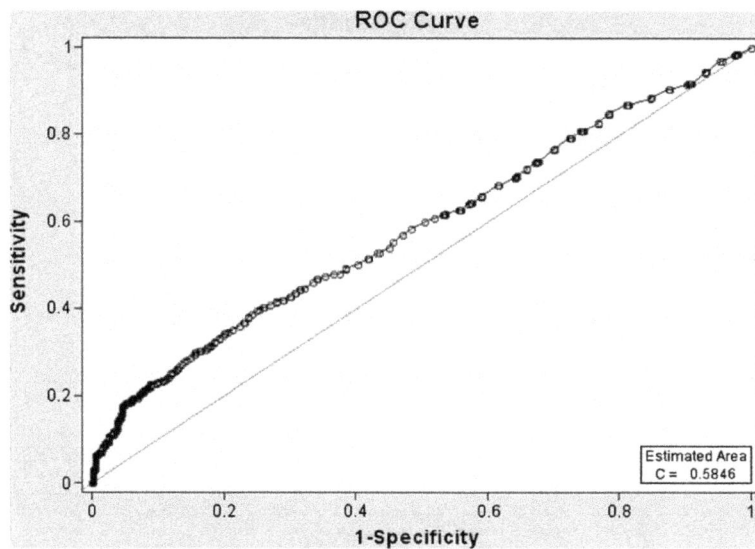

Figure 1 Diagnostic statistics = ROC curve of PSA Alone - Method 1.

Our study has limitations. Men followed by the VA may be subjected to a less or more stringent screening with respect to PC than are other men in the general U. S. population and therefore may not be representative to non-VA healthcare system patient populations. In addition, certain laboratory biomarkers had incomplete data which lead to the exclusion for analysis and interpretation. Although clinicians often obtain a complete blood count (CBC), basic metabolic panel (BMP), and urinalysis (UA) at the time of PSA screening, certain assays (e.g. PT/aPTT, and Folate) are not routinely included in these panels. Both PT and aPTT are used to evaluate the coagulation system, with increasing levels of both being an independent predictor of disseminated intravascular coagulation (a systemic condition seen occasionally with metastatic PC) [12]. A high plasma levels of Folate has been previously reported as both protective and as a risk factor for PC development [13]. Given the plausible links to PC, they warrant further investigation.

Although each prostate biopsy was evaluated by two or more trained pathologists, the possibility that misclassification of disease status (i.e. patients who have PC were classified as 'no PC') does exist. Given that the

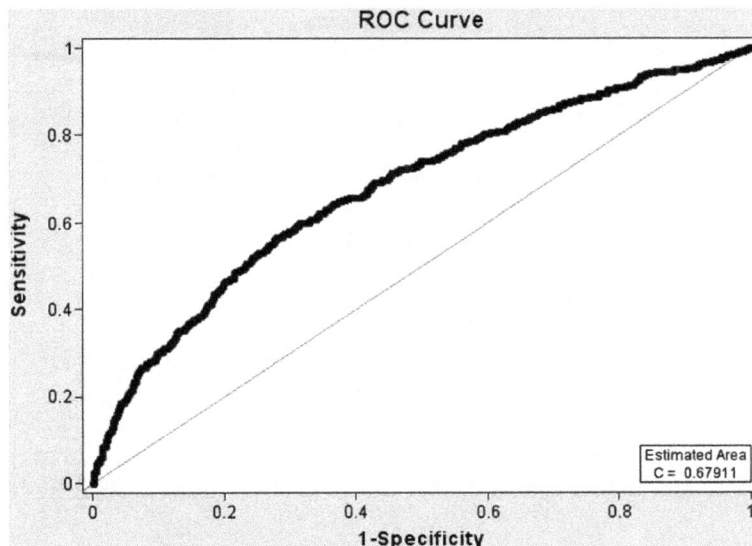

Figure 2 Diagnostic statistics = ROC curve of PSA + lab biomarkers - Method 1.

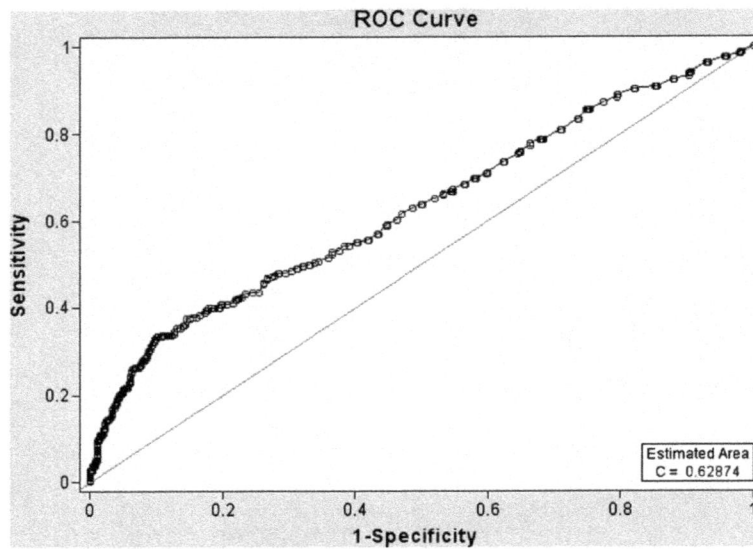

Figure 3 Diagnostic statistics = ROC curve of PSA Alone - Method 2.

outcome variable (PC yes or no) is determined by the results of a prostate biopsy, and that the biopsies themselves are a sampling of the entire prostate, there is a chance that the biopsy did not contain cancerous cells, yet the prostate itself does. However it is unlikely that an individual would be categorized as having PC if the carcinoma was not present on histological sample. It is more likely that a patient with PC is misclassified as not having PC, which would drive the results towards the Null hypothesis.

Other variables were not available for analysis. Information on PC family history was lacking in patient notes; and family history on any medical condition was available in less than 50% of the study participants. In addition, tobacco, alcohol use, and socio-economic status were unavailable for analysis.

A case–control design was utilized in this study. This type of design was employed as PC cases and suitable comparison subjects were identified and compared with respect to their lab values and prior exposures. While this design provided greater statistical efficiency, the potential for uncontrolled confounding and selection bias exists. Although the PBCDR tool can be used with all ages and PSA values, the lack of prostate biopsies in

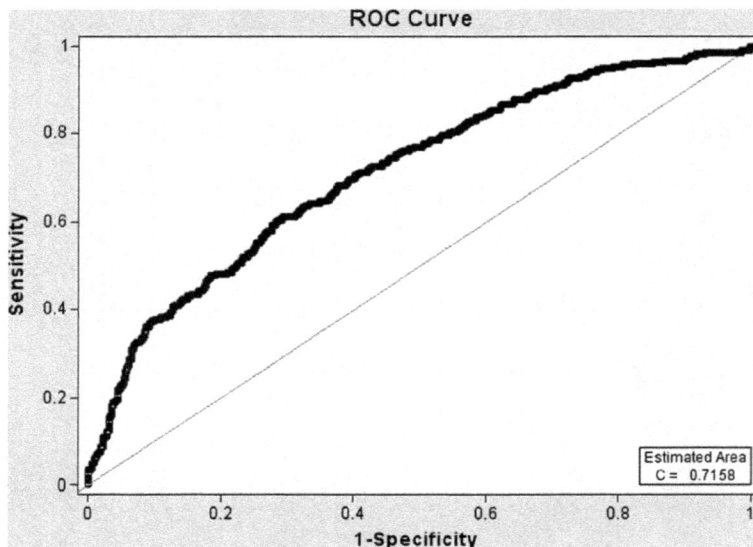

Figure 4 Diagnostic statistics = ROC curve of PSA + lab biomarkers - Method 2.

Table 9 Sensitivity, specificity, PPV, and NPV for probability cut-off points

	Method 1	Method 2
Cut-point 1 (MLE)	Probability .45	Probability .41
Sensitivity	52.1 %	18.3 %
Specificity	74.0 %	96.2 %
PPV	61.8 %	55.3 %
NPV	65.7%	81.9 %
Cut-point 2 (Sen. 90%)	Probability .33	Probability .13
Sensitivity	90.9 %	89.8 %
Specificity	17.6 %	28.0 %
PPV	47.1 %	20.6 %
NPV	70.5 %	91.3 %
Cut-point 3 (Sen. 80%)	Probability .37	Probability .15
Sensitivity	80.5 %	78.2 %
Specificity	37.1 %	45.0 %
PPV	50.9 %	28.7 %
NPV	70.2 %	88.8 %
Cut-point 4 (Spc. 80%)	Probability .48	Probability .23
Sensitivity	39.9 %	45.8 %
Specificity	81.4 %	79.5 %
PPV	63.4 %	36.7 %
NPV	62.6 %	85.0 %

patients with PSA values below 4.0 ng/dl limits evaluating the effectiveness of the PBCDR in this important group.

Despite these limitations, our study has important strengths. This study was completed on a robust sample population (1,378 subjects, of which 616 had PC), and this high proportion of cases increases overall study power and statistical efficiency. This increased study power afforded us the opportunity to stratify on key parameters, such as PC stage and ethnicity. The results are biologically plausible and consistent with existing knowledge. It is accepted that there is a relationship between PC and systemic diseases that occur in the presence of both local and metastatic spread of PC [9]. Moreover, it has been demonstrated that the specified laboratory biomarkers evaluated in this study are highly

Table 10 Comparison of PPV between PSA (> 4ng/dL) and cut-points 1–4 by analysis method

	Method 1	Method 2
Crude PPV	44.7 %	20.6 %
Cut-point 1	61.8 %	55.3 %
Cut-point 2	47.1 %	20.6%
Cut-point 3	50.9 %	28.7 %
Cut-point 4	63.4 %	36.7%

Table 11 Mean value, SD, and 95% CI of lab biomarkers by PC stage

	PC Stage A N=332	PC Stage B N=220	PC Stage C N=48	PC Stage D N=16
*Albumin**				
Mean	4.04	4.00	3.95	3.90
SD	0.38	0.42	0.39	0.42
95%CI	(4.00, 4.08)	(3.96, 4.05)	(3.84, 4.06)	(3.69, 4.11)
*HGB**				
Mean	14.17	13.70	12.59	12.84
SD	1.66	1.87	2.20	14.08
95%CI	(14.00, 14.35)	(13.45, 13.95)	(11.97, 13.21)	(5.94, 19.74)
*RBC **				
Mean	4.69	4.63	4.58	4.50
SD	0.50	0.57	0.44	0.67
95%CI	(4.64, 4.74)	(4.55, 4.71)	(4.46, 4.70)	(4.17, 4.83)
Creatinine				
Mean	1.16	1.15	1.14	1.13
SD	0.56	0.34	0.39	0.20
95%CI	(1.10, 1.22)	(1.11, 1.20)	(1.03, 1.25)	(1.03, 1.23)
*PSA**				
Mean	9.70	14.12	21.85	44.03
SD	11.66	29.27	30.21	48.71
95%CI	(8.45, 10.95)	(10.25, 17.99)	(13.31, 30.39)	(20.16, 67.90)
MCV				
Mean	91.17	90.98	90.23	92.24
SD	5.05	6.11	4.18	4.99
95%CI	(90.63, 91.71)	(90.17, 91.79)	(89.05, 91.41)	(89.79, 94.69)
Bilirubin				
Mean	0.66	0.67	0.65	0.60
SD	0.35	0.35	0.34	0.30
95%CI	(0.28, 1.04)	(0.62, 0.72)	(0.60, 0.70)	(0.45, 0.75)
BUN				
Mean	16.53	17.40	16.00	15.97
SD	6.56	6.73	6.74	4.54
95%CI	(15.82, 17.24)	(16.51, 18.29)	(17.91, 14.09)	(13.74, 18.20)
Platlet				
Mean	226.54	232.50	234.30	235.44
SD	62.26	69.25	68.07	50.76
95%CI	(219.8, 233.2)	(223.4, 241.7)	(215.1, 253.6)	(210.6, 260.3)
WBC				
Mean	7.19	7.13	10.41	7.37
SD	2.42	2.08	1.78	1.84
95%CI	(6.93, 7.45)	(6.86, 7.40)	(9.91, 10.91)	(6.47, 8.27)

* $P < 0.05$.

Table 12 Case example utilizing method 2, cut-point 1

Prob. .41/1-.41 = -0.16	Patients value	Parameter estimate	Pt. value *Parameter estimate	Intercept
HGB	15.2	-0.378	-5.74	-5.10
RBC	4.50	-0.764	-3.44	
Black	(Yes=1) 0	0.361	0.00	
Age	60	0.018	1.08	
PSA	4.3	0.033	0.129	
Creatinine	1.65	-0.601	-0.99	
MCV	90.00	0.050	4.5	
		sum of B*value	2.42	
		Plus intercept=Sum	-2.68	

The probability of this cut-point is .41, therefore the Log OR p/1 – p = .41/1-.41, thus the cut-point is –0.16. (If the number yielded from the equation is above this value, the patient should be referred for prostate biopsy. The patient is a 60 year old, Caucasian male with a recent PSA test value of 4.3 ng/dL. In addition, he had additional lab work to include a HGB, RBC count, MCV, Creatinine, and a negative test for Hematuria. Utilizing method 2, cut-point 1, the Patient's PBCDR total sum is -2.68, which is less than -0.16. Therefore, the recommendation is no biopsy for the patient.

correlated with the systemic diseases related to PC spread [11].

Men with PC have been described as falling into one of four groups, and screening can only really benefit one. The first group consists of men with normally progressing disease that is identified clinically; the second group includes men with PC that advances very rapidly. For the above two groups, screening is of little benefit. The third group contains men with screen-detected PC that would have never advanced to clinically relevant disease; therefore they are exposed to unnecessary procedures and treatments. Lastly, group four contains asymptomatic men who have PC identified through screening and receive beneficial outcomes that otherwise would have been deprived if not for the screening [8]. One difficulty in PC screening is identifying group 4 relative to group 3. The results of this study suggest that the PBCDR might improve our ability to detect PC while also decreasing the number of prostate biopsies. Moreover, the PBCDR seems to be more accurate with PC stages II-IV, providing a novel, simple to implement, inexpensive tool that has the potential to separate more severe PC from indolent PC. This has important implications, especially if PSA is used as a cost effective PC screening program. The overlap of PSA values in men with PC and non-cancerous prostate conditions has been well documented. A thorough physical exam with DRE is the mainstay of PC detection, and a patient's life expectancy and co-morbidities should be considered when developing a unique treatment course of action. However this study provides a glimpse of the potential benefit that these additional lab parameters can provide.

In conclusion, our study results suggest that evaluating certain biomarkers in conjunction with PSA may improve PC prediction prior to biopsy. Moreover, the biomarkers may be more helpful in detecting clinically relevant PC. Follow-up studies should begin with replicating this study

on different U.S. VA patient populations, involving multiple practices, capturing PC family history, and evaluating other biomarkers (such as PSA values lower than 4.0 ng/dl, PT/aPTT and folate) that may assist in improving PC screening efficiency.

Competing interests
The authors declare that they have no competing interests.

Authors' contribution
OTH contributed to the conception, design, analysis, and writing of the manuscript. TJM contributed to the conception, design, and analysis of the manuscript. SWS contributed to the conception, design, and analysis of the manuscript. PRF contributed to the conception, design, and data acquisition. All authors contributed to editing the manuscript and have given final approval of the version to be published.

Acknowledgements
The authors would like to acknowledge and thank Dennis Scofield for his efforts in revising the Tables and Figures imbedded within this manuscript.

Author details
[1]Injury Epidemiology Research Section, Military Performance Division, United States Army Institute of Environmental Medicine, Natick, MA, USA. [2]Department of Environmental and Occupational Health, College of Public Health, University of South Florida, Tampa, FL, USA. [3]Department of Epidemiology and Biostatistics, College of Public Health, University of South Florida, Tampa, FL, USA. [4]Department of Pathology and Laboratory Medicine, James A. Haley Veteran's Administration, Tampa, FL, USA.

References
1. Jones JS: *Managing patients following a negative prostate biopsy*; http://www.renalandurologynews.com/managing-patients-following-a-negative-prostate-biopsy/printarticle/195898/. Last accessed March.
2. Thompson IM, Ankerst DP, Chi C, Goodman PJ, Tangen CM, Lucia MS, Feng Z, Parnes HL, Coltman CA: **Assessing prostate cancer risk: results from the prostate cancer prevention trial.** *J Natl Cancer Inst* 2006, **98:**529–534.
3. Williams SB, Salami S, Regan MM, Ankerst DP, Wei JT, Rubin MA, Thompson IM, Sanda MG: **Selective detection of histologically aggressive prostate cancer.** *Cancer* 2012, **118:**2651–2658.
4. Barry MJ: **Screening for prostate cancer – the controversy that refuses to Die.** *N Engl J Med* 2009, **360:**1351–1354.
5. Andriole GL, Crawford ED, Grubb RL, Buys SS, Chia D, Church TR, Prorok PC: **Prostate cancer screening in the randomized prostate, lung, colorectal,**

and ovarian cancer screening trial: mortality results after 13 years of follow-up. *J Natl Cancer Inst* 2012, **104**(2):125–132.

6. Heidenreich A, Bellmunt J, Bolla M, Joniau S, Mason M, Matveev V, Zattoni F: **EAU guidelines on prostate cancer. Part 1: screening, diagnosis, and treatment of clinically localised disease.** *Eur Urol* 2011, **59**(1):61–71.

7. Schröder FH: **Landmarks in prostate cancer screening.** *BJU Int* 2012, **110**(s1):3–7.

8. Dall'Era MA, Cooperberg MR, Chan JM, Davies BJ, Albertsen PC, Klotz LH, Warlick CA, Holmberg L, Bailey DE, Wallace ME, Kantoff PW, Carroll PR: **Active surveillance for early-stage prostate cancer: review of the current literature.** *Cancer* 2008, **112**(8):1650–1659.

9. Bill-Axelson A, Holmberg L, Ruutu M, Garmo H, Stark JR, Busch C, Johansson JE: **Radical prostatectomy versus watchful waiting in early prostate cancer.** *N Engl J Med* 2011, **364**(18):1708–1717.

10. Basch E, Oliver TK, Vickers A, Thompson I, Kantoff P, Parnes H, Nam RK: **Screening for prostate cancer with prostate-specific antigen testing: American Society of Clinical Oncology provisional clinical opinion.** *J Clin Oncol* 2012, **30**(24):3020–3025.

11. Halabi S, Small EJ, Kantoff PW, Kattan MW, Kaplan EB, Dawson NA, Vogelzang NJ: **Prognostic model for predicting survival in men with hormone-refractory metastatic prostate cancer.** *J Clin Oncol* 2012, **21**(7):1232–1237.

12. Navarro M, Ruiz I, Martin G, Cruz JJ: **Patient with disseminated intravascular coagulation as the first manifestation of adenocarcinoma of the prostate. Risks of prostatic biopsy.** *Prostate Cancer Prostatic Dis* 2005, **9**(2):190–191.

13. Hultdin J, Van Guelpen B, Bergh A, Hallmans G, Stattin P: **Plasma folate, vitamin B12, and homocysteine and prostate cancer risk: a prospective study.** *Int J Cancer* 2005, **113**(5):819–824.

Permissions

All chapters in this book were first published in UROLOGY, by BioMed Central; hereby published with permission under the Creative Commons Attribution License or equivalent. Every chapter published in this book has been scrutinized by our experts. Their significance has been extensively debated. The topics covered herein carry significant findings which will fuel the growth of the discipline. They may even be implemented as practical applications or may be referred to as a beginning point for another development.

The contributors of this book come from diverse backgrounds, making this book a truly international effort. This book will bring forth new frontiers with its revolutionizing research information and detailed analysis of the nascent developments around the world.

We would like to thank all the contributing authors for lending their expertise to make the book truly unique. They have played a crucial role in the development of this book. Without their invaluable contributions this book wouldn't have been possible. They have made vital efforts to compile up to date information on the varied aspects of this subject to make this book a valuable addition to the collection of many professionals and students.

This book was conceptualized with the vision of imparting up-to-date information and advanced data in this field. To ensure the same, a matchless editorial board was set up. Every individual on the board went through rigorous rounds of assessment to prove their worth. After which they invested a large part of their time researching and compiling the most relevant data for our readers.

The editorial board has been involved in producing this book since its inception. They have spent rigorous hours researching and exploring the diverse topics which have resulted in the successful publishing of this book. They have passed on their knowledge of decades through this book. To expedite this challenging task, the publisher supported the team at every step. A small team of assistant editors was also appointed to further simplify the editing procedure and attain best results for the readers.

Apart from the editorial board, the designing team has also invested a significant amount of their time in understanding the subject and creating the most relevant covers. They scrutinized every image to scout for the most suitable representation of the subject and create an appropriate cover for the book.

The publishing team has been an ardent support to the editorial, designing and production team. Their endless efforts to recruit the best for this project, has resulted in the accomplishment of this book. They are a veteran in the field of academics and their pool of knowledge is as vast as their experience in printing. Their expertise and guidance has proved useful at every step. Their uncompromising quality standards have made this book an exceptional effort. Their encouragement from time to time has been an inspiration for everyone.

The publisher and the editorial board hope that this book will prove to be a valuable piece of knowledge for researchers, students, practitioners and scholars across the globe.

List of Contributors

Young Suk Kwon, Parth K. Modi and Amirali Salmasi
Section of Urologic Oncology, Rutgers Cancer Institute of New Jersey and Rutgers Robert Wood Johnson Medical School, The State University of New Jersey, 195 Little Albany Street, New Brunswick, NJ, USA

Yun-Sok Ha
Section of Urologic Oncology, Rutgers Cancer Institute of New Jersey and Rutgers Robert Wood Johnson Medical School, The State University of New Jersey, 195 Little Albany Street, New Brunswick, NJ, USA
Department of Urology, School of Medicine, Kyungpook National University Medical Center, Daegu, Korea

Michael May
Department of Pathology, Robert Wood Johnson Medical School, New Brunswick, NJ, USA

David I. Lee and Elton Llukani
Division of Urology, University of Pennsylvania, Philadelphia, PA, USA

Tuliao Patrick
Department of Urology, College of Medicine, Yonsei University, Seoul, Korea

Jonathan Hwang
Department of Urology, Georgetown University, Washington, DC, USA

Wun-Jae Kim
Department of Urology, Chungbuk National University College of Medicine, Cheongju, Korea

Qiu-Yue Wu1, Na Li, Wei-Wei Li, Tian-Fu Li, Cui Zhang, Ying-Xia Cui and Xin-Yi Xia
Institute of Laboratory Medicine, Jinling Hospital, Nanjing University School of Medicine, 305 East Zhongshan Road, Nanjing 210002, PR China

Jin-Sheng Zhai
Department of Health Care, Jinling Hospital, Nanjing University School of Medicine, Nanjing 210002, PR, China

Nora Eisemann
Institute of Cancer Epidemiology, University of Luebeck, Ratzeburger Allee 160, 23562 Luebeck, Germany

Alexander Katalinic
Institute of Cancer Epidemiology, University of Luebeck, Ratzeburger Allee 160, 23562 Luebeck, Germany
Institute of Social Medicine and Epidemiology, University Hospital Schleswig-Holstein, Campus Luebeck, Ratzeburger Allee 160, 23562 Luebeck, Germany

Sandra Nolte
Medical Clinic, Department of Psychosomatic Medicine, Charité - Universitätsmedizin Berlin, Charitéplatz 1, 10117 Berlin, Germany
Deakin University, 221 Burwood Highway, Burwood, VIC 3125, Australia

Maike Schnoor and Annika Waldmann
Institute of Social Medicine and Epidemiology, University Hospital Schleswig-Holstein, Campus Luebeck, Ratzeburger Allee 160, 23562 Luebeck, Germany

Volker Rohde
Medical Practice of Urology, Auguststr. 4, 23611 Bad Schwartau, Germany
Department of Urology, Pediatric Urology and Andrology, Justus Liebig University of Giessen, Rudolf-Buchheim-Str. 7, 35392 Giessen, Germany

Georgi Tosev, Timur H. Kuru, Johannes Huber, Gerald Freier, Sascha A. Pahernik, Markus Hohenfellner and Boris A. Hadaschik
Department of Urology, University of Heidelberg, Im Neuenheimer Feld 110, D-69120 Heidelberg, Germany

Frank Bergmann
Institute of Pathology, University of Heidelberg, Heidelberg, Germany

Jessica C. Hassel
Department of Dermatology, University of Heidelberg, Heidelberg, Germany

Kazuhiko Nakano, Kenji Komatsu, Taro Kubo, Shinsuke Natsui, Akinori Nukui, Shinsuke Kurokawa, Minoru Kobayashi and Tatsuo Morita
Department of Urology, Jichi Medical University, Yakushiji 3311-1, Shimotsuke, Tochigi 329-0498, Japan

You-Chiuan Chien and Heng-Chieh Chiang
Division of urology, Department of Surgery, Changhua Christian Hospital, No.135, Nansiao St. Changhua city, Changhua county 50006, Taiwan

Ping-Yi Lin
Transplant Medicine & Surgery Research Centre, Changhua Christian Hospital, Changhua, Taiwan

Yao-Li Chen
School of Medicine, Kaohsiung Medical University, Kaohsiung, Taiwan
Department of General Surgery, Changhua Christian Hospital, No.135 Nan-Hsiao Street, Changhua county 50006, Taiwan

Yiannis Philippou
Department of Surgery, Basildon & Thurrock University Hospital, Essex SS16 5NL, UK

Hary Raja and Vincent J. Gnanapragasam
Academic Urology Group, Department of Surgery & Oncology, University of Cambridge, Cambridge Biomedical Campus, Cambridge CB2 0QQ, UK

Shuman Yang and Tianying Wu
Division of Epidemiology and Biostatistics, Department of Environmental Health, University of Cincinnati Medical Center, Kettering Complex, 3223 Eden Ave, Cincinnati, OH, USA, 45267-0056

Bruce Bracken
Department of Surgery, University of Cincinnati Medical Center, Cincinnati, OH, USA

Shuk-Mei Ho
Division of Environmental Genetics and Molecular Toxicology, Cincinnati, OH, USA
Center for Environmental Genetics, University of Cincinnati Medical Center, Cincinnati, OH, USA

Edward Giovannucci
Departments of Nutrition and Epidemiology, Harvard School of Public Health, Boston, MA, USA
The Channing Division of Network Medicine, Department of Medicine, Brigham and Women's Hospital, Harvard Medical School, Boston, MA, USA

Daniele Bianchi and Gabriele Gaziev
School of Specialization in Urology, University of Rome Tor Vergata, Viale Oxford, 81-00133 Rome, Italy

Angelo Di Santo
NeuroUrology Unit, IRCCS Fondazione Santa Lucia, Rome, Italy

Enrico Finazzi Agrò, Roberto Miano and Giuseppe Vespasiani
Department of Experimental Medicine and Surgery, University of Rome Tor Vergata, Rome, Italy

Stefania Musco
Neuro-Urology Unit, Careggi Hospital, Florence, Italy

Karin Sørig Hougaard and Harald Hannerz
The National Research Centre for the Working Environment, Lersø Parkallé 105, DK-2100 Copenhagen, Denmark

Ann Dyreborg Larsen
The National Research Centre for the Working Environment, Lersø Parkallé 105, DK-2100 Copenhagen, Denmark
Department of Occupational Medicine, Aarhus University Hospital, Aarhus, Denmark

Kristian Tore Jørgensen
The National Research Centre for the Working Environment, Lersø Parkallé 105, DK-2100 Copenhagen, Denmark
Department of Occupational and Environmental Medicine, Bispebjerg Hospital, Copenhagen University Hospital, Copenhagen, Denmark

Gunnar Vase Toft
Department of Occupational Medicine, Aarhus University Hospital, Aarhus, Denmark

Anne-Marie Nybo Andersen
Department of Public Health, University of Copenhagen, Copenhagen, Denmark

Jens Peter Bonde
Department of Occupational and Environmental Medicine, Bispebjerg Hospital, Copenhagen University Hospital, Copenhagen, Denmark

Morten Søndergaard Jensen
Perinatal Epidemiology Research Unit, Department of Paediatrics, Aarhus University Hospital, Aarhus, Denmark

Yan-Ru Zeng, Chao Cai, Ya-Qiang Huang, Hong-Wei Luo and Qi-Shan Dai
Guangdong Provincial Institute of Nephrology, Southern Medical University, Guangzhou 510515, China

Wei-De Zhong
Guangdong Provincial Institute of Nephrology, Southern Medical University, Guangzhou 510515, China
Department of Urology, Guangdong Key Laboratory of Clinical Molecular Medicine and Diagnostics, Guangzhou First People's Hospital, Guangzhou Medical University, Guangzhou 510180, China
Department of Urology, Huadu District People's Hospital, Southern Medical University, Guangzhou 510800, China
Urology Key Laboratory of Guangdong Province, The First Affiliated Hospital of Guangzhou Medical University, Guangzhou Medical University, Guangzhou 510230, China
Department of Urology, Guangzhou First People's Hospital, Guangzhou Medical University, Guangzhou 510180, China

Yang-Jia Zhuo
Guangdong Provincial Institute of Nephrology, Southern Medical University, Guangzhou 510515, China
Department of Urology, Huadu District People's Hospital, Southern Medical University, Guangzhou 510800, China

Zhao-Dong Han and Ze-Zhen Liu
Department of Urology, Guangdong Key Laboratory of Clinical Molecular Medicine and Diagnostics, Guangzhou First People's Hospital, Guangzhou Medical University, Guangzhou 510180, China

Yu-Xiang Liang
Department of Urology, Guangdong Key Laboratory of Clinical Molecular Medicine and Diagnostics, Guangzhou First People's Hospital, Guangzhou Medical University, Guangzhou 510180, China
Department of Urology, Guangzhou First People's Hospital, Guangzhou Medical University, Guangzhou 510180, China

Cong Wang
School of Pharmacy, Wenzhou Medical University, Wenzhou 325035, China

Hai-Bo Zhao
Department of Urology, The Fifth Affiliated Hospital of Guangzhou Medical University, Guangzhou 510799, China

Hung N. Luu
Division of Epidemiology, Department of Medicine, Vanderbilt Epidemiology Center, Vanderbilt-Ingram Cancer Center, Vanderbilt University School of Medicine, Nashville, TN, USA
Department of Epidemiology and Biostatistics, College of Public Health, University of South Florida, Tampa, FL, USA

Hui-Yi Lin
Biostatistics Program, School of Public Health, Louisiana State University Health Sciences Center, New Orleans, LA 70112, USA

Karina Dalsgaard Sørensen
Department of Molecular Medicine, Aarhus University Hospital, Aarhus, Denmark

Olorunseun O. Ogunwobi
Department of Biological Sciences, Hunter College of The City University of New York, New York, NY 10065, USA

Nagi Kumar, Ganna Chornokur and Catherine Phelan
Department of Cancer Epidemiology, H. Lee Moffitt Cancer Center and Research Institute, Tampa, FL 33612, USA

Giuliano Di Pietro
Department of Cancer Epidemiology, H. Lee Moffitt Cancer Center and Research Institute, Tampa, FL 33612, USA
Department of Pharmacy, Federal University of Sergipe, Rodovia Marechal Rodon, Jardim Rosa Elze, Sao Cristóvão, Brazil

Dominique Jones and LaCreis Kidd
Department of Pharmacology and Toxicology, James Brown Cancer Center, University of Louisville School of Medicine, Louisville, KY 40202, USA

Robert J. Rounbehler
Department of Tumor Biology, H. Lee Moffitt Cancer Center and Research Institute, Tampa, FL 33612, USA

Mihi Yang
Research Center for Cell Fate Control, College of Pharmacy, Sookmyoung Women's University, Seoul, Republic of Korea

Sang Haak Lee and Nahyeon Kang
Department of Internal Medicine, The Cancer Research Institute, College of Medicine, The Catholic University of Korea, Seoul, Republic of Korea

Atsushi Tomioka, Nobumichi Tanaka, Motokiyo Yoshikawa, Makito Miyake, Satoshi Anai, Yoshitomo Chihara, Eijiro Okajima, Akihide Hirayama, Yoshihiko Hirao and Kiyohide Fujimoto
Department of Urology, Nara Medical University, 840 Shijo-cho, Kashihara, Nara 634-8522, Japan

María José Martinez-Zapata1,
CIBER de Epidemiología y Salud Pública (CIBERESP), Madrid, Spain
Institute of Biomedical Research (IIB Sant Pau), Iberoamerican Cochrane Centre, Barcelona, Spain
Universitat Autònoma de Barcelona, Barcelona, Spain

Xavier Bonfill
CIBER de Epidemiología y Salud Pública (CIBERESP), Madrid, Spain
Institute of Biomedical Research (IIB Sant Pau), Iberoamerican Cochrane Centre, Barcelona, Spain
Universitat Autònoma de Barcelona, Barcelona, Spain
Public Health and Clinical Epidemiology Service, Hospital de la Santa Creu I Sant Pau, Barcelona, Spain

Víctor Abraira and Javier Zamora
CIBER de Epidemiología y Salud Pública (CIBERESP), Madrid, Spain
Unidad de Bioestadística Clínica, Hospital Universitario Ramón y Cajal, IRYCIS, Madrid, Spain

Joan Palou
Universitat Autònoma de Barcelona, Barcelona, Spain Fundació Puigvert, Barcelona, Spain

Juan M. Ramos-Goñi
Health Services Research on Chronic Patients Network (REDISSEC), HTA Unit of the Canary Islands Health Service (SESCS), S/C de Tenerife, La Laguna, Spain

Stefanie Schmidt
Department of Experimental and Health Sciences, Universidad Pompeu Fabra (UPF), Barcelona, Spain

Narelle Hanly
Faculty of Health Sciences, The University of Sydney, Sydney, NSW, Australia

Ilona Juraskova and Shab Mireskandari
Centre for Medical Psychology & Evidence-based Decision-making (CeMPED), School of Psychology, The University of Sydney, Level 6, Chris O'Brien Lifehouse (C39Z), Sydney, NSW 2006, Australia

Hicham Charoute, Brahim El Houate, Abdelhamid Barakat and Hassan Rouba
Laboratoire de Génétique Moléculaire Humaine, Département de la Recherche Scientifique, Institut Pasteur du Maroc, 1 Place Louis Pasteur, 20360 Casablanca, Morocco

Yassine Naasse
Laboratoire de Génétique Moléculaire Humaine, Département de la Recherche Scientifique, Institut Pasteur du Maroc, 1 Place Louis Pasteur, 20360 Casablanca, Morocco
Laboratoire de Physiopathologie et Génétique Moléculaire, Faculté des Sciences Ben M'Sik, Université Hassan II, Casablanca, Morocco

Chadli Elbekkay and Lunda Razoki
Laboratoire de Cytogénétique, Département de la Recherche Scientifique, Institut Pasteur du Maroc, 1 Place Louis Pasteur, 20360 Casablanca, Morocco

Abderrahim Malki
Laboratoire de Physiopathologie et Génétique Moléculaire, Faculté des Sciences Ben M'Sik, Université Hassan II, Casablanca, Morocco

Yasushi Nakai, Nobumichi Tanaka, Satoshi Anai, Makito Miyake, Shunta Hori, Yoshihiro Tatsumi, Yosuke Morizawa and Kiyohide Fujimoto
Department of Urology, Nara Medical University, 840 Shijo-cho, Kashihara-shi, Nara 634-8522, Japan

Tomomi Fujii and Noboru Konishi
Department of Pathology, Nara Medical University, 840 Shijo-cho, Kashihara-shi, Nara 634-8522, Japan

Jin-Jia Hu
Institute of Biomedical Engineering, National Cheng Kung University, Tainan 70101, Taiwan

Cheng-Ching Wu
Institute of Biomedical Engineering, National Cheng Kung University, Tainan 70101, Taiwan
Division of Cardiology, Department of Internal Medicine, E-Da Hospital, I-Shou University, Kaohsiung 82445, Taiwan

Hung-Yu Lin
Department of Urology, E-Da Hospital, I-Shou University, Kaohsiung 82445, Taiwan

Li-Fen Lu
Division of Cardiac Surgery, Department of Surgery, E-Da Hospital, I-Shou University, Kaohsiung 82445, Taiwan

Jer-Yiing Houng
Department of Medical Nutrition, Institute of Biotechnology and Chemical Engineering and I-Shou University, Kaohsiung 82445, Taiwan

Yau-Jiunn Lee
Lee's Endocrinology Clinic, Pingtung 90000, Taiwan

Fu-Mei Chung, Teng-Hung Yu and Wei-Chin Hung
Division of Cardiology, Department of Internal Medicine, E-Da Hospital, I-Shou University, Kaohsiung 82445, Taiwan

Chao-Ping Wang
Division of Cardiology, Department of Internal Medicine, E-Da Hospital, I-Shou University, Kaohsiung 82445, Taiwan
School of Medicine for International Students, I-Shou University, Kaohsiung 82445, Taiwan

Shimpei Yamashita, Yasuo Kohjimoto, Takashi Iguchi, Hiroyuki Koike, Hiroki Kusumoto, Akinori Iba, Kazuro Kikkawa, Yoshiki Kodama, Nagahide Matsumura and Isao Hara
Department of Urology, Wakayama Medical University, 811-1 Kimiidera, Wakayama 641-0012, Japan

G. Hatiboglu, I. V. Popeneciu, M. Deppert, J. Nyarangi-Dix, B. Hadaschik, M. Hohenfellner, D. Teber and S. Pahernik
Department of Urology, University of Heidelberg, Im Neuenheimer Feld 110, 69120 Heidelberg, Germany

Sun-Ouck Kim, Seong Woong Na, Ho Song Yu and Dongdeuk Kwon
Department of Urology, Chonnam National University Medical School, Gwangju, South Korea

Ho Seok Chung, Myung Soo Kim, Yang Hyun Cho, Eu Chang Hwang, Seung Il Jung, Taek Won Kang and Dong Deuk Kwon
Department of Urology, Chonnam National University Medical School, 42 Jebongro, Donggu, Gwangju 501-757, Republic of Korea

Suk Hee Heo
Department of Radiology, Chonnam National University Medical School, Gwangju, Republic of Korea

Chan Choi
Department of Pathology, Chonnam National University Medical School, Gwangju, Republic of Korea

Shusei Fusayasu, Koji Izumi, Yumiko Yokomizo, Hiroki Ito, Yusuke Ito, Kayo Kurita, Kazuhiro Furuya, Hisashi Hasumi, Narihiko Hayashi and Masahiro Yao
Department of Urology, Yokohama City University, Graduate School of Medicine, Yokohama, Japan

Takashi Kawahara and Hiroji Uemura
Department of Urology, Yokohama City University, Graduate School of Medicine, Yokohama, Japan
Department of Urology and Renal Transplantation, Yokohama City University Medical Center, 4-57 Urafune-cho, Minami-ku, Yokohama, Kanagawa 232-0024, Japan

Yasuhide Myoshi
Department of Urology and Renal Transplantation, Yokohama City University Medical Center, 4-57 Urafune-cho, Minami-ku, Yokohama, Kanagawa 232-0024, Japan

Hiroshi Miyamoto
Departments of Pathology and Urology, Johns Hopkins University School of Medicine, Baltimore, USA

Mev Dominguez-Valentin, Patrick Joost and Mats Jonsson
Institute of Clinical Sciences, Division of Oncology and Pathology, Lund University, SE-22381 Lund, Sweden

Eva Rambech and Mef Nilbert
Institute of Clinical Sciences, Division of Oncology and Pathology, Lund University, SE-22381 Lund, Sweden
HNPCC-Register, Clinical Research Centre, Copenhagen University Hospital, Hvidovre, Denmark

Christina Therkildsen
HNPCC-Register, Clinical Research Centre, Copenhagen University Hospital, Hvidovre, Denmark

Tanner L Bartholow
University of Pittsburgh School of Medicine, Pittsburgh, PA, USA

Michael J Becich and Uma R Chandran
Department of Biomedical Informatics, University of Pittsburgh School of Medicine, Pittsburgh, PA, USA

Anil V Parwani
Department of Pathology, University of Pittsburgh School of Medicine, Pittsburgh, PA, USA

Vilppu J Tuominen, Jorma J Isola and Tapio Visakorpi
Institute of Medical Technology, University of Tampere and Tampere University Hospital, Tampere, Finland

Paula M Kujala
Department of Pathology, Centre for Laboratory Medicine, Tampere University Hospital, Tampere, Finland

Teemu T Tolonen
Institute of Medical Technology, University of Tampere and Tampere University Hospital, Tampere, Finland
Department of Pathology, Centre for Laboratory Medicine, Tampere University Hospital, Tampere, Finland

Teuvo LJ Tammela
Department of Urology, University of Tampere and Tampere University Hospital, Tampere, Finland

Ben-Ali Habib, Ali Saad and Mounir Ajina
Unit of Reproductive Medicine, University Farhat Hached Hospital, 4000 Soussa, Tunisia

Monia Raffa and Abdelhamid Kerkeni
Research Laboratory of "Trace elements, free radicals and antioxidants", Biophysical Department, Faculty of Medicine, University of Monastir, 5000 Monastir, Tunisia

Fatma Atig
Unit of Reproductive Medicine, University Farhat Hached Hospital, 4000 Soussa, Tunisia
Department of Cytogenetic and Reproductive Reproduction, Farhat Hached, University Teaching Hospital, 4000 Sousse, Tunisia

Nobumichi Tanaka, Kiyohide Fujimoto, Satoshi Anai, Akihide Hirayama and Yoshihiko Hirao
Department of Urology, Nara Medical University, 840 Shijo-cho, Kashihara, Nara 634-8522, Japan

Isao Asakawa and Masatoshi Hasegawa
Department of Radiation Oncology, Nara Medical University, Nara, Japan

Noboru Konishi
Department of Pathology, Nara Medical University, Nara, Japan

Owen T Hill
Injury Epidemiology Research Section, Military Performance Division, United States Army Institute of Environmental Medicine, Natick, MA, USA

Thomas J Mason
Department of Environmental and Occupational Health, College of Public Health, University of South Florida, Tampa, FL, USA

Skai W Schwartz
Department of Epidemiology and Biostatistics, College of Public Health, University of South Florida, Tampa, FL, USA

Philip R Foulis
Department of Pathology and Laboratory Medicine, James A. Haley Veteran's Administration, Tampa, FL, USA

Index